Fourth Edition

Human
Histology

A Textbook in Outline Form

Leslie Brainerd Arey, Ph.D., Sc.D.(hon.), LL.D.(hon.)

Robert Laughlin Rea Professor of Anatomy, Emeritus
Northwestern University

59 Electron Micrographs on Three Plates
398 Illustrations on 22 Plates—in Color
23 Synthetic Diagrams on 22 Plates

1974   **W. B. SAUNDERS COMPANY**
Philadelphia • London • Toronto

W. B. Saunders Company: West Washington Square
                           Philadelphia, Pa. 19105

                           12 Dyott Street
                           London, WC1A   1DB

                           833 Oxford Street
                           Toronto, Ontario M8Z 5T9, Canada

Listed here is the latest translated edition of this book, together with
the language of the translation and the publisher.

Spanish (3rd Edition) — La Prensa Medica Mexicana,
                        Mexico City.

Human Embryology   ISBN 0-7216-1392-6

Print No.:   9   8   7   6   5   4   3   2   1

Preface
to the Fourth Edition

The endorsement of the original edition of this book in the United States and other countries, and its prompt translation into Spanish, were a sufficient earnest of its usefulness to warrant the presentation of second and third editions. In these revisions 398 drawings in color were first assembled into 22 plates, and then 59 electron micrographs on three plates were added to illustrate fine structure.

In the present edition the entire text matter has undergone critical review and revision in the light of new information and altered interpretations that have accumulated steadily in the past six years. The chapter on the cell has been largely rewritten, and those on the tissues have received substantial revisions. Each chapter on the organs has benefitted by significant improvements, although such are naturally more sporadic than those dealing with the cell and tissues. A thoroughgoing effort has been made to improve the clarity of descriptions, even where no new information was involved, and these revisions are continuous throughout the text.

Through the generous co-operation of Dr. Thomas L. Lentz, 23 line drawings have been borrowed from his atlas, Cell Fine Structure. One correlated illustration is reproduced on the reverse surface of each color plate. These idealized diagrams have the advantage of combining all aspects of organizational ultrastructure into one picture.

L. B. AREY

Chicago, Illinois

Contents

Chapter V

The Connective Tissues 44

Chapter VI

The Blood and Lymph 59

Chapter VII

The Development of Blood 67

Chapter VIII

Cartilage 72

Chapter IX

Bone, Bone Marrow and Joints 77

Chapter XX

The Major Glands of Digestion 230

Chapter XXI

The Respiratory System 243

Chapter XXII

The Urinary System 252

Chapter XXIII

The Male Reproductive System 264

Chapter XXIV

The Female Reproductive System 279

A Collection of Electron Micrographs
Illustrating the Ultrastructure
of
Cell-, Tissue- and Organ Specializations

Permission to use portions of published micrographs and of cell drawings has been granted generously by the following authors and publishers:

W. Bloom and D. W. Fawcett, *Textbook of Histology,* Saunders, 1968: Plate I, figs. 1, 6; Plate II, figs. 1, 8 (Hodge and Schmitt), 11 (Jakus), 16, 19 (Hanson and Huxley); Plate III, figs. 1 (Webster), 2 (Fernández-Morán), 7 (Orkand and Palay), 8 (Jones), 11, 13 (Farquhar and Palade), 17, 20 (Jakus).

J. E. Dowling, *Science, 147,* 57, 1965; Plate III, 18.

D. W. Fawcett, *The Cell,* Saunders, 1966: Plate I, figs. 2, 3, 4, 5, 7, 8, 9, 12, 13, 14, 15, 16, 18; Plate II, figs. 3, 4, 6, 7, 10, 14, 15, 18; Plate III, figs. 3, 10, 19.

R. O. Greep, *Histology,* McGraw-Hill, 1966: Plate II, fig. 9 (Dudley and Spiro); Plate III, fig. 4 (Rosenbluth).

C. R. Leeson and T. S. Leeson, *Histology,* Saunders, 1966: Plate I, fig. 17; Plate II, figs. 13, 17 (Huxley), 20 (Huxley); Plate III, figs. 6 (Peters), 15.

T. L. Lentz, *Cell Fine Structure,* Saunders, 1971: Line drawings on reverse of all color plates in the present volume.

J. A. G. Rhodin, *Atlas of Ultrastructure,* Saunders, 1963: Plate II, figs. 2, 5, 12; Plate III, figs. 5, 9, 12, 14, 16, 21.

S. L. Robbins, *Pathology,* Saunders, 1967: Plate I, figs. 10, 11 (Friend).

ELECTRON MICROGRAPHS OF CELL COMPONENTS

Fig. 1. Part of a pancreas cell, showing small chromatin masses within the nucleus and a spongy, nonmembrane-bounded nucleolus. Other features are a double-layered nuclear membrane ('pores' marked by arrows), bordered by endoplasmic reticulum of the cytoplasm. × 16,000.

Fig. 2. A 'pore' in the double-layered nuclear membrane of an erythroblast. × 100,000. A seemingly open pore at moderate magnifications may appear to be closed by a diaphragm at high magnifications such as this.

Fig. 3. The plasma membrane of an intestinal microvillus. × 230,000. The three layers of this typical 'unit membrane' are revealed at this extreme magnification. Left of the membrane is interior cytoplasm of the microvillus; right of the membrane is a secreted surface-coat of glycoprotein.

Fig. 4. Two kinds of endoplasmic reticulum of a liver cell. × 33,000. Left half of the micrograph contains agranular (smooth-surfaced) reticulum; right half contains granular (rough-surfaced) reticulum bearing ribosomes involved in protein synthesis.

Fig. 5. Detail of agranular reticulum from a testicular interstitial cell. × 51,000. Each membrane-bounded cavity constitutes a cisterna. Between cisternae is ground cytoplasm.

Fig. 6. Detail of granular reticulum from a pancreatic alveolar cell. × 85,000. Both closely spaced membranes of a cisternal pair bear ribosomes on their external surfaces.

Fig. 7. Near the top is a centriole-pair (arrows) that was located at one pole of a mitotic spermatocyte. × 15,600. The two hollow cylinders, lying at right angles, are sectioned lengthwise; the shorter one is cut somewhat tangentially. Each cylinder is closed at one end. At arrows are so-called spindle fibers, actually microtubules.

Fig. 8. A centriole-pair (arrows), sectioned lengthwise, from intestinal epithelium. × 41,000. Only two of the nine sets of rod-like tubules show plainly in each centriole.

Fig. 9. A centriole, sectioned transversely, from a pancreatic alveolar cell. × 135,000. Nine so-called fibrils (each actually a triple tubule: a,b,c) are embedded in a dense matrix. The whole constitutes a hollow cylinder.

Fig. 10. A mitochondrion from a duodenal gland is sectioned lengthwise among the endoplasmic reticulum. × 20,000. Cristae subdivide the interior into incomplete compartments.

Fig. 11. The upper half contains a mitochondrion, sectioned transversely, and endoplasmic reticulum from a duodenal gland. Below is part of a Golgi apparatus with a stack of curving, layered cisternae; at the base are several prominent secretion granules. × 20,000.

Fig. 12. Detail of one end of a mitochondrion, sectioned lengthwise, from epididymal epithelium. × 165,000. The inner layer of the double, external membrane folds inward, producing double-layered cristae. Enzymes are located both in this inner membrane and in the adjoining matrix.

Fig. 13. A Golgi apparatus from epididymal epithelium. × 18,000. A lamellar system of curved membranes comprises cisternae; centrally there are small vesicles and larger ones of agranular endoplasmic reticulum. The dense mass at the bottom has the appearance of a secretory granule.

Fig. 14. Detail of part of a Golgi apparatus from a duodenal gland. × 54,000. The lower cisternae are more distended and contain a flocculent material (arrows) like that of the secretory granules (dark body, at bottom). Such synthesized material is concentrated and packaged here.

Fig. 15. A microbody from the liver. × 26,000. These particles are enclosed by a single-layered membrane and often, as here, contain a crystalloid. They are enzyme-rich but their function and relations are problematical.

Fig. 16. Lysosomes from the suprarenal cortex. × 25,000. Each is dense and bounded by a single membrane. They contain hydrolytic enzymes active in digesting ingested substances.

Fig. 17. Detail of cytoplasm from a testicular interstitial cell. × 75,000. Larger circles represent agranular cisternae; tiny circles and parallel lines represent microtubules sectioned across and lengthwise.

Fig. 18. Detail of microtubules, cut transversely, from a spermatocyte. × 158,000.

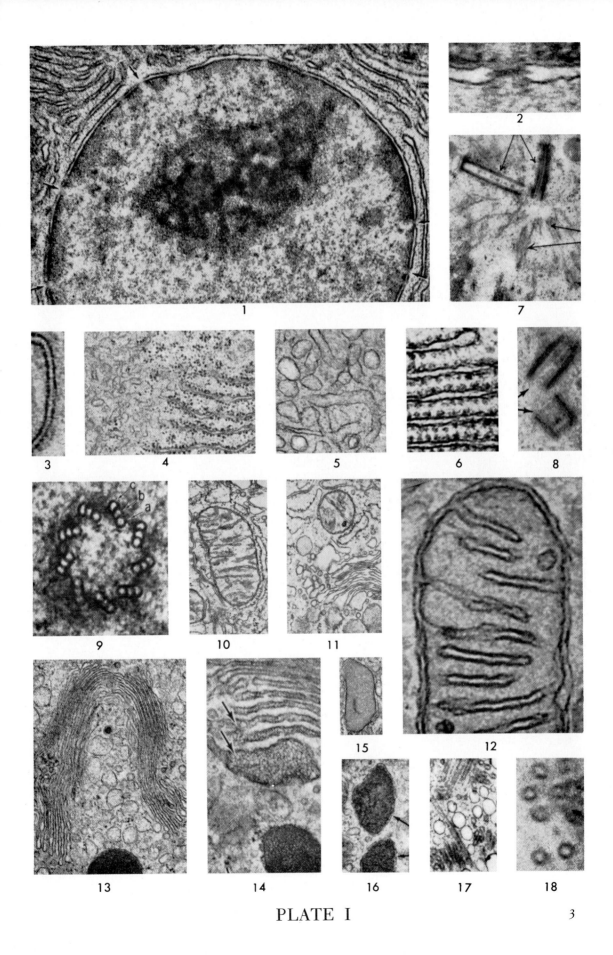

PLATE I

3

ELECTRON MICROGRAPHS OF DIFFERENTIATIONS IN EPITHELIUM, CONNECTIVE TISSUE, BLOOD AND MUSCLE

Fig. 1. Microvilli, sectioned longitudinally, on intestinal epithelium. × 40,000. Below, the cytoplasm is reinforced by fine filaments of the terminal web; they are typically denser than shown.

Fig. 2. Two cilia and a microvillus (Vi), sectioned longitudinally, from tracheal epithelium. × 30,000. Peripheral filaments (Pf) of a cilium originate in a basal corpuscle (Bc) which continues as a filamentous rootlet (R). In the cilium at the right an axial filament shows discontinuously.

Fig. 3. Two cilia, sectioned transversely, from gill epithelium. × 110,000. In each, nine peripheral double 'filaments' (actually tubules) surround two axial, single ones.

Fig. 4. Two desmosomes occur along the slightly separated plasma membranes of two cells in oral epithelium. × 70,000. A dense material (arrow) produces a desmosome by massing on each plasma membrane; tonofilaments in the cytoplasm converge and insert on these masses.

Fig. 5. A terminal bar (T) and desmosome (Des) are located near the tops of two adjoining pancreatic cells. × 34,700. Such a 'tight junction' (T) of the two plasma membranes (Cm) apparently involves actual fusion between them. It seals off the intercellular space; a desmosome does not.

Fig. 6. Infoldings of the plasma membrane at the base of a distal-tubule cell of the bat's kidney. × 32,000. In man the infoldings are much longer and long, slender mitochondria lodge between them. The cell is underlaid by the basal lamina (arrow); this and still deeper collagenous fibrils (asterisk) comprise the total basement membrane.

Fig. 7. The endothelium of a myocardial capillary. × 41,000. Vesicles, illustrating stages in micropinocytosis, occur at the basal surface (arrows), in the interior cytoplasm, and at the luminal surface (at left). A basal lamina, at the right, supports the endothelium.

Fig. 8. A collagen fibril, sectioned lengthwise. × 110,000. The pattern of cross banding repeats regularly at intervals of 0.064μ (or 640 Å). A bracket marks an interval-unit.

Fig. 9. An osteoblast-osteoid junction. × 28,000. Below is the osteoblast margin; above, osteocollagenous fibers bear some dense particles of bone salts and enclose other particles.

Fig. 10. A granule within an eosinophil, near its margin. × 33,000. An equatorially located crystalloid is a characteristic feature of this cytoplasmic granule which is a type of lysosome.

Fig. 11. A blood platelet, next to a capillary wall below. × 11,500. A central granulomere, with dense granules, tends to be enveloped by a clear, nongranular hyalomere (best seen below).

Fig. 12. Portions of two smooth muscle fibers, sectioned longitudinally, from the intestine. × 25,000. Lateral projections adhere in intimate contact (Lc). Some micropinocytotic vesicles occur in both fibers, above the level of fiber junction. Myofilaments are barely visible.

Fig. 13. The border of a smooth muscle fiber from an artery. × 21,000. Above is the sarcolemma; it consists of the plasma membrane (dark line) overlaid by a basal lamina. Just below the plasma membrane, the sarcoplasm contains a few, faint micropinocytotic vesicles.

Fig 14. Myofilaments of smooth muscle (arrow), sectioned transversely, are embedded in sarcoplasm. × 118,000. Such a group of filaments constitutes a bundle, known as a myofibril.

Fig. 15. The marginal region of a cardiac muscle cell, sectioned transversely. × 41,000. The plasma membrane (dark line) is overlaid on the left by a basal lamina; the two constitute a sarcolemma. In the sarcoplasm beneath the plasma membrane a few small, dark tubules of the sarcoplasmic reticulum and some larger vesicles are recognizable. Still deeper in the sarcoplasm are myosin filaments of the A band, sectioned transversely.

Fig. 16. An intercalated disk, at the end-to-end junction of two cardiac muscle cells. × 28,000. The abutting plasma membranes are separated by a narrow space. They interdigitate and bear accumulations of sarcoplasmic dense substance (arrows), on which myofibrils (not shown) insert.

Fig. 17. Myofibrils of skeletal muscle, sectioned longitudinally. × 13,000. One myofibril is bordered, above and below, by a part of another fibril; all show myofilaments faintly. The dark A band is bisected by the pale H band which, in turn, is bisected by the M line. The light I band is bisected by the dark Z line. The portion of the fibril between two Z lines is a sarcomere (S).

Fig. 18. Sarcoplasmic reticulum is displayed as it extends between longitudinally sectioned skeletal myofibrils. × 30,000. At the level of junction of each A and I band occurs a triad of circularly coursing tubules (cut transversely; arrow), two large and one small. Longitudinal tubules connect successive triads. The tiny, circular tubule (at arrow) is the transverse T-tubule.

Fig. 19. The two types of myofilaments of a skeletal myofibril, sectioned transversely in their region of overlap within the A band. × 350,000. Six thin actin filaments group in a regular pattern about a thick myosin filament.

Fig. 20. Myofilament relations shown within sarcomeres of two myofibrils, sectioned longitudinally. × 74,000. Thin actin filaments insert in the Z lines of the sarcomere and extend far between the thick myosin filaments of the A band. In these zones of overlap cross-bridges between filaments can be seen. H-bracket demarks H band, bisecting A band; arrow-line marks I band.

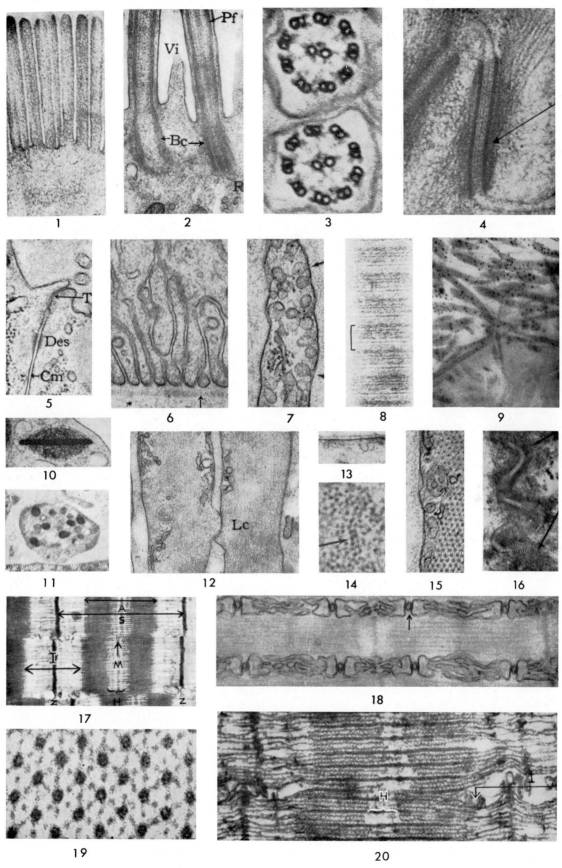

PLATE II

5

ELECTRON MICROGRAPHS OF DIFFERENTIATIONS IN NERVE FIBERS AND VARIOUS ORGANS

Fig. 1. Sample area of a myelinated nerve fiber, sectioned transversely. × 50,000. A basal lamina (arrow) overlies the laminated myelin sheath. At the bottom is axoplasm of the axon.

Fig. 2. Detail of the myelin sheath, sectioned transversely. × 460,000. Dense, uniformly spaced lamellae alternate with somewhat thinner and less dense intermediate layers.

Fig. 3. Interior of an axon, sectioned transversely. × 40,000. Neurofilaments show as dots in a bed of neuroplasm (*i.e.,* axoplasm). Neurotubules do not show.

Fig. 4. Half of a myelinated nerve fiber, sectioned longitudinally through a node of Ranvier. × 18,800. Two neurolemma sheaths (S), bordered by a basal lamina (BM), end in contact at the node (arrow). Myelin lamellae (M) similarly terminate there, but in staggered sequence. Beneath the myelin, at the bottom, is the pale axon whose fibrillations are poorly resolved.

Fig. 5. Part of a neurolemma cell (of Schwann), nearly enclosing two unmyelinated nerve fibers, sectioned transversely. × 38,000. Near the top, a basal lamina (arrow) overlies the thin, dark plasma membrane of the sheath cell. The plasma membrane inrolls to form grooves, in each of which a nerve fiber courses. At the bottom is a part of the nucleus of the neurolemma cell; its double-layered nuclear membrane includes a prominent 'pore' (arrow).

Fig. 6. Detail of the synaptic region between an axon (above) and a dendron (below). × 60,000. Here the two plasma membranes thicken and the axon contains numerous presynaptic vesicles.

Fig. 7. An axonal ending, at the right, in the neurohypophysis; it lies near an associated capillary, at the left (arrows). × 22,000. The swollen ending contains neurosecretory granules.

Fig. 8. The border region between an hepatic cell and sinusoid. × 28,000. Near the top are portions of two macrophages (arrowhead); they belong to the lining of the sinusoid, whose lumen is above. At the bottom is an hepatic cell which projects microvilli into the space of Disse (long arrow, at top). Another arrow, at the bottom, indicates lipoprotein discharging into Disse's space.

Fig. 9. A bile canaliculus, sectioned transversely. × 16,000. Plasma membranes (arrows), bounding two abutting hepatic cells, lie left and right. Local grooves, one on each cell surface, unite to produce a canaliculus; microvilli project into its lumen.

Fig. 10. Detail from a beta cell of a pancreatic islet. × 45,000. Maturation stages of secretory granules (insulin precursors) are indicated by arrows; the ripest granule contains a crystalloid.

Fig. 11. A portion of a capillary wall in the pancreas. × 13,000. A thin region of the endothelium bears extremely thin diaphragms or contains actual pores. An edge of a distorted red blood corpuscle shows in the capillary lumen at the right.

Fig. 12. A portion of an alveolar wall of the lung. × 17,000. An extremely thin squamous epithelium (at left) lines the alveolar lumen. It is separated from the endothelium of a capillary (at right) by merged basal laminas only (arrow); pinocytotic vesicles are in endothelium.

Fig. 13. Detail of the filtration apparatus in a renal corpuscle. × 18,000. Bounding the lumen, at the top, is the endothelium of a glomerular capillary; it bears extremely thin regions, or actual pores (arrows). At the bottom are foot-like processes (pedicles) branching from the visceral layer of capsular epithelium. Between the two epithelia is a combined basal lamina (asterisk).

Fig. 14. The base of an epithelial cell in the proximal tubule of a nephron. × 30,000. At the bottom is the basement membrane (B). Above it, the plasma membrane makes tall infoldings (as at arrow), some produced by flanges from neighboring cells. Similar infoldings in cells of the distal tubule are abundant and long; between some of these, slender mitochondria are lodged.

Fig. 15. Microvilli of a proximal tubule of a nephron, sectioned transversely. × 28,000. The cytoplasmic rodlets are so closely packed that little of the space of the lumen separates them.

Fig. 16. Detail near the periphery of a growing ovarian follicle. × 16,000. A follicle cell (at top) sends coarse processes (Pu) through the pale zona pellucida (asterisk) to reach the surface of the oöcyte (at bottom). The oöcyte projects microvilli (V) only part way into the structureless zona.

Fig. 17. Detail within an interstitial cell of the testes. × 32,000. The cytoplasm contains elongate albuminous crystalloids (arrow) and spheroidal lipid granules.

Fig. 18. Detail from a longitudinal section of the cylindrical outer segment of a foveal cone of the retina. × 52,000. It contains a stack of about 2000 disks, each made of a granular substance folded in a double layer whose interspace shows well only at the margin.

Fig. 19. Detail from an immature pigment granule of the pigment epithelium of the retina. × 180,000. Its structural framework consists of layers of enzymic protein showing fine cross bandings. Progressive melaninization will soon obscure this regular pattern.

Fig. 20. Detail of the corneal stroma, sectioned vertically. × 35,000. Collagenous fibrils are embedded in a cementing substance. Sets of parallel fibrils are arranged in alternating layers.

Fig. 21. Detail from the spiral organ (of Corti). × 4,700. The top of a hair cell includes two sensory hairs rooted in a dense terminal web (arrow). This cell-top is set in the mosaic-like reticular lamina, formed by the terminal webs (asterisk) of supporting cells, left and right.

6

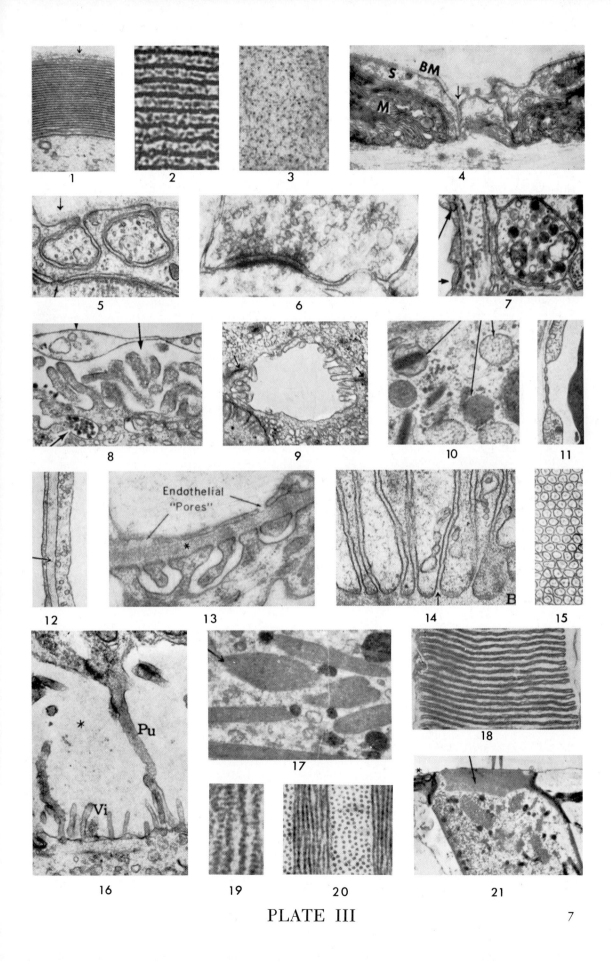

PLATE III

7

ILLUSTRATIVE PLATES

Chapter I

Introductory Topics

Histology treats of the minute structure of living organisms.

Only the most superficial features of tissues and organs are discernible by the naked eye.

Hence the details are 'microscopic' (as opposed to gross, or 'macroscopic' features).

There is an *animal histology* and a *plant histology*, but they differ widely in structural style.

Each records the separate paths taken in adapting to quite different living conditions.

Among animals *comparative histology* covers the animal groups from lowest to highest forms.

The building units (cells and tissues) are much alike in all animals.

But the kinds of organs differ widely from one major group to another.

Each has adapted to the demands of its particular environment.

Vertebrate histology reveals a fairly common plan of organs among its several subgroups.

Yet considerable variation still exists in the structure of individual organs.

Mammalian histology finds a high degree of structural uniformity among its representatives.

Yet striking specializations occur in some animal types.

Example: scent glands; dermal plates of armadillos; stomach of ruminants.

Human histology limits itself to the one species that interests the greatest number of people.

In so doing, the countless minor variations among mammals are disregarded.

I. THE POSITION OF HISTOLOGY

Morphology is the study of the form and structure, in the broadest sense, of living organisms.

It is considered under two divisions:

Embryology deals with the development of form and structure prior to maturity.

Anatomy deals with the structure of the body and the relations of its parts.

Anatomy has two aspects: normal and abnormal.

Abnormal anatomy, or *pathology*, deals with structural changes caused by disease.

Normal anatomy is subdivided into: *gross anatomy;* and *microscopic anatomy.*

The latter is subdivided into: *organology* (organs); *histology* (tissues); and *cytology* (cells).

Note that 'histology' is also used loosely to include all three microscopic categories.

'Textbooks of Histology' treat of cells and organs as well as tissues.

II. THE HISTORICAL BACKGROUND

Early microscopists (Malpighi; Leeuwenhoek; Swammerdam) saw various structural features, but did not recognize or interpret properly their fundamental cellular composition.

Hooke (1665) gave the name *cell* to the walled compartments of dead cork tissue.

Much later the term was extended to include the living contents.

Brown (1831) discovered the nucleus.

But the idea of the cell in this period was still very imperfect.

The '*cell theory*' was asserted by Schleiden (1838) and particularly by Schwann (1839).

He taught that animals were composed of cells as structural and functional units.

Virchow (1863) emphasized the body as a 'cell state,' with specialized categories of cells.

Tissues and organs were described relatively early, as concerns their general features.

In 1841 Henle published the first thorough account of human histology.

Cytology lagged, incidental to the progress of embryological knowledge.

It dates from the discovery of fertilization of the egg by O. Hertwig (1875).

Hence cytology is the infant anatomical science.

Progress has waited on adequate technical methods for revealing cellular composition.

These optical, staining and histochemical methods are still being developed.

The compound light microscope first became effective in 1830 when the image, previously blurred by chromatic aberration, was corrected.

Later, astigmation was eliminated (1876) and the modern instrument evolved.

The electron microscope is a modern invention that enhances detail enormously.

Other advanced techniques also supply important information at a subcellular level.

Molecular biology is a new subscience that utilizes modern, sophisticated, scientific methods.

Its aim is to reveal the characteristics of the molecules of living matter.

Included is information on the form, aggregation and pattern of such units.

III. THE IMPORTANCE OF HISTOLOGY

A base rock of scientific medical practice is an understanding of *normal physiology*.

Physiology is a study of living function (as are also biochemistry and pharmacology).

It is concerned with how cells, singly or in combination, work and react.

But cells and tissues are the unit materials that underlie such activities.

Since structure and function are reciprocals, histology becomes a prerequisite.

Another foundation stone, *pathology*, deals with cells that exhibit deranged functions.

This condition, disease, is accompanied by alterations of cell structure.

But nothing new, either in structure or in function, enters during disease.

Normal functional processes are then merely exaggerated or decreased.

This tends to be reflected in the altered appearance of cells.

Hence a necessary basis of understanding disease is a sound knowledge of the normal.

IV. METHODS FOR EXAMINING TISSUES

A. MICROSCOPE-TYPES AS TOOLS:

Several kinds of microscopes are available for revealing structural details.

1. Bright-field.

This type is the ordinary, compound microscope.

It is often called a 'light microscope' to distinguish it from the electron type.

Its useful power of magnification ceases at about 1200 diameters.

Even more important than greater magnification is the ability to resolve detail better.

That is, the capacity of separating, clearly, points located close together.

The resolving capacity under ordinary conditions is about 0.2 micron (0.0002 mm.).

Objects lying less than that distance apart merge into a single image.

Particles less than that diameter are not recognizable.

2. Phase and interference.

These types employ systems by means of which contrast is created.

Structures, ordinarily not seen, become visible through slight refractive differences.

Use is restricted to the study of living cells and unstained tissues.

Interference microscopy additionally provides quantitative data.

Thickness and refractive index can be established.

3. Polarization.

This type interposes two Nicol prisms (or Polaroid sheets) in the light path.

One prism, when rotated, detects the presence of double refraction in objects.

This demonstrates the presence and orientation of particles too small to be seen.

It permits deductions concerning organization not demonstrable otherwise.

4. *Fluorescence.*

Specimens are examined when fluorescing under invisible, ultraviolet radiation.
Many objects then emit visible light of different colors and qualities.
    Large molecules within cells may be naturally fluorescent and localizable.
    Introduced fluorescent dyes may then bind to specific cell components.
    An antibody, labeled with a fluorescent dye, will attach to its specific antigen.

5. *Dark-field.*

This type employs strong, oblique light that does not enter the objective.
    A vacant field of view then shows merely as a dark background.
Objects present in the field reflect some light into the objective.
    Thus it is possible to demonstrate the presence and shape of particles far below the
        limits of resolution by bright-light microscopy.
        The effect is similar to invisible dust particles that are 'seen' in a strong sunbeam
            traversing a darkened room.
    Also, small, transparent objects can be seen that would be invisible in a glare.

6. *Invisible radiation.*

Images can be formed by rays other than visible light.
    In this instance the image is photographed on a suitably sensitized film.
    A. Ultraviolet Rays.
        The use of quartz lenses and ultraviolet illumination improves resolution.
            Such resolution (0.1 micron) is double that obtainable by visible light.
        Certain cell components absorb ultraviolet light and become demonstrable.
    B. Electron Rays.
        Beams of electrons replace light, and electromagnetic or electrostatic fields replace
            lenses in the relatively recent invention of the electron microscope.
            The final image is visualized on a fluorescent screen and photographed.
        Resolving power has been pushed to 0.001 micron (0.000001 mm.).
            This is 200 times the capability of the light microscope.
        The photographed image may be as much as 50,000 times the original size.
            This image can be profitably enlarged still further.
        A new scanning technique gives a greatly enhanced resolution and depth of field.
            It permits the visualization of three-dimensional structure.
    C. X-Rays.
        Differential absorption by a section produces a focussed, photographable image.
        The negative permits the dry weight of cytological structures to be determined.
        Also, chemical analyses of extremely minute objects can be deduced.

B. Observation of Living Tissue:

1. *Direct observation.*

    A. Some *intact animals* offer favorable materials.
        Examples: protozoa; tail of tadpole; wing of bat; buccal pouch of hamster.
    B. *Quartz-rod illumination* transmits cold light into the interior of organs.
        This medium traps light, conducts it and avoids the coagulation of protoplasm.
    C. *Transparent windows* can be inserted into an animal's ear and left indefinitely.
        Tissue regeneration, vascular activities, etc., can then be observed directly.
    D. *Microdissection needles* can isolate, cut, tear or stretch cells; this is *microsurgery*.
        The needles are activated by a precision, supertype of mechanical stage.
        Capillary tubes can replace needles and inject or suck the cell contents.
    E. *Tissues can be cultured* in plasma and grown indefinitely for continuing study.
    F. *Motion-picture records* aid in the analysis of cellular activities.
        Lapsed-time films demonstrate slower motions at a speeded-up rate.
            Mitosis, phagocytosis, ameboid motion, etc., can be shown to advantage.
        Slow-motion films permit fast action to be analyzed.
            Beating cilia, contracting muscle, etc., can be followed.

2. Staining of unfixed tissues.

A. VITAL STAINING.

Some dyes are neither toxic to living cells nor destroyed by them.

These exist as colloidal particles, rather than as true solutions.

Examples of such vital dyes: trypan blue; India ink; Thorotrast.

Such pigmented substances are injected into the body as dilute suspensions.

They are then removed from the bood stream by phagocytic cells.

These scavenger cells ingest particles and store them in concentrated form.

This colors the phagocytic cells and renders them conspicuous.

B. SUPRAVITAL STAINING.

Other dyes, although toxic, are taken up by cells removed previously from the body.

Such cells are moribund, but may survive for hours.

Examples: mitochondria, stained by Janus green; nerve cells and fibers, by methylene blue; connective-tissue elements (white or elastic fibers; fat or mast cells; leucocytes), by suitable dyes.

This method is limited to special purposes.

C. PREPARATION OF DEAD TISSUE:

1. Fixation.

The primary objective is to preserve protoplasm with the least alteration.

In killing, which produces a coagulation of protoplasm and a separation of solid from liquid, the fixative should accomplish several objectives:

Penetrate quickly, preventing postmortem changes (autolytic; bacterial).

Preserve the living conditions as faithfully as possible.

Render the protoplasm insoluble and harden it.

Increase the affinity of protoplasm for future stains.

Any fixation produces some artificial changes, called *artifacts*.

Carbohydrates and salts are usually removed (as are, sometimes, lipids).

The ability to recognize the more gross induced and unnatural states is indispensable to the proper interpretation of microscopical preparations.

Chemical solutions are most commonly employed as fixing agents.

Typical reagents are: alcohol; formalin; mercuric bichloride; potassium bichromate; acids (acetic; formic; osmic; picric).

But no single fixative possesses all the desirable qualities just listed.

Hence a compromise is made by use of mixtures designed for specific purposes.

Such mixtures are Zenker's fluid; Bouin's fluid; Mueller's fluid; etc.

Nevertheless, all these compound fixatives also give imperfect results.

The freeze-drying technique introduces less alterations than chemicals do.

Tissue is frozen in isopentane (chilled to $-170°$ C.) and dehydrated in a vacuum.

For electron microscopy tiny (0.3 mm.) pieces of tissue are fixed in osmic acid.

Such bits of tissue maintain an appearance close to the living state.

2. Embedding.

The tissue is dehydrated and hardened in alcohol or some other organic solvent.

The withdrawal of water (and its subsequent replacement by embeddng material) tends to distort further the natural appearance of protoplasmic structures.

Next it is 'cleared' (*i.e.*, made translucent) in a reagent, such as xylol (or ether).

These fluids are soluble both in alcohol and in melted paraffin (or nitrocellulose).

This permits paraffin (or nitrocellulose) to infiltrate the tissues.

Finally the specimen is encased in a block of solid paraffin (or nitrocellulose).

For electron microscopy, fluid plastic is infiltrated and then polymerized to a solid.

3. *Sectioning.*

Thin slices of the impregnated and blocked tissue are cut with a microtome.
The thickness is usually between 2 and 10 microns (0.002−0.010 mm.).
Sections are then affixed to a slide and the paraffin dissolved away.
Nitrocellulose or other semitransparent media may be left intact.
For electron microscopy, sections as thin as 0.02 micron are cut on a special microtome.

4. *Staining.*

Staining in contrasting colors brings out the structural details still further.
The coloring ability of most dyes resides in either their acid or basic radical.
If in the anion, the dye is called acid; if in the cation, it is called basic.
In general, cellular components are either acid or basic in nature.
Those that are acid (*e.g.,* nuclear chromatin) stain with basic dyes.
Such components are said to be *basophilic.*
Those that are basic (*e.g.,* various kinds of cytoplasm) stain with acid dyes.
Such constituents are said to be *acidophilic.*
These reactions make selective, differential staining possible.
Special methods are necessary to demonstrate certain cell components.
Some constituents may attract both dyes (or stain by their interaction product).
The granules of neutrophilic leucocytes exemplify this behavior.
In electron microscopy there are differences in electron scatter by cell components.
These differences substitute for staining by producing contrasts.

5. *Mounting.*

Stained sections are placed on a slide in a gummy medium that eventually hardens.
This material has approximately the same refractive index as glass.
The preparation is then covered with a thin wafer of glass.
For electron microscopy, sections are floated onto a thin plastic film.

D. MISCELLANEOUS TECHNIQUES:

1. *Teased* and spread bits of tissue are examined fresh or after supravital staining.

2. *Maceration* softens binding material and thus isolates cells, tubules, lobules, etc.

3. *Microincineration* of tissue slices leaves ash that retains fine structural details.
Some minerals can then be identified within cells in exact locations.

4. *Centrifuging* gives information on the relative weights of cell constituents.
It shows the displaceability of parts, consistent with continued life.
It can separate cell components from a ground-up tissue homogenate.
These graded isolates can then be studied and analyzed.

5. *Autoradiography* is a technique that demonstrates the fate of substances fed or otherwise introduced into an animal.
The substances are ones used by cells and labeled with a radioactive isotope.
The labeled material is incorporated into appropriate tissues of the body.
A section of the affected tissue is placed in contact with a photographic emulsion.
Development shows the location and concentration of radioactivity.
This method can demonstrate syntheses, the process of secretion, the deposit of formed products, and can indicate turn-over times in metabolism.

6. *Microchemical testing* by qualitative analytical methods on local areas is possible.
A large number of organic and inorganic constituents, and numerous enzymes, can be identified, localized and sometimes quantitated by suitable tests.
Such biochemical procedures, done on sectioned tissues, constitute *histochemistry.*
Methods employed are physical, chemical and immunofluorescent.

7. *Microspectroscopy* provides information obtainable by several methods.
   Visible light, ultraviolet light and x-rays are used.
   Absorption spectra identify and show the distribution of specific substances.
   The dry mass of cell components can be measured with exactitude.

8. *X-ray diffraction* employs a crystal-grating of molecular dimensions.
   Its application is limited to crystalline, laminar and linear structures.
   An enormously magnified diffraction pattern is recorded photographically.
   The presence, spacing and orientation of molecules can be deduced.
       It supplies a concept of three-dimensional patterns within molecules.
   It permits certain chemical analyses of objects to be made.
       These may be only a few cubic microns in size.

9. *Micro-electrodes,* used as tubules, can measure potential differences.
   In this way the variance between the inside and outside of cells can be found.

V. THE UNITS OF MEASUREMENT

The small size of microscopical structures requires special units of measurement.
The unit used in work done with the ordinary light microscope is the *micron.*
   Its symbol is μ (the Greek letter mu).
   Its length is 0.001 mm., or 1/25,000 inch.
   The human red blood corpuscle can often be used as a visual measuring stick.
       It can usually be found in stained sections; the diameter is about 5 μ.
The greatest dimension of mammalian cells tends to range between 10 and 30 μ.
   Yet some are very small; certain brain cells measure only 4 μ.
   On the other hand, some nerve cells extend for inches, or even feet.
A smaller unit, sometimes employed, is the *millimicron.*
   It is 0.001 μ and its symbol is mμ.
Extreme magnifications, as in electron micrographs, make use of a still smaller unit.
   Borrowing is made of the *Ångstrom unit,* originally used by physicists.
   This is 0.0001 μ; its symbol is Å.

Chapter II

Protoplasm

"*Protoplasm* is the material basis of life" (Thomas Huxley).

It is the living, essential substance of which all animals and plants are made.

Protoplasm occurs in living organisms as unit masses called *cells*.

A cell is a mass of protoplasm, named *cytoplasm,* containing a central kernel of differently specialized protoplasm named the *nucleus*.

The cytoplasm is bounded by a specialized border, the *plasma membrane* (or *cell membrane*).

I. PROPERTIES

In order to study protoplasm intimately, it must be killed by fixation.

This, however, entails the precipitation and coagulation of proteins; hence changes enter.

1. *Physical characteristics.*

Protoplasm is semifluid, viscid, ductile, and more or less transparent.

It is an aggregate of crystalloids and colloids.

More precisely, it is an aqueous solution holding complex colloids in suspension.

It is also a reversible sol-gel system.

It is predominantly fluid, but capable of becoming more viscous.

At death, or on fixation, an irreversible gelation occurs.

2. *Chemical constitution.*

Analysis shows the presence of C, O, H, N as the major constituents of protoplasm.

In smaller amounts P, S, Mg and Ca occur decreasingly, in that order.

Heavy metals, such as Fe, occur and many other elements are present as traces.

These constituents combine into proteins, carbohydrates, lipids and salts.

As such they are associated intimately in a watery medium.

Considerable progress has been made in demonstrating the presence of specific chemical substances and their exact locations within cells and tissues.

Important to cell structure and function are *macromolecules*.

They are constructed from simpler units that are linked by repeated bondings.

The vital qualities of protoplasm correlate with macromolecular properties.

These macromolecules fall into three main categories:

Polysaccharides include glycogen and important mucopolysaccharides.

Among the latter are chondroitin sulfates and hyaluronic acid.

Proteins consist of amino acids joined in an exact peptide sequence.

Included are structural proteins, enzymes and some hormones.

They participate in the greatest variety of protoplasmic activities.

Nucleic acids engage in protein syntheses, and store the capability for so doing.

Deoxyribonucleic acid (DNA) occurs chiefly in the nucleus.

Ribonucleic acid (RNA) occurs in both the nucleus and the cytoplasm.

Water comprises 75 per cent of the slightly alkaline protoplasm.

It acts as a solvent, as a participant in biochemical reactions and as a determiner of various relations assumed by macromolecules; it is a genuine component.

It is calculated that a single cell contains trillions of molecules.

II. STRUCTURE

Living protoplasm is a colorless, colloidal jelly in which granules, threads and fluid droplets are sometimes demonstrable even with the ordinary light microscope.

Many of these visible objects are nonliving products of cell activity.

Fixed protoplasm tends to vary in appearance, depending on the reagents used.

Acid fixatives favor precipitation into granules or fibrils.

Neutral fixatives favor a more homogeneous coagulation.

A net-like *spongioplasm* and more homogeneous *hyaloplasm* are commonly obtained.

This relatively gross change from the living state is clearly artifactual.

Living protoplasm, at best, shows only as a granular gel under the light microscope.

Yet even a clear, apparently structureless protoplasm consists of both gelled and fluid protein-components, demonstrable with the electron microscope.

The fibrillar proteins of the general cytoplasm constitute important structural components.

Nevertheless, fibrillar proteins disperse at times and later return to a fibrillar state.

They are responsible for the reversible sol-gel behavior of cytoplasm.

The cytoplasm is notable for the presence of abundant, membrane-lined spaces.

The electron microscope demonstrates these as the so-called *endoplasmic reticulum.*

It also demonstrates granules (*ribosomes*) both on the membranes and free in cytoplasm.

Various micromolecular aggregations comprise a group of constituents known as *organelles.*

Many metabolic processes take place in them, rather than in the general cytoplasm.

III. VITAL ACTIVITIES

Protoplasmic components are stereo-isomerically associated and combined in such a manner that the resulting complex acquires the characteristics of life.

Whether protoplasm could be synthesized, and life be created artificially, is debated.

Four general categories of visible activity are recognizable in living protoplasm.

A. MOTILITY:

1. *Protoplasmic streaming.*

Internal streaming of cytoplasm may occur within a relatively immobile cell.

This is well illustrated in the rotatory movements within some plant cells.

Less rapid and more irregular shiftings occur in various animal cells.

These are best appreciated when viewed in lapsed-time motion pictures.

2. *Ameboid movement.*

This is a type of progression achieved by flowing or rolling over a substrate.

The cytoplasm extends a pseudopodial process and then flows into it.

Example: ameba; leucocytes; macrophage.

The exact method of pseudopod formation is, however, not surely known.

Local activity of the peripheral cytoplasm accomplishes *phagocytosis*.

This response may or may not be associated with ameboid movement.

The cell membrane cups about a particle and encloses it.

The enclosed portion of the total membrane then detaches.
> In this way the particle becomes intracellular within a membrane-bounded vesicle.
Phagocytosed material includes: bacteria; red corpuscles; dye particles; soot.
A comparable process ingests tiny fluid droplets or particles of macromolecular size.
> This activity has been named *pinocytosis*.

3. *Ciliary and flagellate lashing.*

Cilia are hair-like protoplasmic processes that vibrate in rhythmic sequence.
> They are numerous and relatively short, acting like oars or lashes.
> Example: mobile ciliate protozoans; stationary epithelial sheets.
Flagella are longer and often stouter; they are few to a cell, or even single.
> Example: flagellate protozoans; spermatozoa.

4. *Contractility.*

Shortening and thickening characterize this type of protoplasmic activity.
Most common and distinctive is a shortening limited to one axis.
> This is illustrated in some protozoans and coelenterates.
> It reaches its highest expression in true muscle fibers.

B. IRRITABILITY:

Protoplasm has the capacity to receive stimuli and set up an impulse.
> An impulse is a wave of excitation passing through protoplasm.
> The ability to transmit an impulse constitutes the property of *conductivity*.
Various kinds of stimuli are able to educe such excitation.
> Example: mechanical; thermal; chemical; photic; electric.
All cells are irritable, but the quality is best developed in nerve cells.

C. METABOLISM:

Included are all the transformations of energy and matter accomplished by protoplasm.
It presents two phases — one constructive, the other destructive.
> Some components of the body are broken down and replaced at short intervals.

1. *Anabolism.*

During digestion, food is split into simpler stuffs (*e.g.,* glucose; glycerine; fatty acids; amino acids); these products are absorbed and transported by the blood and lymph.
Some substances are stored as such (*e.g.,* glucose; fat).
Other substances are built into complex products (*e.g.,* secretions; cellular enzymes).
> Even protoplasm itself is synthesized, both for replacements and for growth.
> Hydrolytic synthesis and reduction are involved; energy is utilized and stored.
One type of growth results from protoplasmic synthesis in excess of maintenance.
> This method of *internal growth* is a distinctive feature of living organisms.
> By contrast, nonliving things (*e.g.,* crystals) grow by *accretion* (*i.e.,* external additions).

2. *Catabolism.*

Energy is released by breaking down and burning up materials (*cellular respiration*).
> In this process cellular enzymes serve as biologic catalysts.
> Hydrolysis and oxidation of stored products are the chief processes involved.
> Protoplasm itself is largely spared from catabolic destruction.
The end-products are unutilizable wastes; these are eliminated from the body.
> *Excretion* is a sifting out from the circulation of such residual waste products.
> > Also excess materials (*e.g.,* water; salts; glucose; hormones) are removed.

D. REPRODUCTION:

Protoplasm is able to perpetuate itself through processes of growth and subdivision.
Growth results chiefly from constructive metabolism and the synthesis of new protoplasm.

New cells arise from the halving of pre-existing cells; this is called *cell division.*
An understanding of cell division depends on a knowledge of cell structure.
For this reason descriptions will be deferred until later (p. 27).

IV. THE CORRELATION OF ACTIVITIES

Motility and irritability are primarily functions of the cytoplasm.
Metabolism and reproduction are functions primarily controlled by the nucleus.
These statements are corroborated when a large protozoan is cut into two parts.
A part consisting wholly of cytoplasm moves and responds to stimuli.
But after a time it dies, incapable of anabolism, growth or reproduction.
A part containing the nucleus regenerates, metabolizes and reproduces.

Chapter III

The Cell

Studies of cell structure (and correlations with cell function) comprise the subject of *cytology*.
The *cell* is the structural and functional unit of the body.

It is a minute (and usually definitely circumscribed) mass of protoplasm.

Most obvious is the *cytoplasm* which contains a central kernel, the *nucleus*.

A delicate *plasma membrane*, or *plasmolemma*, forms a peripheral boundary to the cytoplasm.
All cells also contain several kinds of *organelles* within the cytoplasm.

These specializations are distinctive structural units that perform specific functions.

Among them, animal cells are characterized by having a division body (*centrosome*).
Study shows that the cell is not simple, but extremely complex in its structure and activities.
Functionally the cell is characterized by the ability to assimilate, synthesize, grow, reproduce and
respond to external stimuli.

I. CELL GENERALITIES

1. Shape.

The primary, fundamental shape of isolated cells is spheroidal.
Example: contracted leucocyte; egg cell; fat cell.
Specialization alters the shape of some cells profoundly.
Example: stellate nerve cell; spindle-shaped muscle cell.
Contact with a surface promotes flattening of a cell.
Mutual pressure produces a faceted surface, as in a mass of soap bubbles.
Such cells tend to be 14-sided, thus providing the most effective packing.
A section, cut through a 14-sided solid, usually shows six sides.
In practice, this is the commonest shape seen in sections of massed cells.
Sections of compact fat illustrate this fact well.
Modified shapes accompany specialized activities and stresses.
Example: discoid; columnar; pyramidal; spindle; stellate.
An unstable, changeable shape is characteristic of some cells.
Example: ameba; leucocyte; macrophage.

2. Polarity.

The constituent parts of a cell often exhibit a definite spatial arrangement.
This is with respect both to each other and to the cell as a whole.
When the cell is elongate, the nucleus becomes ovoid to cigar-shaped.
The nucleus then lies in the long axis of the cell.
The location of the nucleus may be correlated with the position and orientation of various
other cell components.
In cuboidal to columnar cells the nucleus takes its position nearer the base.
Certain cell-components then may lie still nearer the base.
Example: synthesizing material (ergastoplasm) of gland cells.
Other cell-components locate above the nucleus, nearer the top.
Example: centrosome; Golgi apparatus; secretion granules.
Still other cell-components may orient in the long dimension of the cell.
Example: mitochondria; tonofibrils.
Such spatial relations illustrate how a cell may possess structural polarity.

3. *Size.*

Only rarely are cells visible to the naked eye; they are then 'macroscopic.'
Example: many eggs (but mammalian eggs are barely visible).
Some cells are greatly elongated; they then become extremely slender.
Example: a muscle cell may be an inch long; a neuron may be a yard long.
Extremely large cells are commonly called *giant cells.*
They may have only a single nucleus within abundant cytoplasm.
Example: megakaryocyte of bone marrow.
When there are several to many nuclei, such cells are called *multinucleate cells.*
This commonly results from the fusion of cells originally separate.
Example: osteoclast; skeletal muscle fiber.
Such a merged product is also named a *syncytium.*
Cell size differs somewhat among the several vertebrate groups.
Amphibians have the largest cells; mammals have rather small cells.
There is no correlation between the size of an animal and the size of its cells.
The cells of an elephant are scarcely larger than those of a mouse.
Cells and their components are measured in micra or Ångstroms (p. 14).

4. *Numbers.*

The size of an animal is determined by the number of its cells rather than by their size.
Colonial protozoa may consist of a cluster containing but few cells.
Rotifers have less than 1000 cells.
The total number in a mouse, man or whale is prodigious.
In the cerebral cortex the number of nerve cells is said to be 9,200,000,000.
The red blood corpuscles of an average-sized man total 25,000,000,000,000.

5. *Specializations.*

Cells develop differences in structure correlated with the acquirement of specific function.
Example: muscle cells specialize for contractility; nerve cells, for conductivity; gland
cells, for secretion; fibroblasts, for support.
Such specialization entails a loss of other potentialities that existed earlier.
That is, differentiation progressively narrows multiple possibilities to one fate.

II. THE CYTOPLASM

The *cytoplasm* is a specific kind of protoplasm.
It includes all of the protoplasm of a cell, except that of the nucleus.
It differentiates locally in ways that produce many kinds of important specializations.

A. PLASMA MEMBRANE (or Cell Membrane).

The cytoplasmic boundary is a condensed peripheral film, the *plasma membrane.*
It is very thin, about 0.008 μ, and only a few molecules thick.
The light microscope sometimes reveals it, in slanting sections, as a line.
The electron microscope resolves a middle zone, bounded by two denser layers.
It also reveals extensive infoldings of the membrane in some cells.
This type of three-layered membrane is called a *unit membrane.*
It consists of a lipid film, bounded at each surface by adsorbed protein molecules.
It is a semipermeable living membrane, essential to cell life.
It determines what exchanges occur by osmosis, and what by active transport.
It is active in phagocytosis, pinocytosis and particle ejection (p. 16).
If broken locally, cytoplasm may extrude; but repair tends to follow.
Too great an injury, mechanical or chemical, leads to cell death.

Microdissection proves the cell membrane to be quite elastic.
>It is also tougher and more resistant than the general cytoplasm internal to it.
Outside the plasma membrane there may be a nonliving reinforcement.
>Such products of cell metabolism are characteristic of plants, bacteria and eggs.
Animal cells in general bear a surface-covering of glycoproteins, the *cell coat.*
>It serves as an adhesive, holding cells together, and probably has other functions.

B. Cytoplasm Proper:

The extreme periphery of some cells is specialized as a clear *ectoplasm,* whereas the more internal and granular protoplasm is called *endoplasm.*
>Example: ameboid cells; some eggs; apical zone of intestinal lining.
>Body cells, in general, do not show this distinction clearly.
Ectoplasm is a clear zone; it is gelated, more refractive and free of organelles.
Endoplasm, by contrast, is more fluid, granular and mobile.
>Its relatively structureless ground-substance contains various constituents.
>>Living, specialized components are called *organelles.*
>>Nonliving components are designated as *inclusions.*
Mature cytoplasm is commonly acidophilic; it then colors with acid stains (*e.g.,* eosin).
>Cytoplasm, however, may be basophilic or neutrophilic.
>>Basophily is associated with the presence of ribonucleic acid in specialized granules.
>>Such cytoplasm, or local region, colors with basic stains (*e.g.,* hematoxylin).

C. Organelles:

These are definite, localized specializations of the living cytoplasm.
>They are permanent constituents of a cell that act as 'cell organs' with important functions.
>They persist during cell division; some, at least, definitely self-replicate.
>Most of the details concerning them have been revealed by the electron microscope.

1. *Plasma membrane.* See page 20.

2. *Ribosomes.*

Cytoplasm frequently displays material that stains deeply with basic dyes.
>Such includes the easily demonstrable *Nissl bodies* within nerve cells and the basally located *ergastoplasm* of some gland cells.
Electron microscopy shows the stainable material to consist of extremely fine granules.
>These *ribosomes* are composed of protein-bound ribonucleic acid.
>This acid is responsible for the basophilic response of the granules.
Some ribosomes lie free in the general ground substance of cytoplasm.
>They are sites of replenishment of proteins used in cytoplasmic activities.
Others attach to sets of cytoplasmic membranes, the *endoplasmic reticulum.*
>They are sites of synthesis of proteins to be expelled from the cells as secretions.
Ribosomes are extremely abundant in some cells and relatively scarce in others.
>(They also occur in the nucleus, and especially arise in the nucleolus.)

3. *Endoplasmic reticulum.*

The cytoplasm contains a system of closely set, channels bounded by unit membranes.
>They take the form of fluid-filled tubules, flat sacs (*cisternae*) or isolated *vesicles.*
>Tubules and sacs branch freely and anastomose with similar membranous units.
The external surface may be studded with ribosomes (*granular endoplasmic reticulum*).
>Such 'rough-surfaced reticulum' makes proteins that are expelled as secretions.
By contrast, the membrane may lack ribosomes (*agranular endoplasmic reticulum*).
>Such 'smooth-surfaced reticulum' functions variously in different types of cells.
The system is at places continuous with the plasma- and nuclear membranes.
Endoplasmic reticulum functions in syntheses: it also acts as a transport system.
>Other activities relate to diffusion barriers, ionic gradients and bioelectric potentials.

4. Golgi apparatus.

This complex is demonstrable in the living cell by phase microscopy or vital staining.
    It then appears as a system of clear canals.
    It is a structural entity since it can be displaced bodily by centrifuging.
Osmic acid or silver impregnation likewise demonstrates a network of blackened canals.
The complex is often localized above the nucleus, and even about the centrosome.
    But it may be scattered or dispersed widely in the cytoplasm (*e.g.*, nerve cells).
    Its appearance varies in different cell types, and also with cell activity.
Electron micrographs show stacks (often curved) of smooth-surfaced flat saccules.
    These bound a region bearing variably sized vesicles and secretion granules.
    Small vesicles occur also on the outer (often convex) surface of the stacks.
Functions of the Golgi apparatus in many types of cells are unknown (or largely so).
    Nevertheless, some relations can be deduced where secretions are protein.
Protein, synthesized in the endoplasmic reticulum, moves within its canals.
    Transported as droplets (in *transfer vesicles*), it is concentrated in the complex.
    Such 'granules' are packaged within membrane-bounded vesicles, and are ejected.
Synthesis of polysaccharides seems to take place within the complex itself.
In intestinal absorption, lipid accumulates briefly in the cisternae of the complex.
The Golgi complex is a self-perpetuating organelle during mitotic cell division.

5. Cell center (or centrosome).

This small, gelated body tends to occupy a central position within the animal cell.
    Yet it is commonly displaced by the nucleus or by synthesized cytoplasmic products.
    It is often inconspicuous in resting cells, but becomes prominent during mitosis.
        At this time a globular *centrosphere* and radiating *astral rays* may be seen.
The light microscope resolves two deeply staining particles within the centrosomal mass.
The electron microscope shows that each particle is a pair of closely associated bodies.
    Each component of a pair is named a *centriole,* and the two are called a *diplosome.*
    A centriole is a cylindrical structure, shaped like a barrel with one closed end.
        The 'staves' of the barrel are nine rod-like fibrils, loosely arranged.
        Each 'fibril' is compound, consisting of three parallel, interconnected tubules.
    The two cylinders of a centriole-pair stand perpendicular to each other, T-fashion.
Both the centrosome and its astral rays (tiny tubules) have been seen in living cells.
    The total mass can be pushed about by the needle of a microsurgery apparatus.
The complex as a whole is a dynamic center, important during cell division (p. 27).
    The centriole is the only cytoplasmic organelle that reproduces itself exactly.
    In ciliated cells centrioles replicate, each becoming a *basal body* of a cilium.

6. Mitochondria.

These numerous organelles are distributed, and sometimes localized, in the cytoplasm.
    Special techniques stain them, both in fresh tissues and in fixed sections.
    The dark-field and phase-contrast methods also demonstrate them in living cells.
Mitochondria range in shape from spherules to rods; the average length is about 5 μ.
    Also their external shape and internal structure vary in different cell-types.
    Their number correlates with the metabolic activity of different cell-types.
Mitochondria consist of a fluid *matrix* contained within a triple-layered *sheath.*
    The inner layer of this *unit membrane* makes thin infoldings into the matrix.
        This produces numerous transverse shelves named *cristae.*
        The number and length of cristae vary with the amount of enzymic work done.
Specific enzymes are located in the matrix and on the inner membrane (and its cristae).
    Some relate to the Krebs cycle and to the synthesis of amino acids and lipids.
    Others direct respiratory processes and provide energy for many metabolic activities.
        A chief result is furnishing energy-rich adenosine triphosphate to the cell.
Some DNA and RNA have been identified in the matrix-substance, and studied.
Mitochondria are semi-independent, controlling some of their own vital activities.
    Included are syntheses, DNA replication, reproduction by binary fission, and growth.
Their life-span is about one week, but the method of replacement is unsettled.

7. Lysosomes.

These are membrane-bounded vesicles, spheroid in shape; most are electron dense.
They have little or no internal organization, but imprison various acid hydrolases.
They merge with membranous vesicles that contain particles engulfed into the cell.
    This material, originally ingested by phagocytosis or pinocytosis, is then digested.
    If indigestible, like lipofuchsin pigment, it is stored in the cytoplasm.
On cell death the released enzymes bring about the autolysis of the containing cell.
Lysosomes probably originate in the Golgi complex, much like secretory granules.

8. Miscellaneous organelles.

Filaments occur in the cells of epithelium, muscle, nerve and neuroglia.
    Functions are related to movement and, presumably, to support.
Microtubules occur generally in cells, but have varied and uncertain significance.
    Example: mitotic spindle; components of neurofibrils, cilia and centrioles.
    A dense aggregation at the apex of some epithelial cells is the *terminal web.*
    Suggested functions relate to the maintenance and change of cell shape.
Microbodies are membrane-bounded spheroids, found only in a few cell-types.
    They are finely granular, and rich in peroxidase and some other enzymes.
(Not all representatives in these categories have a clear claim as living organelles.)

D. Inclusions:

Both metabolic products and ingested substances are nonliving occupants of the cytoplasm.

1. Secretory granules.

They are characteristic features of glandular activity, particularly in epithelium.
Their identification as precursors of secretion products is well established.
    Their history is cyclic, paralleling that of the gland cell.
    In life they are semifluid glubules, whereas on fixation they coagulate into granules.
Some of these membrane-bounded globules give rise to enzymes; others to mucus, etc.
Their association with the Golgi apparatus was discussed in a previous paragraph.

2. Nutritive substances.

A. Proteins.
    Cytoplasm is largely protein, but none seems to be 'free' as an inclusion.
        Yet some of the 'vital store' can be catabolized when nutrition is deficient.
    On fixation, proteins precipitate as granules.
B. Carbohydrates.
    The carbohydrate reserves of the body are almost exclusively glycogen.
    The richest sites of storage are in cells of the liver and skeletal muscles.
        In life glycogen probably occurs in solution as tiny fluid droplets.
        Fixation precipitates its submicroscopic particles.
            It then takes the form of compound granules.
C. Lipids.
    This reserve occurs most prominently as globules within specialized cells.
        There may be separate globules, or a single fat pool in each cell.
            They are not membrane-bounded, and merely occupy vacuoles.
        Such fat-stores dissolve out of fixed tissues unless rendered insoluble.
    Some of the lipid is invisible and is spoken of as 'masked' or 'bound.'
        It either is very finely dispersed or is combined with proteins.
D. Yolk.
    Lipoproteins may be present in the form of yolk spheres.
    They are characteristic of eggs, and hence of the yolk sac of many embryos.
        Cells of the gut of some vertebrate embryos contain yolk for a while.

3. Pigments.

Pigment is synthesized by various cells of the body (*e.g., melanoblasts*, etc.).
> The chief types are *melanin, hemoglobin* and *lipofuchsin.*
> They are, in order, light-absorptive, oxygen-binding, and wear-and-tear products.

Some cells take up and store pigment, but do not make any.
> Such cells are *chromatophores* (*e.g.,* pigment cells of the iris of the eye).
> Of the pigments stored, some (*e.g.,* carotene) come from plants eaten as food.

4. Bodies of uncertain significance.

Crystals sometimes occur, apparently protein in nature.
> Example: interstitial cells of the testis; B-cells of pancreatic islets.

Specific granules (such as *microbodies*) occur in some cells and stain distinctively.

5. Vacuoles.

These cytoplasmic cavities are, for the most part, storage cavities.
> Example: fat droplets; glycogen droplets.
> When the contents are given up or digested, a vacant space may become apparent.

Such vacuoles are different from shrinkage artifacts produced by faulty fixation.
Still different are cavities produced by degenerative and postmortem changes.

6. Foreign substances.

Extraneous materials may come to lie within the cytoplasm.
> These have been taken up by phagocytosis and similar ingestive activities.
> Example: bacteria; cellular debris; dusts; lead accumulations.

E. Functional Correlations:

The cytoplasm contains the specialized units that carry out most of the work of the cell.
> This ranges through the functions discussed previously as 'vital activities' (p. 16).

Of course, the nucleus plays a direct or indirect role in some of these actions (p. 26).
> But the factory and its machinery are almost exclusively the cytoplasm.

III. THE NUCLEUS

Near the center of the cell is a prominent body, known as the nucleus.
> The Latin word *nucleus* or the Greek word *karyon* signifies 'the kernel of a nut.'
> Hence nucleo- and karyo- are used in combined words referring to the nucleus.

A. Number:

Usually there is but one nucleus to a cell.
Sometimes two occur; such cells are *binucleate.*
> Example: some epithelial cells of the liver; of the bladder; of gastric glands.

Moreover, several to many nuclei may occur; such cells are *multinucleate.*
> Example: skeletal muscle fibers; giant cells of developing bone; some ganglion cells.

B. Shape and Size:

Usually the nucleus is globular to ovoid, somewhat in conformity with cell shape.
> Cytoplasmic inclusions may temporarily flatten or otherwise distort the nucleus.

Other shapes occur in special cell types.
> Example: elongate (smooth muscle); crescentic (monocyte); lobate (neutrophil).

Nuclear size is related to cell size, and is uniform in the same cell type.

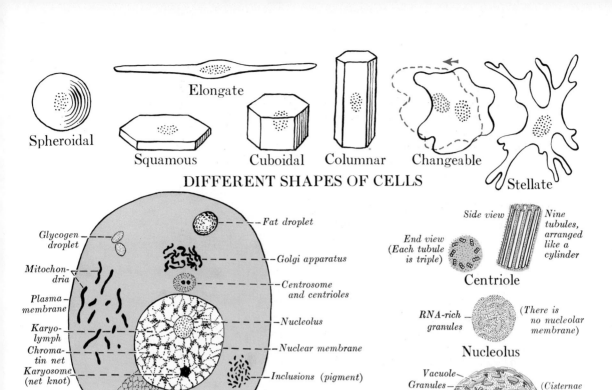

DIFFERENT SHAPES OF CELLS

Spheroidal · Elongate · Squamous · Cuboidal · Columnar · Changeable · Stellate

CELL STRUCTURE (Ordinary microscopy)

Glycogen droplet — Fat droplet — Golgi apparatus — Centrosome and centrioles — Nucleolus — Nuclear membrane — Inclusions (pigment) — Water vacuole

Mitochondria — Plasma membrane — Karyolymph — Chromatin net — Karyosome (net knot) — Cytoplasm detail

DETAILS (Electron microscopy)

Centriole
Side view · Nine tubules, arranged like a cylinder
End view (Each tubule is triple)

Nucleolus
RNA-rich granules · (There is no nucleolar membrane)

Golgi apparatus
Vacuole · Granules · Microvesicles · Cisternae · (Cisternae are flat endoplas. saccules)

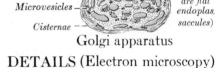

CELL DETAILS (Electron microscopy)

Plasma membrane — Lysosome (hydrolytic enzymes) — Ground cytoplasm — Ribosomes (RNA-rich granules) — Chromatin (DNA-rich granules) — Mitochondria (oxidative enzymes) — Crista — Paired membranes of endoplasmic reticulum (saccules or tubules) — Nuclear membrane

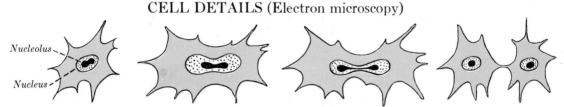

Nucleolus — Nucleus

STAGES SAID TO ILLUSTRATE AMITOSIS

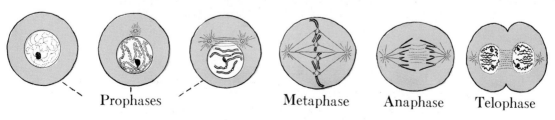

Prophases · Metaphase · Anaphase · Telophase

STAGES OF MITOSIS IN ANIMAL CELLS

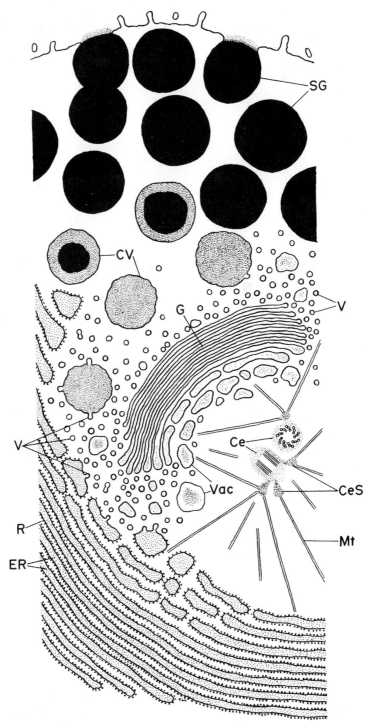

CYTOPLASMIC CONSTITUENTS. Centrioles (Ce) are cut across and lengthwise; associated are centriolar satellites (CeS), from which microtubules (Mt) radiate. Nearby is a Golgi complex (G), which is a stack of smooth double membranes, associated with small vesicles (V) and large vacuoles (Vac). Rough endoplasmic reticulum (ER) bears ribosomes (R); synthesized proteins reach the Golgi through pinched-off vesicles (V, at left). Condensing vacuoles (CV) concentrate the product into secretory granules (SG). Discharge occurs when the membrane enclosing a granule fuses with the plasma membrane.

C. GENERAL CHARACTERISTICS:

Descriptions are usually based on the appearance of the so-called resting cell.

This term refers to the relatively stable period between cell divisions.

Actually, at this time (the *interphase*) the ordinary functions of a cell are being performed.

A living nucleus is usually more of a gel and more refractile than the cytoplasm.

The micro-needle can move the nucleus about in the cytoplasm.

The nucleus has a lower specific gravity than the ground cytoplasm.

It is plastic under pressure, but on release regains its shape.

It is often more viscous than cytoplasm and gels quickly when cut.

The nuclear protoplasm, as a whole, is named *nucleoplasm* or *karyoplasm*.

A generalized nucleoplasmic ground-substance is called *nuclear sap* (or *karyolymph*).

Interspersed in the nuclear sap are a globular *nucleolus* and a mesh of *chromatin*.

If the chromatin meshwork is well spaced, the nucleus is said to be *vesicular*, or pale.

If the nucleus is shrunken and the chromatin condensed, it is said to be *pycnotic*.

Chromatin, as seen, comprises the visible parts of 46 rod-shaped *chromosomes*.

This *diploid* number is the sum of two single (*haploid*) sets of 23 chromosomes.

A single set was furnished by each parent at the time of fertilization.

The nucleus is bounded by a thin *nuclear membrane*, also called a *nuclear envelope*.

D. DETAILED STRUCTURE:

When viewed with the ordinary microscope, the living nucleus appears homogenous, except for the presence of a much smaller nucleolus within it.

But phase contrast or ultraviolet light may demonstrate the chromatin meshwork.

The nuclear protoplasm (*nucleoplasm*, or *karyoplasm*) specializes into four distinctive parts.

1. Nuclear membrane (or nuclear envelope).

The light microscope reveals this envelope as a sharply demarcated, limiting membrane.

It is seven times thicker than the plasma membrane that encloses the cytoplasm.

The apparent thickness, as seen, is enhanced greatly by adhering chromatin.

The electron microscope demonstrates two thin membranes, separated by a space.

The outer membrane is continuous at places with the endoplasmic reticulum.

Also the two layers of the total membrane meet and appear to merge at intervals.

This seemingly leaves tiny circular openings, the *nuclear pores.*

Such would provide communication between nucleus and cytoplasm.

But in some instances, at least, the 'pore' is spanned by a thin diaphragm.

Microdissection proves the nuclear membrane to be tough and definitely elastic.

When it is punctured, the loss of nuclear contents leaves a wrinkled 'bag.'

2. Nuclear sap (or karyolymph).

This is a feebly staining, clear matrix, more viscous than the ground cytoplasm.

The electron microscope shows that it is finely granular, containing 'dispersed' chromatin.

It is a colloidal solution, holding the uncoiled, invisible portions of chromosomes.

3. Chromatin.

This substance was so named because it is so easily stained with dyes; 'chroma' means color.

Its acidic nature gives it an affinity for basic dyes, such as hematoxylin.

In the interphase stage of the cell, the visible chromatin appears as a meshwork, rather than as recognizable separate chromosomes.

Most prominent are deeply staining clumps called *karyosomes*, or *chromatin knots*.

These angular masses are portions of chromosomes arranged in tight coils.

Such masses (*heterochromatin*) are said to be relatively inactive metabolically.

Thinner threads of chromatin (extended coils) link up the larger masses.

Additional chromatin occurs, too extended and pale-staining to be ordinarily recognizable.

It is this loosely coiled *euchromatin* of chromosomes that is active in syntheses.

The complete set of 46 chromosomes is present, as such, during the interphase.

Individuality is retained, even though each is largely uncoiled and swollen.
(More concerning chromosomes will be found under *mitosis*, p. 27.)
One of the two X (or sex) chromosomes of the female remains compact during the interphase.
This *Barr body* is identifiable in nuclei of epithelial cells as a prominent mass.
It lies alongside the nuclear membrane, and is in an inactive state.
This mass (or its absence in the male) is useful in diagnosing doubtful sex.

4. *Nucleolus.*

This 'little nucleus' is conspicuous only in nuclei with a sparse chromatin meshwork.
It is small, eccentric in position, and there may be more than one.
It has a rounded, smooth contour (in contrast to karyosomes), but no enclosing membrane.
Externally there is a protein spongework bearing basophilic granules (RNA).
This surrounds a central, denser mass of paler-staining substance.
The nucleolus is in contact with a particular region of an associated chromosome.
Its loop retracts during early mitosis and the nucleolus disappears from view.
But later this region acts as the *nucleolar organizer*, and the nucleolus reappears.
In life the nucleolus is highly refractile and sharply defined.
It is more displaceable by centrifuging than other nuclear components.

5. *Chemical composition.*

The important components of the chromatin and nucleolus are the *nucleoproteins.*
These consist of nucleic acids combined with complex proteins.
Nucleic acids are complex structures that include a pentose sugar.
The exact type of sugar subdivides the nucleic acids into two main groups.
Deoxyribonucleic acid (abbreviated to DNA) occurs chiefly in chromatin.
It also occurs centrally in nucleoli and in mitochondria.
Ribonucleic acid (RNA) occurs in nuclei (largely in nucleoli) and cytoplasm.
It exists as three different functional kinds (see below).
Responses to dyes depend on the dominance of nucleic acid or protein.
Chromatin is strongly basophilic because of its high content of DNA.
It is stained selectively (purple-violet) with the Feulgen technique.
The nucleolus is also commonly basophilic, but because of preponderant RNA content.
Some of this is a structural component and some (ribosomes) is adherent peripherally.
The nucleolus may become acidophilic to stains when RNA is deficient.
This permits the protein component of the nucleoprotein to dominate in stainability.

E. FUNCTIONAL CORRELATIONS:

The nucleus is necessary to life, growth, differentiation and reproduction.
It directs the work of the cytoplasm, and especially constructive metabolism.
Protein synthesis depends on stored 'information' encoded on nuclear DNA.
A plan for each synthesis is arranged along the helical strands of chromosomes.
This is impressed template-fashion on *messenger RNA* synthesized in the nucleus.
Messenger RNA and a specific *transfer RNA* serve as intermediaries between DNA of the
nucleus and the responding RNA of cytoplasmic ribosomes.
They 'instruct' the latter about the particular protein to be synthesized.
The nucleus is also essential to cell reproduction and heredity-transmission.
The mechanism of heredity is identified with the presence of *genes*.
These are located along the chromatin-strands in definite order and position.
Their influence is exerted in producing properly timed syntheses in the cytoplasm.
The nucleolus is large when proteins are being synthesized actively.
It is small, or lacking, in cells not engaged in such syntheses.
These facts imply that the nucleolus is the source of RNA for ribosomes.

IV. CELL DIVISION

Three methods of cell division are recognized: *amitosis, mitosis* and *meiosis.*
After cells divide, the smaller daughter cells grow until they reach their size-norm.
    Growth-limits are set by individual ratios between cell surface and cell volume.
    This constant reflects the capability of surface intake to care for internal mass.
Each cell also tends to maintain a norm in the ratio of cell size to nuclear size.

A. Amitosis:

    The term *amitosis* (no thread) refers to the incidental role played by chromatin.
        'Direct cell division' is another designation of the process.
    The method is one in which nucleus and cytoplasm constrict and separate directly.
        It is an inexact halving in which the important chromatin is not divided evenly.
    The incidence of amitosis is controversial; many alleged cases are spurious.
        Living cells have been observed to stretch, but never to separate completely.
        Binucleate cells are not reliable proof of an uncompleted direct division.
    It is said that some transitory, specialized or moribund cells do utilize amitosis.
        But this method never occurs in young, unspecialized cells or in germ cells.

B. Mitosis:

    All cells pass through interphasic and mitotic periods at some time in their course.
        The *interphase* designates the stage between successive *mitoses.*
            During this period the cell performs its ordinary biochemical functions.
                Its duration in different cell types ranges from hours to months.
                Some cells (*e.g.,* nerve cells) never divide after the fetal period.
    Mitosis, also called *indirect cell division,* is the normal method of cell proliferation.
        Activities involve the nucleus (*karyokinesis*) and cytoplasm (*cytokinesis*).
        In this method chromatin threads (*chromosomes*) play a most important role.
    Reproductive and embryonic cells utilize mitosis to insure a precise distribution of genes.
        In this way the body acquires cells accustomed to the mitotic method of division.
    For descriptive convenience, five stages (phases) in the cycle are recognized.
        These are somewhat arbitrary subdivisions of a continuous cyclic process.

1. Interphase.

    Individual *chromosomes,* in the number characteristic for the species, are present.
        Yet they are largely uncoiled, and hence not recognizable as total entities.
            The still visible parts resemble a mesh, with some prominent lumps.
            Despite this, a characteristic sequence and spacing of *genes* is maintained.
    During the interphase the DNA, and hence each gene, replicates exactly.
        In doing this, each chromosome acts as a template-pattern.
        The result is a 'double chromosome'; each member is a *chromatid.*
            The previous set of 46 human chromosomes become 92 chromatids.
    The *centrioles,* commonly called a *diplosome,* are really two pairs.

2. Prophase.

    (The more terminal events are often designated as the *prometaphase.*)
    A. Changes within the Nucleus.
        As a start, the loose spiral of each chromatid progressively becomes a tight coil.
            This shortening (and thickening) may reduce the length by 95 per cent.
            The coilings are so tight that a single, solid chromosome seems to result.
                Actually each apparent chromosome consists of two chromatids in contact.
        The *nuclear membrane* fragments and disappears from sight.
        The *nucleolus* also disperses as its associated chromosomal loop retracts.
        All chromosomes move toward the equatorial plane of the cell.

B. CHANGES WITHIN THE CYTOPLASM.

The cell tends to become spherical.

The double pair of centrioles separates into two single sets of centrioles.

About each set may appear a so-called *aster* (*i.e.*, star) that stains poorly.

This is a system of achromatic, microtubular radiations called *astral rays*.

Each centriole-aster complex migrates toward an opposite pole of the cell.

Flowering plants lack centrioles and asters; many mammals lack asters.

A bundle of delicate microtubules, the *spindle,* arises between the asters.

In the production of rays and spindle-tubules the centrioles act as organizers.

3. Metaphase.

Chromosomes reach the equator of the cell and group on the spindle, at its periphery.

The chromosomes are arranged radially; each is still a pair of chromatids.

The arrangement (like the spokes of a wheel) is called the *equatorial plate.*

Spindle tubules attach to each chromatid at a special constricted region.

The two chromatids are separate except at this spot, the *centromere.*

At the end of the metaphase the centromere divides, one for each chromatid.

The individual chromatids then become wholly separate.

Each chromatid thereafter is considered to be a daughter chromosome.

4. Anaphase.

The pairs of daughter chromosomes move apart, beginning at the centromeres.

In this way the separate, new chromosomes become clearly apparent.

The human number in each set again totals 46.

The migration of both chromosome sets, toward opposite poles, continues to completion.

They act as if they were repelled, or pulled on by the microtubules of the spindle.

5. Telophase.

A. NUCLEAR RECONSTRUCTION.

The processes of the prophase now occur in reverse.

Chromosomes lose their condensed state, partially uncoil and swell.

The visible end-result is the formation of a new 'chromatin meshwork.'

A new *nuclear membrane* organizes, using neighboring endoplasmic reticulum.

The nucleolus reorganizes about a particular region of a special chromosome.

B. CYTOPLASMIC DIVISION.

In animals the cytoplasm constricts in the equatorial region.

Following a figure-8 stage, the two daughter cells become separate.

In plants, with rigid-cell walls, a *cell-plate* appears midway along the spindle.

The centriole-pair of each daughter cell duplicates, thus restoring the double set.

Other organelles (and inclusions) become distributed to the daughter cells.

The apportionment is random but fairly equal.

Duration of a mitotic cycle.

The total period varies with animal types, different tissues, physiological state and age.
The following are examples of timing in active cells, as observed in tissue cultures:

Mitotic stage	Embryonic mesenchyme	Fibroblasts
Prophase	10-15 minutes	30-60 minutes
Metaphase	2-3 "	2-10 "
Anaphase	3-4 "	2-3 "
Telophase	7-15 "	3-12 "
Interphase	37-97 "	30-120 "

C. MEIOSIS:

This specialized division occurs at one stage in the development of reproductive cells (p. 266).

Its purpose in man is to reduce the double set of 46 chromosomes to single sets of 23.

Such a single set then passes into each spermatozoön or egg.

This process insures that the fertilized egg acquires only the double set of 46.

Hence the chromosome number does not double in each generation.

D. KARYOTYPE:

Cells can be cultured and their mitoses halted with a drug (colchicine) at the metaphase.

Such cells, swollen and squashed flat, show chromosomes well separated.

Individual chromosomes can then be sorted into 23 matched pairs.

Criteria include size, shape and lengths of the two 'arms' diverging from the centromere.

Arranging pairs in progressive sequence produces the *karyotype* of a species.

Human chromosome pairs can be assigned to seven groups with confidence.

Further identifications within a group are much less certain.

Certain human anomalies are known to correlate with specific chromosomal aberrations.

A chromosome may be missing, partial, extra, or otherwise defective.

V. CELL AGING AND DEGENERATION

The term *cytomorphosis* denotes the series of successive changes undergone normally by a cell during its total life-span.

Although the changes are continuous, four main stages can be recognized.

1. *Embryonal stage.*

Cell division is active; nuclei are large; cytoplasm is relatively scanty and lacks visible signs of differentiation.

Example: embryonic cells; germinal layer of epidermis.

2. *Stage of specialization and maturity.*

Maximal *differentiation* in form, structure and function occurs.

These changes involve chiefly the cytoplasm and its elaborated products.

Also interstitial substance is sometimes laid down between cells.

Occasionally cells *dedifferentiate* and return to a former, less specialized state.

Example: cartilage into mesenchyme; sites of regeneration.

Under proper conditions such reverted cells can redifferentiate.

In doing this, some think they may adapt to new environmental conditions.

3. *Stage of regression.*

Alterations appear in the character of both the nucleus and cytoplasm.

The cell undergoes degenerative changes that characterize *senescence*.

The ordinary and distinctive functions of a cell wane and finally fail.

4. *Stage of death and removal.*

Cell death ensues when the vital processes of protoplasm cease.

As an accompaniment, the protoplasm becomes irreversibly coagulated.

A microscopic sign of death is the diffuse vital staining of nucleus and cytoplasm.

Cells are ultimately lost by shedding, dissolution or phagocytosis.

The course leading to cell death by degenerative processes is called *necrobiosis*.

With a fulfilled life-span it is a normal, inevitable phase in the history of a cell.

All such retrograde phenomena are different from postmortem, degenerative changes.

In the latter, *autolysis* (due to intracellular enzymes) is the causative agent.

Postmortem degeneration occurs quickly in some tissues, slowly in others.

Also the rate of change is governed by temperature.

There are several types of necrobiotic processes leading to cell death, or *necrosis:*

    A. CYTOLYSIS.

        Protoplasmic viscosity decreases; cells liquefy, swell and burst.

    B. COAGULATION.

        Protoplasmic viscosity increases, and irreversible gelatin occurs.

    C. PYCNOSIS.

        The nucleus contracts; chromatin condenses to one or more heavily staining clumps.

    D. KARYOLYSIS.

        The nucleus and its chromatin lose their stainability and disappear, as if dissolved.

        (The loss of colorability by cell constituents, in general, is *chromatolysis.*)

    E. KARYORRHEXIS.

        The nucleus fragments and scatters.

Some cells have a transitory existence; others last part or all of the total life-span.

    Example: intestinal cell, few days; epidermal cell, several weeks; neuron, many years.

Aging of tissues and organs, with discernible changes, is a normal feature of the life-span.
It enters at different times and proceeds at different speeds.

    Some organs run their course and regress before birth.

        Example: yolk sac; mesonephros.

    Others become obsolete and start their degenerative course at birth.

        Example: superseded, fetal blood vessels; fetal cortex of suprarenal gland.

    Still others decline in adolescence or middle age.

        Example: thymus; ovary.

    Most organs, even when impaired, continue to function even into old age.

With increasing age the amount of amorphous intercellular substance is reduced.

    Changes occur in collagenous and elastic fibers; bones rarefy.

An appreciation of the importance of understanding the aging process is recent.

    Out of it has emerged the science of *gerontology* (or, including treatment, *geriatrics*).

PART **II**

General Histology

Foreword on the Origin and Nature of Tissues

The study of tissues is *histology* in the strict sense of that term.
But *Histology*, as commonly used, includes the consideration of cells and organs as well.
    Hence the term *General Histology* can be employed to denote tissue structure alone.
    This term then contrasts with *Special Histology*, which is a synonym of *Organology*.
        These terms denote the subscience dealing with the arrangement of tissues in organs.
        Special Histology also examines adaptations of tissues for specific organ-purposes.

Tissues and organs are understood best in the light of their development.
    These topics belong to the science of *Embryology*.
    Accordingly, only a few basic facts concerning the origin of tissues will be mentioned.
A ripe egg, when fertilized by a sperm cell, divides repeatedly into smaller cells.
    These *cleavage cells,* or *blastomeres,* segregate into three superimposed *germ layers.*
    From its position each layer receives a descriptive name, as follows:
        Ectoderm (external); *mesoderm* (middle position); *entoderm* (internal).
The germ layers produce an embryo by processes of folding, localized growth, etc.
    Among these products are the early rudiments of the various organs of the body.
        Such then differentiate into the *tissues* that characterize the developing organs and parts.
    This process of tissue specialization is called *histogenesis.*
    Histogenesis produces four chief groups of tissues:
        1. Epithelia arise from all three germ layers.
        2. Supporting tissues arise from mesoderm.
        3. Muscular tissues arise from mesoderm.
        4. Nervous tissues arise from ectoderm.
A *tissue* is defined as a group of similar cells (together with their cell products), specialized in a common direction and set apart for the performance of a common function.
    Also, the cells of any particular kind of local tissue have the same embryonic origin.
    Certain associated elements play a subordinate but useful role.
        These auxiliaries stand in sharp contrast to the predominant, characteristic cells.
        Such elements are connective tissue, blood vessels and nerve fibers.
Tissues are the practical building materials that fashion the various organs.
    A sound understanding of tissues is more fundamentally useful than is organ structure.
    This is because organ activities, normal and abnormal, are those of their component tissues.
The four major types of tissues are structurally and functionally distinct.
    1. Epithelium.
        These are sheet-like coverings, with one surface free and the other attached.
    2. Supporting tissues.
        Their fibers perform connecting, binding and supporting functions.
        Their cells perform a variety of activities.
    3. Muscle.
        These cells respond to stimulation by producing oriented, contractile movements.

4. Nerve.

This tissue is highly irritable; it conducts waves of excitation as nerve impulses.

Two other types are often, in a loose sense, designated as tissues.

This is because of their wide occurrence as components of organs.

One is *'vascular tissue,'* really simple organs in structure (p. 127).

Another is *'lymphoid tissue,'* a complex of two tissue elements (p. 142).

Hence in diagnosing tissues, only four major possibilities have to be considered.

There are some subtypes of each, but these are variant differentiations.

The role of fluids in the composition and functioning of the body is important.

Water comprises 70 per cent of the body weight of man.

Obviously some tissues (blood; muscle) contain much more water than others (fat; bone).

Protoplasm is 75 per cent water.

Part of the water is free, but much is bound to other components of the protoplasm.

As a whole, the intracellular fluid constitutes 50 per cent of body weight.

In general, living cells are bathed to some extent with fluid or a watery jelly.

These extracellular fluids are: blood; lymph; cerebrospinal fluid; tissue fluid.

Of supreme importance is the relation existing between cells and the extracellular fluid, residing in the tissue spaces and derived largely from the blood plasma.

This interstitial fluid constitutes 15 per cent of body weight.

Through it nutritive materials and oxygen reach the cells.

Also through it waste products from cell catabolism reach the blood and lymph.

Firmer substances than watery fluids may be deposited upon a cell surface.

Similar material may also be deposited as an interstitial substance that embeds cells or fibers.

This nonliving, formed material is named *ground substance*.

Chapter IV

The Epithelial Tissues

An *epithelium* is a sheet of cells that covers an external surface or lines an internal surface.
  The component cells are in intimate contact-relation with each other.
  Typically one of its surfaces is free, facing against either air or fluid.
      This exposed surface ranges from an expansive sheet to a tiny, microscopic tubule.
  The other surface almost always rests upon a vascularized, connective-tissue bed.
  A small amount of intercellular, formed substance occurs between adjacent cells.
      This material is so inconspicuous that the tissue appears to be nothing but cells.
Directly beneath an epithelium, and attached to it, is a (usually thin) *basement membrane*.
  This sheet of noncellular material serves to support and bind down the epithelium.
Epithelia frequently send downgrowths into the underlying connective tissue.
  Most of these are actual diverticula (*i.e.,* blind tubes) that specialize as glands.
  In a few instances they become a detached, solid mass.
      These may convert into solid cords (*e.g.,* parathyroid; suprarenal cortex).
      Contrariwise, the solid mass of the primordial thyroid gland cavitates secondarily.
The free surface of the epithelial sheets is frequently increased by folds (*e.g.,* stomach), finger-like
      elevations (*e.g.,* intestinal villi), inpocketings (*e.g.,* glands) and cell-fringes (microvilli).
Beginners sometimes misinterpret certain conditions encountered in sections.
  An epithelium that is folded or collapsed, so that free surfaces are brought into contact, will
      seem to lack an obvious free surface.
  Artificial clefts or shrinkage spaces, commonly occurring in connective tissue, may give the
      appearance of a cavity more or less bordered by flat or stretched cells.
  Solid 'islands' of epithelium are often seen, surrounded by connective tissue.
      These are almost always glancing slices of epithelial folds, glands, etc.

I. OCCURRENCE AND TYPES

A. OCCURRENCE:

  In general, epithelium occurs wherever free surfaces exist in relation to an organism.
      The free surface may be expansive.
          Example: epidermis; gut lining; body-cavity lining.
      The free surface may be limited, and the bounded cavity is then small to tiny.
          Example: small blood vessels; ducts and tubules of glands; liver cords.
  A few special free surfaces of the body are not lined by a true epithelium.
      Example: joint cavities; bursae; cavity of brain and spinal cord.

B. CLASSIFICATION:

  The basis of classification is cell layering and cell shape.
  The three main groups are named in accordance with the presence of one layer, or of several to
          many layers:
      1. Simple epithelium: one layer thick.
      2. Pseudostratified epithelium: staggered cell-heights give a false appearance of layering.
      3. Stratified epithelium: several to many layers are superposed.
  Pseudostratified epithelium has no subgroups of consequence.
  Simple and stratified epithelia have three important subgroups each.

In simple epithelium these minor groups are classified on the basis of cell shape.

1. *Simple squamous epithelium;* the cells are flat plates.
2. *Simple cuboidal epithelium;* the cells have about the same height as width.
3. *Simple columnar epithelium;* the cells are taller than they are wide.

In stratified epithelium the minor groups are classified on the basis of the shape of the superficial cells at the free surface.

1. *Stratified squamous epithelium;* the superficial cells are flattened.
2. *Stratified cuboidal epithelium;* the superficial cells are approximately cubical.
3. *Stratified columnar epithelium;* the superficial cells are elongated prisms.

Special names are given, for convenience, to two epithelia of wide occurrence.

Actually these are merely simple epithelia, characteristic of definite locations.

Endothelium is the simple squamous lining of the heart, blood vessels and lymphatics.

Mesothelium is the simple squamous lining of the several body cavities.

Mesenchymal epithelium is another special name sometimes used.

It denotes the simple layer of squamous cells that lines certain spaces.

Such spaces arise as clefts in the embryonic mesenchyme.

These spaces are: subdural and subarachnoid spaces; perilymphatic spaces of the ear; anterior chamber of the eyeball.

This type is structurally indistinguishable from mesothelium.

False epithelium is a name sometimes given to the membrane that encloses the cavities of joints and bursae.

It is a layer made of collagenous fibers and scattered, flattened fibroblasts.

Hence it is not epithelium, but an exposed connective-tissue surface.

Epithelioid is an adjective applied to layers of cells that imitate epithelium.

Example: connective-tissue osteoblasts and odontoblasts, arranged as sheets in developing bone; ependymal cells, lining the cavity of the brain and spinal cord.

II. CHARACTERISTICS OF THE EPITHELIAL TYPES

A. SIMPLE EPITHELIUM:

1. *Squamous.*

It was formerly called 'pavement epithelium' because of its thin, covering nature.

The cells are scales or plates, definitely broader than they are thick.

A. OCCURRENCE.

Body cavities (mesothelium).

Cardio-vascular and lymphatic systems (endothelium).

Smallest ducts of many glands.

Terminal respiratory ducts and air sacs.

Membranous labyrinth (except sensory areas); tympanic cavity.

Kidney tubules (in part).

Mesenchymal epithelium (see above).

B. ARRANGEMENT.

The component cells are flat plates, joined to make a simple sheet.

A pan-full of fried eggs is a fairly faithful model of this arrangement.

The cell body is often expansive in comparison to its nuclear extent.

Centrally the cells are thicker because the nucleus bulges there.

Cell borders are often prominently serrated and interlocking.

C. APPEARANCE IN SURFACE VIEW.

The cell outline is commonly hexagonal; the whole sheet is a mosaic.

There is a geometrical reason for this, since six circles can be circumscribed about a central circle; mutual pressure makes hexagons.

Mesothelial cells are polygons with all diameters approximately equal.

Endothelial cells are typically elongated polygons, commonly diamond-shaped.

D. APPEARANCE IN VERTICAL SECTION.

('Vertical section' is in a plane perpendicular to the surface and base.)

Cell boundaries are frequently indeterminable with ordinary stains.

Cells, when cut through the nucleus, appear as slender spindles

Nuclei usually are relatively far apart, and are often the most conspicuous feature.

They cause the thin epithelial disk to bulge locally.

Cells, cut so as to miss the nucleus, vary in thickness and particularly in length.

This depends on the distance of the sectioned slice from the nucleus.

2. Cuboidal.

The cells are short prisms; they have a top, bottom and, commonly, six sides.

Since a vertical section approximates a square, this type became named 'cuboidal.'

The name 'cubical' was used formerly, but the shape is rarely an exact square.

Actually, all intermediates occur between squamous and columnar types.

Hence there is the problem of naming borderline types.

'Low cuboidal' and 'low columnar' are the terms used by many histologists.

A. OCCURRENCE.

Many glands; portions of their ducts.

Pigmented epithelium of retina; epithelioid covering of choroid plexus.

Germinal layer of ovary; rete testis; lens (front surface); iris (back surface).

B. ARRANGEMENT; APPEARANCE IN SECTIONS.

The cells are arranged like cubical blocks in a mosaic.

In surface view or horizontal section the cell outline tends to be hexagonal.

Cell diameters are less than the longest diameter in the squamous type.

In vertical section the pattern is that of a row of approximate squares.

Nuclei are practically centered, and hence make an evenly spaced row.

3. Columnar.

The component cells are distinctly taller than they are wide.

A. OCCURRENCE.

Stomach and intestine; gall bladder.

Many glands; portions of the ducts of some glands.

Uterine tube and uterus.

Small bronchi; large bronchioles.

B. ARRANGEMENT; APPEARANCE IN SECTIONS.

The cells are prisms, set on end and closely packed.

The arrangement resembles the grouping of the 'cells' of a honeycomb.

In surface view the cell outline is most commonly hexagonal.

In horizontal section the pattern is like that in surface view.

Nuclei may or may not show, depending on the level of the section.

In vertical section the pattern is that of a row of rectangles.

The nuclei lie at one general level.

Usually this is below the middle of the cell.

Sometimes, however, crowding displaces nuclei into a staggered row.

The nuclei may even occur at two levels.

The cells are frequently pyramidal in shape.

This is due to folds or curves in the epithelium.

Example: tubules; thick-walled sacs; alveoli of glands.

Note that all three types of epithelium appear much alike in surface view or horizontal section; that is, they are arranged in an hexagonal mosaic.

It is the vertical section that identifies the three types by shapes.

4. Specialized types.

Simple epithelium (usually columnar) frequently undergoes specializations.

There are four lines of such distinctive specialization.

A. GLANDULAR.

Details of these types are given in the chapter dealing with glands (pp. 164-169).

1. *Unicellular.*

Generalized secretory cells (example: stomach lining).

All cells in the epithelial sheet have the ordinary columnar shape.

Goblet cells (example: in intestinal lining).

Individual cells swell with secretion, distorting adjacent cells.

2. *Multicellular.*

Invaginations produce tubules, thick pear-shaped dilatations (alveoli or acini) or actual sacs.

Cells assume a pyramidal shape, with their broader ends as bases.

B. CILIATED.

The cells bear tiny protoplasmic lashes, or *cilia* (p. 39).

Example: nasal cavity; bronchi; uterine tube; uterus.

C. PIGMENTED.

The cells contain colored pigment granules (p. 24).

Example: pigment epithelium of retina.

D. NEURO-EPITHELIUM.

Some columnar cells are specialized for sensory reception.

Example: receptive cells of smell, taste, and hearing (pp. 295, 297, 309).

B. PSEUDOSTRATIFIED EPITHELIUM:

This type was formerly confused with stratified columnar epithelium.

Actually there is a deceptive appearance of stratification.

However, maceration separates the cells and shows the true relations.

It is then seen that there is a closer resemblance to simple epithelium.

That is, cells vary in height and many do not reach the free surface.

But all rest on the basement membrane.

1. *Occurrence.*

Larger ducts of glands opening onto a stratified epithelial surface.

Nasal cavity; much of pharynx; trachea; bronchi.

Much of male urethra; some of female urethra.

Most of male sexual duct.

2. *Arrangement.*

In a fully specialized epithelium, three cell types occur:

(a) Basal cells; (b) fusiform cells; (c) columnar cells.

All these cells rest on a basement membrane.

Their upper ends extend to varying heights in the order just listed.

The columnar cells alone reach the free surface.

They are commonly ciliated; frequently some are goblet mucous cells.

Nuclei of the three cell types may lie at fairly distinct levels.

Most regular in this regard are the nuclei of the basal cells.

The majority of nuclei lie well below the middle level of the total layer.

It is not clear whether or not the cell-types represent growth stages.

In many regions the fusiform cells (of intermediate length) are lacking.

Such an epithelium consists of columnar and basal cells only.

3. *Appearance in sections.*

Cell boundaries of the basal cells are usually quite easy to see.

Columnar cells are often reasonably distinct as they approach the surface.

It is the middle level that is crowded and confused.

Hence fusiform cells are difficult to demonstrate as entities.

Sometimes a middle stratum of nuclei furnishes a practical aid.

These belong to fusiform cells and to some columnar cells.

Also the total number of nuclei in the middle level is often greater than might be expected were a third cell type not present as fusiform cells.

The basal halves of columnar cells and fusiform cells are crowded (hence slender) as they extend toward the basement membrane.

They are easiest to trace when cells are shrunken and somewhat separated.

Simple columnar epithelium sometimes deceptively resembles pseudostratification.

Its nuclei may be crowded (somewhat alternatingly) into different levels.

Also its cells, cut slantingly, seem to lie in more than one layer.

C. STRATIFIED EPITHELIUM:

This type contains truly superposed cells.

The subtypes are named according to the shape of the surface cells alone.

1. *Stratified squamous.*

A. OCCURRENCE.

Wherever there is exposure to friction, mechanical insult or drying.

Skin; conjunctiva (in part); cornea; external acoustic meatus.

Mouth; esophagus; anal canal.

Urethra (near outlet); vagina.

B. LIMITS OF STRATIFICATION.

The layering may vary from a few layers to dozens or scores of layers.

Example: corneal epithelium, few layers; epidermis, many layers.

C. ARRANGEMENT.

This type is usually draped over connective-tissue papillae.

It is this condition that gave epithelium its name — 'upon nipples.'

The deepest cells are soft, delicate and are arranged in one layer.

Their shape is cuboidal to low columnar.

Cells at a higher level are polygonal in outline, and larger.

So-called intercellular bridges (*desmosomes*) bind them together.

Shrinkage gives the cell border a prickly or spiny appearance.

The more superficial layers are progressively flattened by pressure.

At the surface, the flattened cells may become dead scales.

Epidermis is a 'dry epithelium' whose superficial cells undergo cornification.

The upper layers contain keratin granules, and the nucleus has disappeared.

This type of epithelium shows well the several stages of cytomorphosis (p. 29).

All internal epithelia, simple to stratified, are 'wet epithelia.'

Stratified squamous occurs where protection is needed, but not absorption.

Nuclei are retained in the superficial, largely uncornified cells.

D. APPEARANCE IN SECTIONS.

The layering and the gradual flattening (and spreading) of cells are diagnostic.

In cornified epithelium the upper layers may separate or shred irregularly.

Boundaries of the caked cells are often obscure.

2. *Stratified cuboidal (including 'transitional').*

A. OCCURRENCE.

Testis tubules; vesicular (Graafian) follicles of ovary.

Ducts of sweat glands; sebaceous glands.

Intermediate zones, such as in the urethra, anal canal and conjunctiva.

Urinary tract from kidney into urethra (so-called transitional epithelium).

B. ARRANGEMENT; APPEARANCE IN SECTIONS.

Typically there is a superposition of increasingly larger polyhedral cells, with the superficial cells taking a somewhat more cuboidal shape.

Mostly this type occurs in special situations, but best known is the epithelium of the urinary tract commonly called *transitional epithelium.*

This example is, by far, the most widespread in its distribution.

c. TRANSITIONAL EPITHELIUM.
The name is inappropriate and without real meaning.
It is a plastic epithelium, whose appearance varies with stretching.
It is not indented by papillae; there is no obvious basement membrane.
In a relaxed epithelium the cells are about six layers deep.
The basal cells are small, polyhedral elements.
The middle layers of cells are larger, and often club- or pear-shaped.
The surface cells are bloated and cuboidal, with bulging convex tops.
The lower surface of a superficial cell bears several indentations.
Into these pits fit the clubbed ends of the cells next below.
Distention of the bladder stretches and thins the epithelium markedly.
The cells may slip by, then reducing the layering to two or three cells.
The sheet then looks more like a stratified squamous type.
The cells have few interconnections, thus facilitating slippage.

3. Stratified columnar.

A. OCCURRENCE.
Pharynx (in part); larynx (in part).
Urethra (in part); conjunctiva (in part).
Excretory ducts of salivary and mammary glands (in part).
(In general, where columnar or pseudostratified epithelium meets stratified squamous epithelium.)
B. ARRANGEMENT; APPEARANCE IN SECTIONS.
The surface cells are columnar and sometimes ciliated.
The intermediate cells, when present, are irregular polyhedrons.
The basal cells are cuboidal to low columnar.
The occurrence of this type in mammals is limited and localized.
In sections it cannot be distinguished surely from pseudostratified epithelium.
(Also, simple columnar epithelium, cut slantingly, has an appearance resembling either stratified columnar or cuboidal.)

III. THE GENERAL CHARACTERISTICS OF EPITHELIAL CELLS

Many epithelial cells qualify as rather typical cells.
Only the general features will be treated in the present topic.
Details of specialized types will be treated under glands, neuro-epithelium, etc.

A. NUCLEUS:

This conforms to the shape of its particular cell.
In squamous cells it is a flattened disk.
In cuboidal cells it is spheroidal.
In columnar cells it is ovoid to elongate.

B. CYTOPLASM:

It tends to be much like that of a generalized cell, as already described (pp. 20-24).
The usual organelles are represented; tonofibrils are common, and prominent in some cells.
Secretion precursors and storage products are sometimes encountered.

C. POLARITY:

Epithelial cells are organized differently at their free and attached ends.
Such differences are inherent in a sheet-like arrangement of cells.
They are most clearly seen in simple columnar epithelia.
There is a basal attached surface, and an apical free surface.
The *basal surface* is usually less specialized.

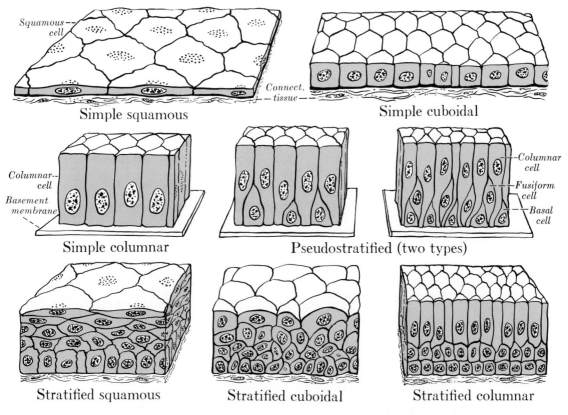

Simple squamous

Simple cuboidal

Simple columnar

Pseudostratified (two types)

Stratified squamous

Stratified cuboidal

Stratified columnar

CLASSIFIED TYPES OF EPITHELIUM

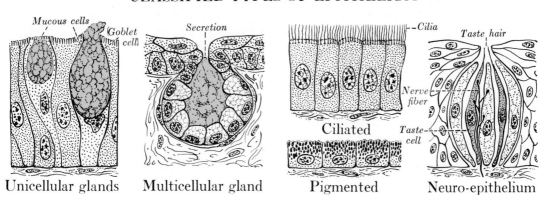

Unicellular glands

Multicellular gland

Ciliated

Pigmented

Neuro-epithelium

TYPES OF SPECIALIZED EPITHELIUM

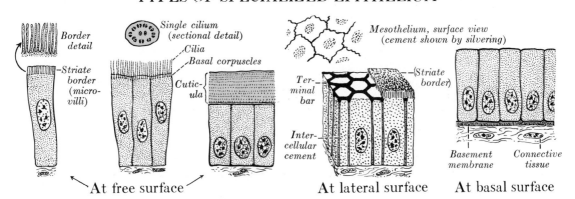

At free surface

At lateral surface

At basal surface

DIFFERENTIATIONS AT CELL SURFACES

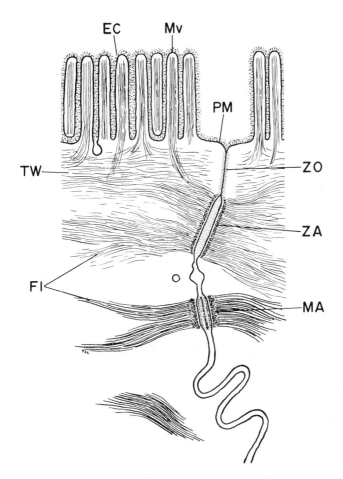

EPITHELIAL CELL APEX. The plasma membrane (PM) ensheathes microvilli (Mv) into which extend filaments of the terminal web (TW). The free surface bears a filamentous surface coat (EC). Adjoining cells are sealed by tight junctions (ZO) and supported by tonofilaments (Fl) which converge on the dense material of desmosomes (MA); a variant junctional type (ZA) receives filaments of the terminal web (TW).

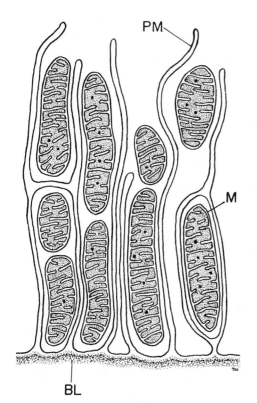

EPITHELIAL CELL BASE. The plasma membrane at the cell base rests on a dense, filamentous basal lamina (BL). Extensive infoldings of the plasma membrane (PM) characterize cells engaged in active transport of ions and fluids. In such cells mitochondria (M) often occur, between folds, in vertical alignments.

It is the receptive side through which nutriment comes from nearby vessels.

The *apical surface* is more highly specialized.

It is directly subject to external influences.

Here microvilli and cilia are elaborated.

The position, above the nucleus, of metabolic products (*e.g.*, secretion precursors), centrioles and Golgi apparatus is an expression of cellular polarity.

Some gland cells are further polarized by a ribosomal concentration below the nucleus.

In columnar cells, the nucleus tends to take a more basal position.

Rod-shaped mitochondria orient in the long dimension of the cell.

In some cells they aggregate distally; in others, basally.

In some cells they are both filamentous in form (near top) and granular (near base).

D. CYTOSKELETON:

The cell receives support from tough filaments contained in the cytoplasm.

One type is a compact layer of fine filaments known as the *terminal web*.

It lies just beneath the free surface of the cell.

Other filaments are the *tonofibrils* that come into relation with lateral surfaces.

They converge on the desmosomes (p. 40) and insert on them.

IV. DIFFERENTIATIONS AT THE SURFACES OF CELLS

Epithelial cells have different kinds of functional surfaces.

These are best illustrated in simple epithelium where there are three such surfaces.

1. Free surface: either exposed to air or bathed by fluids.

2. Lateral surface: actually any surface in contact with other cells of the same kind.

3. Basal surface (or attached surface): resting on a basement membrane.

In stratified epithelia no cell can possess more than two of these surface-relations.

Exposed cells have *1* and *2*, as listed above; intermediate cells, *2*; basal cells, *2* and *3*.

A. FREE SURFACE:

1. Cytoplasmic specializations.

Several different kinds of elaborations have been developed by cells where exposed.

A. SURFACE COAT.

There may be a '*fuzzy (or fluffy) coat*', containing extremely few filaments.

Its substance is a glycoprotein that colors with the PAS stain.

Ascribed functions are protective, barrier and trap activity.

B. MICROVILLI.

These are tiny rod-like processes that project freely above some cells.

Their number to a cell ranges from only a few to 3000.

Some are inconspicuous, short stubs; others are relatively long (1.5 $\mu\pm$).

With the light microscope the longer type appears as a *striate-* or *brush border*.

The thickness of these processes is less than 0.1 μ.

Hence they are resolved well only by the electron microscope.

Centrally there is a core of cytoplasm that may contain supporting filaments.

These are anchored in the *terminal web* (when present) in the cell proper.

The core is bounded externally by a continuation of the plasma membrane.

A 'fuzzy,' glycoprotein coat covers and supports some microvilli.

Functions are related to absorption, secretion and sensory reception.

C. CILIA.

These are lashing protoplasmic processes that vary in length (5–10 μ) and fineness (0.2 μ).

Cilia (literally, eyelashes) may number several hundred to a cell.

If there are from one to several extremely long ones, each is a *flagellum* (*i.e.*, whip).

1. *Occurrence.*

Respiratory tract; uterine tube; uterus; efferent ductules of testis.

2. *Structure.*

A cilium is a slender thread of cytoplasm enclosed by a plasma membrane.

These cell-extensions are thicker than microvilli, and usually much longer.

The light microscope reveals them only as delicate threads.

Internal details are demonstrable solely by the electron microscope.

Their ultrastructure is the same in all animals (even invertebrates).

The cytoplasm contains longitudinal tubules, commonly designated *filaments.*

There are two single filaments, located axially.

These are encircled by nine pairs, each a double or twin filament.

Each cilium arises from a granule just beneath the surface of the cell.

This is a modified centriole named a *basal corpuscle,* or *basal body.*

So-called *stereocilia,* as in male sex ducts, are actually giant microvilli.

3. *Movement.*

In mammals cilia beat toward outlets of the body, moving fluids onward.

The stroke consists of a stiff, vigorous lash and a flexible, slower recovery.

Cilia may beat simultaneously or in regular sequence.

Thus a wave is propagated and fluids are moved onward.

The transport of mucus is as fast as 0.5 mm. per second.

Recurring rhythms produce wave after wave of motion.

A ciliated sheet, in surface view, resembles a wind-swept field of grain.

Ciliary activity is independent of nervous control.

The mechanisms of the stroke and co-ordination are not surely known.

2. Secreted plates.

These are more or less solid formed-substances, secreted by the cytoplasm.

They lie on an epithelial surface and can be detached from it; they are *cuticulae.*

Commonly they become impregnated with a hard substance of some kind.

Example: clam shell (lime); beetle shell (chitin).

Even mammals have some representatives of this specialization.

Example: lens capsule; tectorial membrane of ear; enamel of developing tooth.

B. LATERAL SURFACE:

'Lateral,' as used, means any cell surface not at the extreme top or base of an epithelium.

Along such surfaces provision is made to enhance cell coherence.

This is because the cells, of themselves, have little tensile strength.

They require aid in resisting forces that would tend to tear them apart.

1. Intercellular cement.

Cohesion of these cells has long been attributed to a plastic cementing substance.

In fact, there is a minute cleft between the facing surfaces of epithelial cells.

This intercellular space contains a readily extractable muco-polysaccharide.

It is akin to the surface coat, already described (p. 39).

Yet to what extent this 'cement' promotes cellular cohesion is not known.

At least, wandering cells and nutrient fluids can penetrate into the clefts.

Cell boundaries can be outlined prominently by a deposit of silver granules.

This follows a soaking in silver nitrate and exposure to sunlight.

Such blackening, however, is not wholly attributable to the presence of cement.

2. Desmosomes.

These interconnections occur wherever there is special need for cellular cohesion.

They are especially conspicuous between facing cells of the deeper epidermis.

Yet details are only resolved with the electron microscope.

At places the facing plasma membranes are united by denser, intercellular material.

Internally, each membrane is reinforced with an electron-dense, fibrillar mass.

From this mass of *tonofibrils* individual strands radiate back into the cytoplasm.

A tonofibril is a bundle composed of much finer *tonofilaments*.
In a sense, a desmosome consists of two separate halves; single ones are known.
The former idea of cytoplasmic continuity at these *'intercellular bridges'* is false.
Dissection tests show that the desmosome is truly a point of strong attachment.
The official term for such a local, adhering spot is *macula adherens*.

3. Terminal bars.

A ring-like band encircles the tops of simple cuboidal and columnar cells.
This lies just beneath the free surface, closing off the intercellular space.
The sealing effect is proved when collected fluid cannot escape between cells.
Also external fluids enter such cells only through their top surface.
These stainable *terminal bars* were long described as condensed cement.
Electron micrographs, however, show them as zones where cells unite.
The distinctive peculiarity of a bar is in being a 'tight junction,' close to the free surface.
Here the plasma membranes of contiguous cells actually fuse.
The plane of section determines the appearance as seen with the light microscope.
The part cut will show as a dot, bar or polygonal ring.
The 'terminal bar' is officially designated as a *zonula occludens*.
It is often one component of a larger composite, the *junctional complex*.
This also includes a nearby *macula adherens*, or desmosome.

4. Interlocking contours.

Some epithelial cells have their facing surfaces thrown into ridges and grooves.
These corrugations fit together like the pieces of a jigsaw puzzle.
Mechanical resistance to shearing forces is an obvious 'explanation' for interlocking.
But, also, complicated foldings are presumably significant in fluid transfers.

C. BASAL SURFACE:

Special means of support prevent both the dislocation and disruption of epithelia.

1. Basement membrane (membrana propria).

Anchorage of all epithelia is by a *basement membrane* that serves as an intermediary.
It attaches both to the epithelium above and to general connective tissue beneath.
The membrane varies greatly in thickness in different locations in the body.
In some places (*e.g.*, trachea) it is so thick as to be seen without staining.
Elsewhere (*e.g.*, skin; intestine) it may be so thin as to escape notice.
In general, the membrane is refractory to coloring with ordinary stains.
The membrane is compound; it consists of two different components.
Next to the epithelium is a nearly amorphous layer, less than 0.1 μ thick.
There is evidence that this *basal lamina* is an epithelial collagenous product.
In some epithelia adhesion is to half desmosomes on the plasma membrane.
The deeper component contains a meshwork of reticular fibers.
These fibers are embedded in amorphous ground substance of the lamina.
This mucopolysaccharide becomes demonstrable with the PAS staining technique.
The reticular fibers are demonstrable with special silver staining.
The usefulness of the basement membrane as a support and limiting layer is obvious.
In addition, it acts as a semipermeable filter for metabolites.

2. Papillary interlock.

Stratified squamous epithelia bear pits or grooves on their basal surface.
Into these project elevations (papillae) of the underlying connective tissue.
Such interlocking of papillae and epithelium holds the epithelium in place.

3. Plasma-membrane infoldings.

Infoldings of the cell membrane may be numerous, even extending far into the cytoplasm.

This specialization is related to a function of fluid-transport by the cell.
Example: kidney tubule; choroid plexus of the brain.

V. THE RELATIONS OF EXTRANEOUS ELEMENTS TO EPITHELIUM

1. Blood vessels.

Capillaries do not penetrate into the epithelium proper; it is, therefore, avascular.
Exceptions are found in the cochlear epithelium and the egg follicle.
Hence fluids escape from the vessels, join the fluids of the tissue spaces, cross the basement membrane, and seep along the spaces between epithelial cells.
This is the pathway used for epithelial nutrition, respiration and excretion.
The vascular supply to thick, stratified epithelium is made easier by the presence of finger-like, connective-tissue papillae.
These indent the epithelial sheet and may carry blood capillaries far 'into' it.
Yet the capillaries still remain outside the basement membrane.
In other words, the epithelium is merely draped over these vascular papillae.

2. Nerve fibers.

Fine fibers may pierce the basement membrane and pass between epithelial cells.
Such fibers are receptive (sensory) or excitatory (motor) in function.

3. Wandering cells.

Migratory cells may pass between epithelial cells, and some emerge at their tops.
Example: leucocytes in intestine and vagina; pigmented cells in epidermis.
How cells can squeeze through tight junctions (terminal bars) is not known.

VI. EPITHELIAL REPLACEMENT AND REPAIR

Epithelia are subject to wear and replacement, but at different rates.
Epidermal and intestinal cells are shed continuously.
The lining epithelium of the intestine is replaced every few days.
Cells of respiratory passages, protected cavities and glands are replaced infrequently.
Hence some cells of a layer must retain the capacity of cell division.
In a stratified epithelium these are the basal cells, and some higher cells also.
Daughter cells get pushed gradually to the surface by those formed later.
In a simple epithelium the newly divided cells naturally lie side by side.
In certain epithelia, such as glands, the proliferative regions are restricted.
Daughter cells may then gradually shift far from their site of origin.
Epithelia are also capable of repairing losses produced by trauma, disease, etc.
Although their cells are normally immobile, those near the injury become activated.
Their gliding movements alone are adequate to cover defects of fair size.
Mitosis is a secondary phenomenon in point of time.
It may add new cells to the denuded region.
It also restores cell losses to adjacent regions that furnished the migratory cells.

VII. THE FUNCTIONS OF EPITHELIUM

Epithelial cells specialize for different kinds of functional activities.

The details of these structural modifications will be treated later, in relation to the organs in which they occur.

In general, epithelia that secrete, absorb, resorb, dialize and filter are single-layered.

Their height (squamous to columnar) is correlated with functional efficiency.

Pseudostratified epithelia engage in secretion, ciliary transport and sensory reception.

The layering of stratified epithelium limits it largely to the function of protection.

Yet epidermis buds off glands and produces nails and hair.

1. Protection.

The effects of mechanical insult or noxious substances are minimized.
Epidermis, mouth and vagina furnish examples of protection against mechanical trauma.
The bladder lining furnishes protection against the hypertonic excretory-wastes in urine.
The total body is enveloped in a casing of cornified dead cells.
In this way the body is protected against drying, absorbing and bacterial invasion.

2. Transport.

Mucus and particulate matter are transported along epithelial surfaces.
This is achieved by the ciliated epithelia of respiratory and genital ducts.
Fluids may traverse the total layer of some epithelia.
Example: kidney tubule; capillary endothelium.

3. Secretion.

Cells synthesize products and pass them out of the body or into the blood.
This sequence characterizes all glandular activity, both exocrine and endocrine.

4. Excretion.

Certain cells filter from the blood the wastes that were produced elsewhere.
Urine, sweat and carbon dioxide illustrate such excreted filtrates.

5. Absorption.

Cells are permeable to certain substances in solution.
Lungs pass oxygen; intestines absorb nutriment; kidneys recapture sugar from raw urine.

6. Lubrication.

Mechanical chafing of part on part does not occur normally within the body.
Secreted mucus is a principal agent used as a lubricant (*e.g.*, rectal mucus).
The serous fluid in the body cavities prevents undue friction of their mesothelial linings.
That is, viscera play smoothly against each other and against the body wall.

7. Sensory reception.

Some cells of an epithelium specialize as intermediaries in nervous transmission.
Certain cells of taste buds, olfactory epithelium and the ear perform this function.
They even develop delicate, hair-like receptive processes.

8. Reproduction.

Certain cells are set aside for the sole purpose of species-perpetuation.
These cells are produced in the ovary and testis, which are glands that 'secrete' cells.

Chapter V

The Connective Tissues

Connective tissue, cartilage and bone share in performing certain mechanical functions.
They connect and anchor parts, and give support to the body and its organs.
Without them the body could not maintain a distinctive form.
Hence this larger group is sometimes given an inclusive name, the *supporting tissues*.
All the supporting tissues are notable for the presence of nonliving *formed substance*.
This material, located between the cells, varies in amount and firmness.
Yet its abundance is the feature that characterizes the group as a whole.
In many ways, at least, it is the most important part of these tissues.
All the supporting tissues have *cells* interspersed in the intercellular substance.
There are different kinds of cells; in some tissues they are relatively sparse.
These varied cells also have important functions of different kinds.
In all supporting tissues, *fibers* occur as one constituent of the synthesized formed substance.
They lie in an amorphous *ground substance*, semifluid to solid in consistency.
Fibers and ground substance, together, are often designated as *matrix*.
The origin of fibers in connective tissue, cartilage and bone was disputed for many years.
The controversy hinged on whether they are extruded cytoplasmic specializations or extracellular differentiations within a nonliving ground substance.
The dominant view is that cells secrete the substance out of which fibers differentiate.
Fibers then appear as such, extracellularly, by a process of polymerization.
Sometimes 'connective tissues' has been used as synonymous with 'supporting tissues.'
In a better, narrow sense the former applies to the obviously fibrous, binding tissues.
This excludes essentially rigid, supporting tissues, such as cartilage and bone.

I. EMBRYONAL TISSUES

Two subtypes are usually recognized, but they are only the early and late phases of a temporary tissue occurring normally in prenatal development.
These are important also because they reappear in wound healing and as tumorous new growths.

A. MESENCHYME:

1. *Occurrence.*

It is the typical, unspecialized packing-tissue of the early weeks of embryonic life.
Subsequently it disappears as such when its cells enter into tissue differentiation.

2. *Structure.*

Mesenchyme is a spongy and delicate tissue, filling-in between layers and parts.
It consists of cells and an intercellular ground substance.
A. MESENCHYMAL CELLS.
Their shape ranges from stellate (star-shape) to fusiform (spindle-shape).
Cytoplasm is scanty, but the nucleus is relatively large and pale.
Cells appear to join by their processes, thereby forming a syncytium.
There is, however, only an intimate contact, but not fusion.

    B. GROUND SUBSTANCE.

        In the earliest stages of development this is simply a coagulable fluid.

        Later it becomes a mucoid jelly that contains fine, scanty fibrils.

           This condition passes imperceptibly into the type called *mucous tissue.*

        Young mesenchyme is a generalized tissue whose further differentiation produces the supporting tissues, vascular tissues, blood and smooth muscle.

3. Appearance in sections.

        Young mesenchyme takes the form of a network of stellate cells.

           The nucleus is vesicular and relatively large; the cytoplasm is scanty.

           The interspaces between cells commonly appear to be empty.

               This is because the ground substance is unstained or has been extracted.

        Old mesenchyme grades into the characteristics of mucous tissue (see beyond).

4. Functional correlations.

        Typically these cells are transient elements, awaiting differentiation.

           They become the cells of supporting tissues, vascular tissues and muscle.

        A minority are retained as reserve elements and persist in adult tissues.

           On demand these multipotential cells can differentiate in various directions.

B. MUCOUS TISSUE:

1. Occurrence.

        It occurs transiently in the normal development of all connective tissues.

        Elsewhere its sole representative is the *Wharton's jelly* of the umbilical cord.

           In this fetal appendage the packing tissue never progresses further.

        In adult vertebrates it occurs in the cock's comb and in the 'sex skin' of the monkey.

2. Structure.

        Typical mucous tissue is a gelatinous, semifluid mass.

           A jelly comprises most of the bulk of the tissue.

        Cells and scanty fibers are strewn throughout the jelly.

        There are no intrinsic blood vessels, lymphatics or nerves.

    A. CELLS.

        The distinctive cell is a *fibroblast*, with wing-like processes.

           In end view it may appear stellate; in side view, spindle-shaped.

           Many of the processes touch (but do not fuse) with those of neighboring cells.

           The cell tends to flatten itself on the surface of fiber bundles.

        Macrophages (phagocytes) and migratory lymphocytes are encountered rarely.

    B. GROUND SUBSTANCE.

        In the fresh condition it is homogeneous, like a slippery jelly.

        Chemically it contains much muco-polysaccharide and gives the mucin reaction.

           It stains deeply (and metachromatically) with toluidine blue.

    C. FIBERS.

        They vary in abundance with the age of the tissue.

        Fine *collagenous fibrils* aggregate in compound bundles called *fibers* (p. 49).

        Other fiber types (reticular; elastic) are lacking.

3. Appearance in sections.

        The abundant jelly substance is a highly distinctive feature.

           With most of the ordinary stains it colors palely.

                Reducing the aperture of the microscope enhances visibility.

                Yet some stains (thionine; Mallory) demonstrate it satisfactorily.

           Shrinkage commonly produces gaps in the jelly.

        Fibers vary in number and size with the age of the specimen.

           In the first half of pregnancy those of the umbilical cord are fine and scanty.

           In the last half of pregnancy they become coarser and more numerous.

           In the vicinity of the umbilical vessels they group in wavy fiber-bundles.

4. *Functional correlations.*

As a stage in the development of fibrous tissues, mucous tissue serves usefully.

During this period it provides a temporary, fibro-gelatinous packing substance.

In the umbilical cord it furnishes a yielding bed for the flexing umbilical vessels.

In repair processes, young fibrous tissue duplicates the mucous-tissue condition as an intermediate stage of progress in the restoration of supporting tissues.

II. CONSTITUENTS OF THE ADULT CONNECTIVE TISSUES

The connective tissues, in general, contain characteristic constituents with distinctive qualities.

The representation of these varies widely in the individual members of the group.

For this reason it is advantageous to discuss these constituents in some detail before entering into a consideration of the peculiar features of each tissue-type.

Such a preliminary discussion concerns cells, fibers and intercellular substances.

A. CONNECTIVE-TISSUE CELLS:

Ordinary sections, with routine staining, show the details of many cells poorly.

Nuclei stain satisfactorily, but cytoplasmic details are often unsatisfactory.

1. *Reserve mesenchymal cells.*

Many authorities maintain that cells of this 'embryonic' type persist in the adult.

They resemble fibroblasts but tend to be smaller.

In loose connective tissue they usually lie along the wall of blood vessels.

When stimulated, these primitive cells can differentiate into various cell types.

Such responses are appropriate to local environmental conditions.

This capacity is responsible for producing, under certain conditions, *metaplasia.*

It means the replacement of a tissue by a different kind of tissue.

In this process no adult cell or tissue changes directly into a different type.

(Yet friction can make falsely stratified epithelium truly layered.)

2. *Reticular cells.*

The *reticular cells* are stellate elements in intimate relation with reticular fibers.

They have considerable, weakly basophilic cytoplasm and a large, pale nucleus.

Thin cytoplasmic extensions appear to merge with those of other cells.

The true relation, however, is one of intimate contact, not continuity.

Some of these elements are the so-called *primitive reticular cells.*

They resemble embryonic mesenchyme rather closely.

They are not phagocytic, and can differentiate into diverse cell-types.

Those specializing to produce reticular fibers are akin to fibroblasts.

Other, larger elements are *phagocytic reticular cells.*

They have differentiated further than the primitive (more mesenchymal) type.

In so doing they have lost some of their earlier developmental potentialities.

These cells are *fixed macrophages;* they are actively phagocytic.

Such a fixed macrophage may become a *free macrophage* under certain conditions.

For example, when bacteria or other particulate matter are numerous.

(Additional information concerning macrophages, and a larger category (the *reticulo-endothelial system)* to which phagocytic reticular cells belong, will be found on p. 48).

3. *Fibroblasts.*

These cells are responsible for the formation of ground substance and fibers.

In a mature tissue they are almost immobile, and are often called *fibrocytes.*

Yet, following tissue injury, they become active and form new fibers.

They are large, long, flat, branching cells; they appear spindle-shaped in edge view.

Nuclei are ovoid, pale (because of finely granular chromatin) and larger than any other in connective tissue; one or two nucleoli are conspicuous.

The cytoplasm of mature cells is sparse, nearly homogeneous and stains palely.

In sections it is often obscure, so that nuclei are chiefly seen.

The cytoplasm of young cells is granular, basophilic and more abundant.

Fibroblasts are the commonest cell of areolar tissue and the only cell of tendon.

Endothelial cells (especially their nuclei) resemble them, but occur only in vessels.

4. Macrophages.

Among the many other names proposed, *histiocyte* is also frequently used.

These cells are most abundant along small blood vessels in richly vascular areas.

In loose connective tissue they are second only to fibroblasts in numbers.

The cell outline is irregular, but the cell processes are usually short and blunt.

Normally these cells are immobile and stretched along collagenous fibers.

For this reason they are often called *fixed macrophages*.

They then resemble fibroblasts, except for having smaller darker nuclei.

Yet when activated by inflammation they can become free and ameboid.

Such wandering *free macrophages* have well-outlined, abundant cytoplasm.

The nucleus is oval (often indented), but smaller than that of a fibroblast.

Chromatin forms a coarse pattern, so that the nucleus stains darkly.

Nucleoli are present, but not as conspicuous features.

Macrophages are highly endowed with the ability to ingest particulate matter.

Most remarkable is their capacity for taking up ultramicroscopic particles.

For example, colloidal carbon and acid colloidal dyes, such as trypan blue, are phagocytosed and stored in membrane-bounded, cytoplasmic vesicles.

This greedy response distinguishes them sharply from all other cell types.

Macrophages are important agents of defense by acting as scavengers.

They engulf loose blood, bacteria, dead cells and foreign bodies (p. 16).

Ingested organic material is digested by cytoplasmic enzymes (in lysosomes).

Inert foreign substances may remain stored indefinitely.

Example: soot particles deposited by macrophages in the lung.

Macrophages mobilize under the stimulus of inflammation and at its site.

This is apparently brought about in several ways.

Part of the increase is the result of mitoses among macrophages.

Important additions come from the activation of fixed macrophages.

Further recruits are transformed monocytes that leave the blood stream.

Tissue macrophages are one component of the so-called *reticulo-endothelial system* (p. 48).

5. Plasma cells.

They are normally rare, except in serous membranes, in the lining of the respiratory and intestinal tracts and in lymphoid tissue.

They are also plentiful in regions of chronic inflammation.

Plasma cells represent a special differentiation of the lymphocyte-line.

The nucleus is spheroidal and located well off-center in the cytoplasm.

Its clumped chromatin tends to be arranged peripherally like spokes of a wheel.

The cytoplasm is deeply basophilic and more abundant than in small lymphocytes.

An area near the nucleus remains pale and unstained.

This is the region of the Golgi complex and centrosome.

Plasma cells are rich in endoplasmic reticulum, studded with ribosomes.

This protein-synthesizing apparatus produces most, at least, of the antibodies.

6. Mast cells.

These elements occur sparsely, often along the course of small blood vessels.

They are fairly large cells, but have relatively small, pale, spheroidal nuclei.

The cytoplasm is crowded with coarse, deeply basophilic secretory granules.

These stain well with basic aniline dyes, but not with hematoxylin.

The cell membrane ruptures readily during fixation and liberates the granules.
The granules are highly refractile and rather soluble in water.
Hence they are not preserved in ordinary sections of tissues.
These tissue basophils are entirely distinct from the basophils of the blood.
They produce *heparin,* an anticoagulant, and *histamine,* a vasodilator.

7. Leucocytes.

Lymphocytes and monocytes may outwander into connective tissue.
Some of these, however, arose in connective tissue and have remained there.
Yet they can enter the circulation and sometimes do so.
Eosinophils emigrate from the blood stream into connective tissue.
They are numerous in the lactating breast and in the respiratory and gastro-intestinal tracts; they accumulate beneath absorptive membranes.
Neutrophils, in particular, escape from capillaries in regions exhibiting inflammation.
In general, leucocytes perform their chief functions in loose connective tissue.
Some of these functions are summarized on p. 64.

8. Fat cells.

These conspicuous elements are normal components of areolar tissue.
They occur singly, or in clusters arranged along small blood vessels.
They are special cells resembling fibroblasts, but they store fat.
Fat appears first as droplets which later merge into a common, fluid pool.
Hence, adult cells are usually bloated with a huge vacuole filled with fat.
These elements will be considered further under the topic of adipose tissue (p. 53).

9. Chromatophores.

Pigmented cells (*chromatophores*) occur in the skin, pia mater and choroid of the eye.
The cell body, containing brown *melanin granules*, extends into cytoplasmic processes.
Some cells (*melanocytes*) synthesize pigment; others (*melanophores*) phagocytose it.
Known functions of melanin are limited to its role in absorbing light rays.

B. The Reticulo-Endothelial System:

This is a macrophage system, all of whose cells possess phagocytic power.
A criterion for inclusion in this category is the ability to take up particles of colloidal dyes.
Only some of the cells are reticular cells and none are true endothelium.
Members of this system include: cells lining the sinusoids of bone marrow and liver; reticular cells of lymph nodes, spleen and less well-organized lymphoid differentiations; macrophages of loose connective tissue; emigrated monocytes of blood.
Probably the microglia of the nervous system also should be included.
They arise, like the others, from mesenchyme.
These widely distributed cells act to protect the body through phagocytosis.
Ingested materials are: bacteria; dead cells; tissue debris; foreign substances.
These are removed from the blood, lymph and tissue-fluids.

C. Connective-Tissue Fibers:

Three kinds of fibers occur in adult connective tissue.
Two kinds (collagenous; elastic) are wholly different both physically and chemically.
The third type (reticular) is a variant of the ordinary collagenous fiber.

1. Collagenous fibers.

Another name, sometimes used because it is colorless, is *white fiber*.
It is notable for being a compound fiber, composed of still finer fibrils.
The total fiber is demonstrably a product of fibroblastic activity.
A. General Features.
Collagenous fibrils are fine threads (0.3 to 0.5 μ), visible with the light microscope.
The fibrils run parallel courses which are actually more or less wavy.
Individual fibrils are of indefinite length and do not branch or unite.

Groups of fibrils are held together by a cementing substance.

A *collagenous fiber* is a bundle, composed of a variable number of fibrils.

Hence the size of a fiber-bundle depends on the number of fibrils in it.

Bundle thickness ranges from 1 to 12 μ in loose connective tissue.

A fiber-bundle is said to be encased in a thin covering of cementing material.

Bundles frequently branch and recombine, forming a network.

This arrangement is brought about by clusters of fibrils leaving one bundle and joining other bundles (as do wires in a cable-complex).

B. PHYSICAL PROPERTIES.

A fresh collagenous fiber is opaque, with a dull, pearly appearance.

That is, it is colorless (white) and has a low refractive index.

Pulling on a wavy fiber merely straightens it, without significant stretching.

Its resistance to a further pulling-force is remarkable (several kg/mm^2).

When it yields, it breaks and frays irregularly, like a rope.

Electron micrographs prove that fibrils are composed of still finer *microfibrils*.

These 'unit fibrils' are 0.02–0.1 μ thick, and are uniform at any given site.

Each is composed of fundamental macromolecules, called *tropocollagen*.

These are elongate threads, measuring 0.28 by 0.0014 μ (ratio, 200:1).

They lie side-by-side, with staggered overlaps of one-fourth a length.

This produces a cross-banding that repeats every 0.064 μ.

The parallel arrangement of microfibrils in a fibril is responsible for the birefringence shown under polarized light.

Tropocollagen, the structural unit, consists of three polypeptide chains.

These intertwine in a helix, and one is out of phase with the others for a distance of 0.28 μ, which is the length of the tropocollagen microfibril.

Fibroblasts synthesize these structural units and secrete them.

Liberated into the ground substance they polymerize into microfibrils.

C. CHEMICAL CHARACTERISTICS.

These fibers consist of an albuminoid, *collagen*, which gives them their name.

Boiling dissolves the fibers into a colloidal solution of 'animal glue.'

(This explains the name, collagen, which means 'glue producing.')

Animal glue is really gelatin, which gels on cooling.

Weak acids and alkalies cause fibers to swell markedly.

They swell unevenly and become transparent.

Strong acids and alkalies dissolve the fibers.

Long action of weak solutions will do the same.

This action is the basis of maceration processes.

The dissolution frees structures supported by white fibrous tissue.

Fibers are readily digested by an acid solution of pepsin (gastric juice).

On the contrary, they resist the enzymes of pancreatic juice.

Fibers dissolve in cold, neutral salt solutions, liberating tropocollagen molecules.

When such a solution is incubated at body temperature, fibrils are re-polymerized, with the typical banding restored.

Tannic acid converts collagen into a tough, insoluble product.

This reaction is the basis of the tanning of leather.

There is no specific stain for collagenous fibers.

However, acid aniline dyes stain them strongly; eosin stains them fairly well.

The Mallory or Masson stain is a good practical test for these fibers.

The aniline-blue or light-green component colors them brilliantly.

2. *Elastic fibers.*

The cell type responsible for the deposition of these fibers is not known.

It would seem that it should be a special type of fibroblast.

A. PHYSICAL PROPERTIES.

Elastic fibers are always solitary in loose tissue, never occurring in bundles.

They branch and anastomose abundantly, thereby forming a network.

In life they are stretched and under tension.

Stretching to 1.5 times its relaxed length causes a fiber to break.

The force required is one-tenth that for a collagenous fiber of equal size.

Severed fibers break squarely across, like a rubber band.

They then retract and curl in a loose spiral.

With advancing age these fibers lose their resiliency.

A fiber tends to be coarser (up to 1.0 μ) than a collagenous fibril (0.3 to 0.5 μ).

Most, however, are definitely thinner than average collagenous fibers.

Only electron micrographs of the highest resolution yield any fiber detail.

An amorphous material (*elastin*) embeds the more peripheral microfibrils.

When fresh, a fiber appears microscopically as a bright thread.

This appearance is due to its high refractivity.

Fresh, massed fibers have a yellowish color.

Hence they are sometimes called *yellow fibers*.

B. CHEMICAL CHARACTERISTICS.

The fiber contains *elastin*, an albuminoid with distinctive qualities.

Elastin resists boiling water, dilute acids or alkalies, and gastric juice.

The enzyme *elastase*, present in pancreatic juice, digests the fiber readily.

Ordinary stains demonstrate elastic fibers poorly or erratically.

Orcein or resorcin-fuchsin stains them deeply and electively.

With aging, elastin degenerates into *elacin*, with loss of resiliency.

3. *Reticular fibers.*

A. PHYSICAL PROPERTIES.

These fibers branch and unite in a fine meshwork, or reticulum.

They are of different sizes, but all are relatively thin (0.2 to 1.0 μ).

Each represents a bundle of *microfibrils* like those in a collagenous fiber.

Reticular fibers are inelastic and have features in common with collagenous fibers.

In many locations the two blend and become continuous.

Most important is banding with the same periodic spacing (0.064 μ).

This means that the molecular arrangement is identical in both.

At best, only a minor chemical difference (tyrosin lack?) exists.

B. CHEMICAL CHARACTERISTICS.

Reticular fibers are often obscured in sections by other, crowding elements.

Ordinary stains show them poorly or not at all.

However, special silver techniques blacken them prominently and specifically.

Hence these fibers are called *argyrophilic*.

By contrast, the same silver techniques do not blacken collagen fibers.

They merely tinge them yellow to brown.

Also the PAS technique stains reticular fibers but not collagenous fibers.

Since a significant chemical difference between the two fiber types is lacking, it is logical to ascribe unlike responses to dissimilar physical qualities.

The silver staining of reticular fibers has been attributed to thin fiber-size.

A thin fiber has a larger surface in comparison to its mass.

Also each component fibril is coated with a glycoprotein sheath.

This amorphous coat may be responsible for PAS and silver staining.

Reticular fibers are the first connective-tissue fibers to appear in development.

They are still abundant in fetuses and the newborn.

But, as time goes on, many take on collagenous-fiber characteristics.

Some, however, remain permanently at the 'reticular' stage.

Such fibers can be interpreted as immature, arrested collagenous fibers.

In wound healing, fibers of the reticular type are the first to develop.

Gradually they thicken and become typical collagenous fibers.

D. AMORPHOUS SUBSTANCES:

1. *Ground substance.*

Connective-tissue fibers and cells are embedded in an amorphous *ground substance*.

When fresh, it is optically homogeneous and transparent.

Hence it can be seen only when placed in media with a different refractive index.
It is extracted by ordinary fixatives, so is not seen in ordinary sections.
It can, nevertheless, be preserved by the freeze-drying method, and then stained.
Ground substance varies in consistency between a semifluid and a colloidal jelly.
Such variations occur with activity, aging and injury.
It stains poorly or not at all with ordinary dyes.
Toluidine blue stains ground substance (metachromatically) a purple tone.
This response indicates the carbohydrate nature of the ground substance.
Two such carbohydrate components (acid muco-polysaccharides) are known.
Their viscosity is markedly decreased by enzymes, such as *hyaluronidase*.
This permits substances to spread faster through the tissues.
It is possible that still other unidentified glycoproteins are represented.
Fibroblasts are concerned in the production of the amorphous ground substance.
They contain granules that are the precursors of this material.

2. *Tissue fluid.*

This liquid is a transudate derived from the plasma within blood vessels.
It constitutes one-third of the total body fluid and is important functionally.
Tissue fluid contains proteins, crystalloids, metabolic products and gases.
Under certain conditions it can exist in part as a free fluid within tissue spaces.
The extent to which such spaces and fluid exist normally is not surely known.
When there is tissue injury or inflammation, a rapid accumulation is obvious.
It seems that much water is bound to the ground substance in a colloidal state.
Dissolved substances diffuse through such an aqueous phase of the colloid.
Ground substance helps in maintaining a proper water and electrolyte balance.

III. THE LOOSE CONNECTIVE TISSUES

This group of adult tissues is characterized by the loose arrangement of its fibers.
A distinction between loose and dense, however, is arbitrary in some instances.
The members of this group include: reticular tissue; areolar tissue; adipose tissue.

A. RETICULAR TISSUE:

1. *Occurrence.*

In some regions reticular fibers are associated intimately with *reticular cells*.
They help to form the framework of lymphoid organs, bone marrow and liver.
They occur in the linings of the stomach, intestines, trachea and bronchi.
This association of cells and fibers constitutes reticular tissue.
In other regions reticular fibers are associated with *fibroblasts*.
Example: fat cells; smooth muscle; capillaries; stroma of various organs; at junctions
between collagenous fibers and epithelia; basement membranes.
This association is not 'reticular tissue' in the strict sense of that term.

2. *Cells.*

Reticular cells (p. 46) and *fibroblasts* (p. 46) are the cellular elements.
The phagocytic reticular cells are a part of the *reticulo-endothelial system* (p. 48).

3. *Fibers.*

Reticular fibers are arranged as a fine lattice-work of branching threads.
Most of the protoplasmic processes of reticular cells are related to the fibers.
Such processes wrap about or extend in intimate contact along the fibers.
Lymphocytes and other cells occupy the interstices of the meshwork.

4. *Appearance in sections.*

Reticular cells and fibers are obscured in many densely populated organs.
Also ordinary stains do not color reticular fibers.

Hence their identification depends on special staining techniques.

In preparations, stained routinely, this tissue is seen less clearly and satisfactorily than any other type of adult tissue.

In open regions (*e.g.*, lymph nodes) it appears as a network of highly stellate cells.

Cell processes are long; some may seem to join those of other cells.

Occasionally the cytoplasm contains phagocytosed particles.

The arrangement resembles embryonic mesenchyme, but 'adult' tissues adjoin.

The nuclei are relatively smaller, and the cytoplasm more abundant.

The interspaces are commonly clogged with lymphocytes.

5. *Functional correlations.*

Reticular fibers make delicate connecting and supporting frameworks.

Beneath epithelia they enter into the composition of basement membranes.

Primitive reticular cells produce lymphocytes and macrophages (and others?).

Phagocytic reticular cells play important roles as scavengers and as agents of defense against bacteria.

B. Areolar Tissue:

The word 'areolar' refers to the 'little areas,' or spaces, occurring within this tissue.

It is a loosely arranged, fibro-elastic connective tissue.

It displays a greater variety of cells and fibers than any other connective tissue.

1. *Occurrence.*

Areolar tissue is the most widespread of all the connective tissues.

Gross dissection is largely a matter of freeing other things from areolar tissue.

It is encountered to some extent in every microscopical section of the body.

It fastens down the skin and other membranes, conducts vessels and nerves, and binds together muscles and their component parts.

It supplies a general bedding-substance (*stroma*) in the interior of many organs.

Wherever organs or parts enjoy some mobility, areolar tissue occurs as a stretchy, anchoring and embedding medium.

It also serves as a packing material, filling in the unused spaces between organs.

2. *Gross appearance.*

To the naked eye areolar tissue looks whitish to translucent.

It is soft, pliable, slippery, stretchy and easily displaceable.

With a hand lens it appears cobwebby; the fibers interlace loosely.

3. *Structure.*

Areolar tissue consists of a ground substance that contains various kinds of cells and two principal kinds of fibers.

A. Ground Substance.

This is an amorphous jelly (mucopolysaccharide), holding coagulable tissue fluid.

It is often described as occurring in sheets (*lamellae*).

But even its existence is difficult to demonstrate microscopically.

This is because it is extracted during the preparation of tissues.

B. Cells.

All the cells previously described (pp. 46-48) may be encountered.

The two commonest by far are *fibroblasts* and *macrophages*.

C. Fibers.

Collagenous fibers are far in excess, from the standpoint of total bulk.

These compound bundles branch and recombine; their ends cannot be found.

Elastic fibers also show a continuous branching network, without free endings.

In typical areolar tissue they are relatively inconspicuous.

Reticular fibers are also represented to some degree.

They occur where areolar tissue borders upon other structures.

Notable is a contribution to basement membranes and tiny blood vessels.

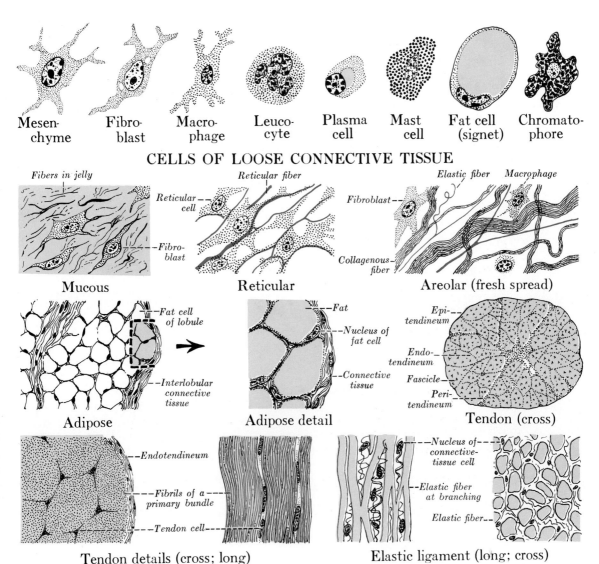

Mesen-chyme | Fibro-blast | Macro-phage | Leuco-cyte | Plasma cell | Mast cell | Fat cell (signet) | Chromato-phore

CELLS OF LOOSE CONNECTIVE TISSUE

Mucous   Reticular   Areolar (fresh spread)

Fibers in jelly — *Reticular fiber* — *Elastic fiber* — *Macrophage*

Reticular cell — *Fibro-blast* — *Fibroblast* — *Collagenous fiber*

Adipose   Adipose detail   Tendon (cross)

—Fat cell of lobule — —Interlobular connective tissue — —Fat — —Nucleus of fat cell — —Connective tissue

Epi-tendineum — Endo-tendineum — Fascicle — Peri-tendineum

Tendon details (cross; long)   Elastic ligament (long; cross)

—Endotendineum — —Fibrils of a primary bundle — —Tendon cell— — Nucleus of connective-tissue cell — Elastic fiber at branching — Elastic fiber—

TYPES OF CONNECTIVE TISSUE

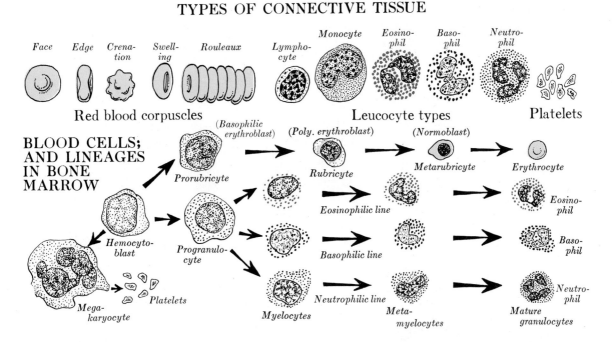

Face | Edge | Crena-tion | Swell-ing | Rouleaux | Lympho-cyte | Monocyte | Eosino-phil | Baso-phil | Neutro-phil

Red blood corpuscles   Leucocyte types   Platelets

BLOOD CELLS; AND LINEAGES IN BONE MARROW

(Basophilic erythroblast) — *(Poly. erythroblast)* — *(Normoblast)*

Prorubricyte   Rubricyte   Metarubricyte   Erythrocyte

Hemocyto-blast   Progranulo-cyte

Eosinophilic line   Eosino-phil

Basophilic line   Baso-phil

Megakaryocyte   Platelets   Myelocytes   Neutrophilic line   Meta-myelocytes   Mature granulocytes   Neutro-phil

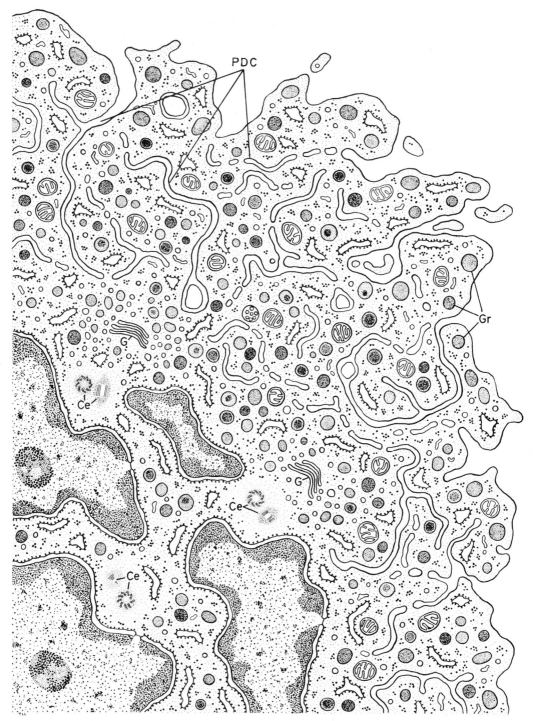

MEGAKARYOCYTE DETAIL. Portions of the multilobed nucleus are at the left and base. Pairs of centrioles (Ce) occur between nuclear lobes, and small Golgi complexes (G) are nearby. Rough endoplasmic reticulum is sparse, but free ribosomes are numerous. Vesicles coalesce into extensive channels (PDC) that join the surface membrane and set free cytoplasmic fragments, the blood platelets.

4. Appearance in sections.

There is no apparent plan to the interweaving tissue arrangement.
> Shrinkage markedly reduces the interspaces of the living tissue.
> The total tissue of the slice has a 'hashed' appearance.

Collagenous fibers, cut in random planes, intermingle without order.
> They stain satisfactorily with ordinary acid dyes.
> Fibers cut more or less lengthwise appear as wavy bands.
>> If well fixed, their component fibrils show as fine, longitudinal threads.
>>> Acid fixatives cause fibrils to swell; their discreteness is then lost.
> Fibers, cut across, present angular areas of irregular sizes and shapes.
>> With good preservation the component fibrils show as dots.
>> If swollen by fixatives, the sectioned fiber appears as a homogeneous disk.

Elastic fibers are shown poorly or not at all by ordinary stains.
> If identifiable they resemble dots or short rods, smaller than white fibers.

Cells are squeezed in between fibers; only their nuclei are prominent.
> The cytoplasm is usually deformed and not well seen.

Ground substance is not demonstrable in ordinary preparations.

5. Functional correlations.

A. MECHANICAL.
> Areolar tissue both provides support and permits some mobility.
>> Displacement and stretching are followed by a return to the original position.
> Thus it holds various tissues, organs and organ components in place.
>> Yet it permits considerable play between such parts.
> It provides pathways for vessels and nerves.
> It acts as a packing material between parts of the body, both large and small.

B. TRANSPORT OF METABOLITES.
> Nutrient substances, gases and wastes traverse the interval between capillaries and the sites where tissue metabolism takes place.
> Tissue fluid is the carrier of these substances.
> The ground substance does not present a barrier to this transport.

C. DEFENSE.
> Ground substance seems to act as a barrier against the spread of bacteria.
>> Its success in defense is in inverse relation to the ability of certain bacteria to form an enzyme that tends to liquefy this jelly.
> Macrophages, and outwandered neutrophils and monocytes, mobilize on occasion.
>> Noxious substances, formed locally, are neutralized and destroyed by them.
>> Foreign bodies, micro-organisms and degenerating cells are ingested.

D. REPAIR.
> Reserve mesenchymal cells can produce specialized cell types.
> Fibroblasts repair injuries produced by mechanical insult or disease.
>> They may even erect barriers against disease and wall-off foreign bodies.
> The process of repair (wound healing) repeats fiber-formation, as in embryos.
>> The synthesis of collagen is dependent on the presence of vitamin C.

C. ADIPOSE TISSUE:

Areolar tissue, in general, contains scattering fat cells.

Regions dominated by aggregations of these cells are designated *adipose tissue*.

Since fat is a storage tissue, its amount varies with the nutritional state of the individual.
> It totals about 10 per cent of body weight; masses are, in a sense, *fat organs*.

1. Occurrence.

Fat is abundant beneath the skin, where it constitutes the *panniculus adiposus*.
> (This insulating layer is not present in mammals with a hairy coat.)

Other collections occur: around the kidneys and suprarenals; in the mesenteries and mediastinum; in the grooves of the heart; in bone marrow; in the cervical, axillary and inguinal regions.

The regional distribution of fat in men and women is different.

This suggests a genic and gonadal endocrine influence on fat deposition.

It is absent from the nervous system, lungs, eyelids, ear, dorsum of hand and penis.

2. Development and involution.

Small droplets of fat accumulate in certain cells of the fetus (and of the adult).

Interpretation of these storage cells is not beyond dispute.

A majority view them as specific *lipoblasts*, differentiated from mesenchyme.

This could explain the absence of fat wherever fibroblasts are plentiful.

Such cells tend to collect along small blood vessels, and especially capillaries.

They enlarge, withdraw their processes, and round up.

Further growth of the fat droplets is followed by their coalescence.

This produces a bloated cell, containing a single, large globule of fat.

The cytoplasm is thereby reduced to a thin, enveloping layer.

The nucleus is pressed to the periphery and flattened.

Numerous fat cells tend to arise at a definite site, in close relation to other groups.

In time of need, stored fat is given up through a reversal of the storage-events.

Fat leaves a cell (as it also enters) not as fat, but as fatty acids.

As the fat is lost, the cell reverts to a type that resembles a fibroblast.

Such a depleted cell is capable of again storing fat.

After losing fat, some cells may remain rounded and contain watery vacuoles.

This is a type of atrophy, and the cells are named *serous fat cells*.

Certain adipose pads of the body retain their fat tenaciously.

These give up fat only after long starvation.

Example: orbit; joints; palm; sole.

3. Structure.

Fat is an atypical connective tissue, specialized for particular purposes.

It is the cells, rather than interstitial substance, that dominate the scene.

They comprise most of the tissue-bulk and impart its characteristic features.

A *fat cell* is a large, clear spherule that measures up to 120 μ in diameter.

The fresh cell is highly refractive, bright and glistening.

The fat of primates has a yellow color, due to lipochrome pigments.

The cytoplasm is a thin shell, somewhat more abundant about the flattened nucleus.

It contains an oil drop which is not bounded by a cytoplasmic unit membrane.

A glycoprotein coat and a fine network of reticular fibers envelop each cell.

Chemically, fat consists of a mixture of glycerides and fatty acids.

Fat is insoluble in water and cold alcohol.

It is soluble in ether, chloroform, benzol and xylol.

Hence fat has usually been dissolved out of sections prepared for study.

A vacant cavity is then left within the cytoplasm.

However, fat is rendered insoluble and retained by formalin fixation.

Several staining agents color the fatty component of adipose tissue.

The dye named Sudan IV stains frozen-sectioned tissue red.

If this dye is fed to an animal, its fat (and milk) become pink.

Yet there are no simple, specific stains for neutral fat.

Osmic acid preserves and blackens both fat and myelin.

Sudan Black is an excellent fat stain that also colors other lipids.

Scattering fat cells, free from mutual pressure, retain a spherical shape.

Compact fat differs, in that its cells are mutually compressed and deformed.

Between the fat cells are compressed connective-tissue cells, reticular- collagenous- and elastic fibers, and capillaries.

Closely packed fat cells make up *lobules* of 'yellow fat,' separated by fibrous *septa*.

A lobule is a territory supplied during its development by a single arteriole.
> The blood supply of adult fat seems to be scanty because cells are so bloated.
> Actually, in relation to cytoplasmic volume the vascularity is rich.
There is no intrinsic nerve supply, although nerves may be found in the tissue.

4. Brown fat.

A peculiar type of fat occurs in certain locations in various mammals.
> Such a fatty mass is light brown in color and has a glandular appearance.
The cells retain a polyhedral shape; the nucleus and cytoplasm are fairly typical.
Fat occurs as numerous separate droplets, distributed throughout the cytoplasm.
> The fat-content is not readily affected by changes in the nutritional state.
> It is, however, depleted rapidly after the hypophysis or suprarenals are removed.
This tissue is physiologically more active in certain regards than is ordinary fat.
> It is distinctly lobulated and highly vascular, but its full significance is unknown.
> Hibernating animals use it as a heat source during their arousal from dormancy.
Brown fat is identifiable in the human fetus, but not surely in the adult.

5. Appearance in sections.

Ordinary sections of yellow fat consist largely of vacant spaces that vary in size.
> Such spaces are bounded by exceedingly thin rims of cytoplasm.
> When the nucleus happens to be included, it also is flattened and thin.
Scattered or loosely arranged cells have circular outlines.
> Sections through the nucleus give a 'signet-ring' appearance.
Compact fat shows crowded cells, pressed into polygons (many are hexagons).
> The nucleus is also distorted by the mutual pressure.
> The tissue between cells is compressed beyond easy recognition.
Compact fat occurs in lobules, bounded by fibrous septa.
> Little or no areolar tissue is seen within the lobule.

6. Functional correlations.

Adipose tissue stores reserve energy — material in the form of neutral fat.
> This is synthesized from glucose, fatty acids or even amino acids.
Fat cells are rich in enzymes and show considerable enzymic activity.
> The stored fat is not a static deposit; there is a fairly rapid turnover.
Fat forms soft elastic pads between organs and parts, holding structures in place.
> Some pads act as shock absorbers.
It serves as a buffer tissue, as in bursae.
Fat is an efficient insulator against cold; that is, body heat is retained.
> This is important to aquatic mammals, as is also its buoyancy.
> It is also important to man, since an insulating hair-coat is lacking.
It has a cosmetic value by padding hollows and softening angles of the body.

D. REGENERATIVE ABILITY:

The loose connective tissues, as a group, repair losses well.
In reticular and areolar tissue the events repeat histogenesis in the fetus.
> Reserve mesenchymal cells proliferate and differentiate into fibroblastic types.
> First a mucinous ground substance is deposited.
> In it new fibers are laid down, reticular and collagenous fibers forming promptly.
>> Elastic fibers reappear slowly, and often incompletely.
>> The formation of collagenous fibers is dependent on the presence of vitamin C.
Fat cells do not divide; new fat cells differentiate from reserve mesenchymal elements.
> Other mesenchymal cells produce the fibrous tissue that embeds fat cells.

IV. THE DENSE CONNECTIVE TISSUES

These tissues have an abundance of compactly arranged fibers, one type being predominant.
> Cells are proportionately fewer than in loose connective tissue; fibers are coarser.

Space available for ground substance and tissue fluid is extremely limited.
(Obviously there are intergrades between loose- and dense fibrous tissue.)
This group can be subdivided, on the basis of fiber direction, into two main categories.

A. INTERWOVEN ARRANGEMENTS:

The fibers are arranged so as to withstand tensions exerted from different directions.
This category has also been designated as 'irregularly arranged' tissue.

1. Tissues predominantly collagenous.

Some fascias are interwoven sheets with irregularly arranged bundles.
Others are incompletely layered, with different, dominant fiber-directions.
Other examples of interlacing, dense tissue are: fibrous *capsules* of organs (spleen; testis);
sheaths (periosteum of bone; epimysium of muscles; dura mater); *septa* and *trabeculae*
(*i.e.*, partitions and beams within organs).
All of these, and especially the most compact types, are notably whitish in color.
The appearance in sections is essentially like that of areolar tissue.
But the arrangement is far more compact and felt-like; cells are compressed.
Functionally, the tissue forms a fibrous, supportive 'skeleton' for organs.
The deep fascias exercise a restraining action, preserving body contours.
These and some other membranes provide areas for muscle attachments.

2. Tissues predominantly elastic.

Scarpa's fascia, of the abdominal wall, is largely an elastic sheet.
Networks of elastic fibers exist as tubular sheets within blood vessels.
In the largest arteries, elastic tissue consolidates into spiraling elastic membranes.
The sheets are perforated by irregular openings and interconnect somewhat.
A latticework is seen well only in sections that parallel the surface.
Functionally, the tubes give with the pound of the pulse, and then relax.

B. PARALLEL ARRANGEMENTS:

This category is sometimes designated as 'regularly arranged' tissue.
The fibers are oriented so as best to withstand tension exerted in one direction.

1. Tissues predominantly collagenous.

The popular example is *tendon*, and this will be described as a type-form.
The great majority of *ligaments* are similarly composed and constructed.
Their organization, however, is not quite so regular as that of tendon.
Aponeuroses are organized like tendon; they are broad expansions of tendon.
Some show layering, with a different 'grain' in adjacent layers.
Other examples of layering are the cornea and some sensory corpuscles.
A. STRUCTURE.
The unit of tendon structure is the so-called *primary tendon bundle*.
This is merely a very large collagenous fiber (30 μ $\pm$) clasped by fibroblasts.
The designation of the fiber as a 'bundle' refers to its compound nature.
That is, the primary bundle is a collection of still finer fibrils.
Primary bundles run parallel, yet slightly wavy, courses.
Slanting anastomoses occur at acute angles, as in ordinary fibers.
Fine elastic networks have been described between bundles.
Tendon cells (fibroblasts) are located between primary bundles.
They are the only type of cell present there; nothing else is seen.
Their cytoplasm is compressed into thin, radiating wings.
These pass between the adjacent primary bundles.
Hence each *lamellar cell* is in a clasping relation to several bundles.
A variable number of primary bundles group together as a tendon *fascicle*.
This compound unit is also known as a *secondary tendon bundle*.

Fascicles are crowded and comprise most of the tendon substance.

Nevertheless, they are separated by some loose connective tissue.

B. TENDON AS AN ORGAN.

Tendons are rope-like cables that attach muscles to bones.

A total tendon is an entity that qualifies as a simple organ.

As such it possesses a distinctive plan of organization.

The entire tendon is composed of a variable number of *fascicles*.

The total number in any instance depends on the size of the tendon.

The whole tendon is ensheathed by a moderately compact fibrous tissue.

This external covering is given the name of *epitendineum*.

In larger tendons there are also radial plates of loose connective tissue.

They converge centrally and divide the tendon into V-shaped areas.

Such coarse radial septa constitute the so-called *peritendineum*.

Finally, the individual fascicles are ensheathed with loose connective tissue.

It serves to separate one fascicle from another.

This ensheathing tissue, as a whole, is named the *endotendineum*.

Some tendons course in osseo-fibrous tunnels (*e.g.*, hand; foot).

Such tendons are contained within a double-walled, fibrous *tendon sheath.*

The cavity of the double, tubular sheath contains a secreted, lubricating fluid.

Bounding the fluid is a vascular sheath-lining, the *synovial membrane.*

The superficial cells are flattened, epithelioid connective-tissue cells.

The inner and outer layers of the sheath are continuous at the ends of the tube.

They are also continuous lengthwise, suspending the tube as a *mesotendon.*

This is a mesentery that carries blood vessels to the tendon.

Vessels and nerves course in the epi-, peri- and endotendineum.

They are sparse and never invade the fascicles.

C. APPEARANCE IN SECTIONS.

1. *Longitudinal Section.*

Each tendon fiber (primary bundle) is a wavy band.

Its appearance is either homogeneous or longitudinally fibrillate.

This depends on whether or not the fixative preserved fibrils faithfully.

Tendon cells occur in rows, squeezed in between the fibers.

Only their elongate nuclei usually show well.

Nothing else is seen between the tendon fibers.

Endotendineal sheaths show at intervals as strips of looser tissue.

2. *Transverse Section.*

A fiber takes the form of a prominent, angular area.

Tendon cells are stellate, with circular (or distorted) nuclei.

The cells are usually greatly shrunken and their processes short.

Often crack-like shrinkage spaces (especially about cells) separate fibers.

In other instances fibers, swollen by technical procedures, tend to merge.

Tendon fibrils, faithfully preserved, show as tiny dots within each fiber.

Commonly, however, the appearance is homogeneous and glassy.

This is due to swelling, produced by chemical fixation.

On focusing, the fiber-areas usually shift position or rotate somewhat.

It is caused by focusing up and down short portions of the wavy fibers.

Loose tissue of the endotendineum does not penetrate into a fascicle.

Tendon fibers and cells are the only things seen within a fascicle.

D. FUNCTIONAL CORRELATIONS.

This group of dense tissues provides tough, inelastic cords, bands or sheets.

Each is constructed so as to satisfy the mechanical requirements imposed.

A tendon is flexible, yet highly resistant to a pulling force.

It has greater tensile strength than a bone of equal size.

A pencil-size tendon can sustain a weight of one-half ton before breaking.

It anchors muscles and completes the pulling action by inserting on bone.

Tendons are also indirectly concerned with sensory reception (p. 294).

2. *Tissues predominantly elastic.*

These are far less numerous than the dense, collagenous type.

Examples: ligamenta flava (of the vertebrae); suspensory ligament of the penis; stylohyoid ligament; true vocal cords; ligamentum nuchae (of quadrupeds).

They are distinctly yellow in color because of their elastic-fiber content.

A. STRUCTURE.

In an elastic ligament the elastic fibers are coarse (up to 5 μ in man).

They run parallel courses, but branch and unite frequently at acute angles.

The elastic ligament is not organized as fully as is tendon.

Nevertheless, the fibers may tend to group into clusters.

Interspaces are occupied by scanty fibroblasts and fine collagenous fibers.

Vessels and nerve fibers are relatively sparse.

B. APPEARANCE IN SECTIONS.

1. *Longitudinal Section.*

An elastic ligament shows as loosely spaced, often coarse bands.

These fibers branch and anastomose at short intervals.

Such connecting fibers are set at acute angles.

Hence the general fiber direction is nearly parallel.

A fiber appears homogeneous and stains poorly in ordinary preparations.

Delicate connective tissue occupies the spaces between fibers.

2. *Transverse Section.*

Fibers are homogeneous areas, often arranged in groups.

The outline of a fiber is angular to rounded.

Delicate areolar tissue surrounds these groups (fascicles).

It also continues into a fascicle and surrounds individual fibers.

C. FUNCTIONAL CORRELATIONS.

Elastic ligaments maintain a state of tension when put on the stretch.

They yield to a pulling force, but recover when the tension ceases.

C. REGENERATIVE ABILITY:

If a tendon or ligament is torn or severed, it can repair the injury.

Fibroblasts and vessels grow in, and new fibers are laid down, properly oriented.

At first the new fibers are fine; subsequently they gradually coarsen.

The original tissue, at the cut ends, plays little or no role in repair.

Autotransplants of tendon or fascia survive; cells live and fibers probably persist.

Homotransplants replace both their original cells and fibers.

Chapter VI

The Blood and Lymph

I. THE BLOOD

Blood is a specialized and somewhat atypical connective tissue.

The ground substance is a fluid, the *blood plasma*.

Fibers make their appearance in the plasma as *fibrin*, but only when blood clots.

Previously they existed, potentially, in solution in the plasma.

Cells of two main types (red and white) are prominent constituents.

Red cells are so colored because they contain the respiratory pigment, *hemoglobin*.

Because of the fluid plasma, blood cells have no fixed positions.

Other visible particles suspended in the plasma are *blood platelets* and *chylomicrons*.

Blood constitutes about 7 per cent of body weight; a 150-pound man contains 5 quarts.

A. ERYTHROCYTES:

These elements are also called *rubricytes, erythroplastids* and *red blood corpuscles*.

In a strict sense the word 'erythrocyte' is inappropriate for mammals.

This is because the mature corpuscle lacks a nucleus and so is not a complete cell.

All vertebrates, other than mammals, have nucleated red cells, elliptical in shape.

In mammals the nucleus has been discarded; this enhances respiratory efficiency.

1. Shape.

In all mammals the shape is that of a biconcave disk.

This shape favors the quick absorption and release of gases.

It also favors a flexibility that permits passage throughout tiny capillaries.

The outline is circular (except in the camel family, where it is oval).

Both surfaces of the disk are depressed, like large dimples, centrally.

Hence in edge view the outline is like that of a plump dumbbell.

Variant shapes occur pathologically, such as 'sickle cells.'

2. Size.

In man the living, undehydrated corpuscle is 8.5 μ in diameter.

In dry smears it measures 7.6 μ, and in sectioned tissues usually about 5.0 μ.

Size variations occur pathologically, both larger and smaller.

Most mammals have slightly smaller corpuscles than man.

The extremes are 9.4 μ (elephant) and 2.5 μ (musk deer).

(The largest erythrocytes in vertebrates occur in salamanders; up to 80 μ).

The total surface area available for respiratory exchanges is impressive.

For human corpuscles this amounts to 4200 square yards.

This area is nearly the size of a football field.

3. Number.

All statistics of frequencies refer to a volume of 1 cu. mm. of blood.

In human males the red-corpuscle count is 5,200,000; in females, 4,700,000.

The total number of corpuscles in an average-sized human is 25 million millions.

Placed in single file they could encircle the earth four times!

A marked decrease in number is encountered in pernicious anemia.

Increases in number follow chronic exposure to high altitudes or to carbon monoxide.

4. Color.

A single fresh corpuscle is pale greenish-yellow; massed corpuscles are red.

In conventionally stained blood smears the corpuscles take a pinkish tint.

5. Structure.

There is a peripheral plasma membrane of the usual extreme thinness (0.005 μ).

It is a lipid-protein complex, making an elastic and semipermeable barrier.

The internal cytoplasm is apparently a homogeneous colloidal sol.

The nucleus and cytoplasmic organelles were lost in the later stages of development.

Hence a corpuscle is an extremely thin bag containing hemoglobin in solution.

About 1 per cent of the corpuscles encountered are not quite mature.

These *reticulocytes* show a network of RNA when stained with brilliant cresyl blue.

6. Physical properties.

A red corpuscle is soft, flexible and elastic.

It is frequently distorted momentarily when squeezing through capillaries.

Yet it is relatively firm, containing 40 per cent solids (muscles, 20 per cent).

Rouleaux are columns of corpuscles, stacked like a pile of coins.

These occur spontaneously in a stagnant circulation or in drawn blood.

The adherence is apparently a surface tension effect.

It can be imitated by greased, weighted corks.

If plasma concentrates by evaporation, *crenation* of the corpuscle occurs.

This is a shriveling which produces a scalloped or prickly contour.

Water passes outward into the more concentrated (hypertonic) plasma.

If the plasma is diluted, the corpuscle imbibes fluid and swells.

Cup shapes become progressively fatter as the hypotonicity increases.

At a certain stage the hemoglobin leaves the corpuscle.

This outward passage of hemoglobin is called *hemolysis* or *laking*.

The pale corpuscle is then called a *blood shadow* or *blood ghost*.

Hemolysis is also accomplished by other agents that injure the plasma membrane.

Example: lipid solvents, such as ether; bile salts; snake venom.

Agglutination (*i.e.*, clumping) of corpuscles is induced by various agents.

Example: acid salt-solutions; glucose solution; agglutinins.

Agglutinins, present in the plasma, furnish the basis for the four blood types.

These are responsible for specific compatibilities and incompatibilities.

7. Chemical composition.

The coloring pigment of red corpuscles is *hemoglobin,* an aggregate of 557 amino acids.

It comprises 95 per cent of the dry weight of a corpuscle.

Hemoglobin is a complex protein, containing iron.

It crystallizes in rhombic plates.

These have characteristic shapes in different mammalian species.

Some lower animals use different metals in their respiratory pigments.

Example: molluscs, copper; tunicates, vanadium (present; respiratory?).

Hemoglobin hydrolyzes into *hematin* and *globin.*

The chloride of hematin is called *hemin.*

It crystallizes in brown rhombic plates, used as a test for blood.

This test, however, does not distinguish human from other bloods.

Hemoglobin can take up and bind 1.3 times its weight of oxygen.

This compound, *oxyhemoglobin,* is easily reduced by the tissues.

The amount carried is decreased in secondary anemias.

8. *Life-span and disposal.*

The life-span of the circulating human red corpuscle is approximately 127 days.
> This means that some 2,500,000 new corpuscles must enter the blood stream every second, while an equal number are lost.

The total picture of normal red-corpuscle destruction is not known.
> Damage is incurred mechanically by buffeting within the blood stream.
>> (During its life cycle a corpuscle travels about 700 miles.)
>
> The plasma membrane is further damaged by constant O_2 and CO_2 transfers.
>> Both buffeting and tension changes facilitate rupture of the membrane.
>
> It is known that whole corpuscles and fragments are engulfed by macrophages.
>> This occurs where there is reticulo-endothelium (liver; spleen; bone marrow).
>> The macrophages break up the hemoglobin into simpler products.
>>> *Bilirubin* is excreted with the bile.
>>> *Iron* is retained and used again in new, developing red corpuscles.

9. *Appearance in sections.*

The corpuscles are acidophilic disks of uniform size, staining pink in smears.
They are usually encountered within the blood vessels of tissues.
> Ordinarily corpuscles do not occur free in the tissue spaces.
>> Their presence there may be due to rough handling in tissue-preparation.

Well-preserved corpuscles are sharply defined disks (or often cups) in shape.
> With delayed or inferior preservation there is agglutination.
> This is marked by the loss of clearly defined corpuscular outlines.

10. *Functional correlations.*

Blood is a fluid carrying a respiratory pigment; in man and most animals, in cells.
> The primary function of blood is to make possible tissue-respiration.
> Although a nucleus lacks, energy is obtained by enzymic oxidation of glucose.

Red corpuscles carry oxygen from the lungs to the tissues, but remain in capillaries.
> In the lungs their hemoglobin combines with oxygen to form *oxyhemoglobin*.
> In the tissues oxygen is given up and the oxyhemoglobin is reduced.

On the return journey they transport carbon dioxide from the tissues to the lungs.
Rh antigen and blood-group antigens reside in the membrane of the red corpuscle.

B. LEUCOCYTES:

The white cells are true cells with ameboid ability; their general name is *leucocyte*.
They are much alike in all the vertebrate groups.

1. *Classification.*

There are two main groups, each with subgroups.
> A. NONGRANULAR LEUCOCYTES.
>> 1. Lymphocytes (25% ±).
>> 2. Monocytes (5% ±).
>
> B. GRANULAR LEUCOCYTES.
>> 1. Neutrophils (65% ±).
>> 2. Eosinophils (3% ±).
>> 3. Basophils (0.5% ±).

Nongranular leucocytes have a few inconstant, nonspecific granules in the cytoplasm.
> All cytoplasmic 'granules,' in life, are actually semifluid droplets.
> The nucleus is spherical to kidney shape.

Granular leucocytes have abundant, specific granules in the cytoplasm.
> The nucleus ranges from two lobes to a series of connected lumps.

2. *Number.*

The average normal limits are 5000 and 9000 per cu. mm. in adults.
> The ratio of white cells to red corpuscles is about 1:700.

The count in children is higher than in adults.

At birth the number is approximately 16,000 per cu. mm.

Marked variations from the normal number occur pathologically.

An increase is *leucocytosis;* more than 12,000 indicates disease.

This increase is then out of proportion for one or more types.

Example: lymphocytes increase in whooping cough; monocytes, in tuberculosis; neutrophils, in pus-forming infections; eosinophils, in allergies and parasitic infestations; basophils, in chickenpox.

A decrease below 5000 is called *leucopenia.*

Example: in typhoid fever.

3. Structural characteristics.

Leucocytes are typical cells, changeable in shape and somewhat resembling amebae.

In fixed preparations their pseudopodia are withdrawn and do not show.

Centrioles, mitochondria, Golgi apparatus and nucleoli are all demonstrable.

None of these cell components shows satisfactorily in stained smears.

In smear preparations, cells flatten and appear larger than in life.

Sizes, as usually stated, refer to their measure in stained smears.

Special stains, applied to smears, give the best blood picture.

These stains contain eosin (acid), and methylene blue (basic).

The methylene blue is in part oxidized into the azures (basic).

Besides these three staining components there is an eosin-azure-methylene blue complex which is neutral.

A. LYMPHOCYTES.

The commonest type by far in normal blood is known as the *small lymphocyte.*

Most of them are slightly larger than a red blood corpuscle.

The cell has a relatively large nucleus, enclosed by a thin layer of cytoplasm.

The nucleus is nearly spherical; its slight indentation may not be noticed.

It is very dense and dark because of heavy chromatin masses.

The cytoplasm is basophilic and stains a clear blue color.

It occasionally contains a few nonspecific, azurophil granules.

Some lymphocytes are nearly twice the size of the ordinary small type.

These larger cells are commonly called *large lymphocytes* (but see p. 142).

They have the same structural characteristic as the small ones.

But there is more cytoplasm in relation to the size of the nucleus.

They are relatively scarce in blood and are regarded merely as older cells.

There are two different functional types of small lymphocytes in the blood.

One arises chiefly in lymph nodes and in other nodular lymphoid tissue.

Its circulating progeny live only a few days.

The other type arises in bone marrow, passes to the thymus and proliferates.

Some live for years and recirculate between blood and lymphoid organs.

B. MONOCYTES.

These cells have also been known as *large mononuclears* and *transitionals.*

They are larger (often twice plus) than a red corpuscle, but vary in size.

The nucleus is ovoid-, kidney-, or U-shaped; these are age-stages.

It tends to be eccentric in position.

The chromatin is distributed in a more delicate network than in lymphocytes.

Hence the nucleus takes a paler stain.

The cytoplasm comprises more than half of the cell.

It stains a grayer or muddier blue than the cytoplasm of lymphocytes.

It may contain few to many dark-staining azurophil granules.

Rarely, intermediate types between monocytes and large lymphocytes occur.

In this instance positive assignment to one group or the other is difficult.

C. NEUTROPHILS.

The diameter is nearly twice that of a red corpuscle.

This size-ratio is also true of eosinophils and basophils.

The nucleus is markedly lobate (usually three, but as many as five, parts).

These masses, connected by thin threads, make irregular patterns (**U** to **S**).

The degree of lobation increases progressively as the cells age.

Some immature '*band cells*' occur, with horseshoe-shaped nuclei.

The chromatin is rather compact and quite dark-staining.

In 3 per cent of cells from females the nucleus has a 'drum-stick' projection.

This mass contains a complete X chromosome, or 'Barr body' (p. 26).

The abundant cytoplasm is closely packed with fine (often inconspicuous) granules.

These stain with neutral dyes, but give up the dye readily.

With blood-stains the color is lilac to lilac-pink.

Additionally, there may be some coarser granules, reddish to purple in color.

D. EOSINOPHILS.

The nucleus is usually bilobed, with a slender connecting isthmus.

Its chromatin is fairly dense; the nucleus stains moderately well.

The cytoplasm constitutes considerably more than half the bulk of the cell.

It is packed with coarse, spheroidal granules, uniform in size.

They stain electively with acid dyes (red to orange with blood-stains).

E. BASOPHILS.

The nucleus is usually elongate and somewhat bent (often S-shape).

It is partially constricted into two or three lobes (less marked than neutrophils).

The chromatin network is more loosely arranged than in eosinophils.

Hence the nucleus is relatively pale-staining.

The nucleus constitutes half the cell bulk, or two-thirds its diameter.

The cytoplasmic granules are spheroidal, coarse and variable in number and shape.

Some characteristically overlie the nucleus and tend to obscure it.

They are water-soluble, and so do not show in routinely preserved sections.

They stain electively with basic dyes (dark blue to purple with blood-stains).

This cell is distinct from the mast cell, but also forms heparin and histamine.

4. Life-span and disposal.

The total length of life is hard to determine because these cells enter the tissue spaces.

The period spent in the blood stream is brief; for some less than one day.

The viable period after leaving the blood stream is uncertain.

Some lymphocytes are recaptured from tissue spaces into lymph and blood.

They seem to continue this alternation indefinitely.

Information is meager or lacking for other types of leucocytes.

Probably macrophages (reticulo-endothelium) of the liver and spleen are the most active agents in removing aging leucocytes from the circulation.

Other leucocytes, outwandered into the connective tissues, disintegrate there.

Example: eosinophils congregate in the walls of the respiratory and gastro-intestinal tracts; neutrophils migrate into inflamed tissue, play a defensive role there and soon die.

Many lymphocytes enter the epithelia of the alimentary and respiratory tracts.

Their fate is presumably degeneration and death.

5. Appearance in sections.

Leucocytes show well-stained nuclei; the cytoplasm rounds up about the nucleus.

The differential staining of cytoplasmic granules is inferior and incomplete.

Stained sections cannot compete with smears for accurate identifications.

6. Functional correlations.

Little beyond the obvious activities of leucocytes is known.

Information is based on experimental and pathological material.

Leucocytes appear to be largely inactive while in the blood stream.

They perform most of their functions outside the vessels in connective tissue.

A. AMEBOID MOVEMENT.

This is a crawling process on a substrate; swimming does not occur.

There is an active front end, producing pseudopodia.

At the temporary rear end there is a passive, trailing tail.

Neutrophils are the most active (up to 33 μ per minute).

Monocytes are only moderately active, while basophils are sluggish.

Lymphocytes are often immobile, but they can become remarkably active.

B. MIGRATORY ACTIVITIES.

There is a constant migration of leucocytes out of blood capillaries.

Some of these cells return into the blood and lymph streams.

Monocytes and neutrophils slip through at the junction of endothelial cells.

Lymphocytes pass through the actual substance of endothelial cells.

Emigration is greatly increased during periods of inflammation.

There is a specific response by granulocytes to chemotactic stimulation.

First neutrophils, and later monocytes, arrive at the site of irritation.

Eosinophils flock to the digestive and respiratory tracts in allergies.

Lymphocytes accumulate in the tissues at sites of chronic inflammation.

C. PHAGOCYTOSIS.

This is the ability to ingest foreign particles, bacteria, cells, etc.

Such activity is far greater outside of vessels than within them.

Neutrophils are especially concerned with ingesting small, discrete particles.

Example: carbon particles; bacteria.

Dead neutrophils become pus cells.

The granules of all three types of granulocytes are *lysosomes* (p. 23).

These liberate hydrolytic enzymes which digest engulfed matter.

Monocytes greedily ingest particulate matter, and coarse masses also.

They are the prime scavengers of cells and tissue debris.

When outside the blood stream they can differentiate into macrophages.

Lymphocytes and basophils are phagocytic to a limited degree.

Eosinophils can become active and destroy antigen-antibody complexes.

D. OTHER PROPERTIES.

All leucocytes increase in number in response to specific stimuli (p. 62).

Some information exists concerning the presence of enzymes in leucocytes.

Oxidases occur in granular leucocytes and monocytes.

Neutrophils contain phosphatases and liberate proteolytic enzymes.

Defense activities include phagocytosis, proteolysis, antibody formation, etc.

Neutrophils provide the first line of defense against invading organisms.

Lymphocytes, eosinophils and basophils are involved in immune phenomena.

C. BLOOD PLATELETS:

1. *Occurrence.*

Blood platelets are cytoplasmic corpuscles that are characteristic of mammalian blood.

Lower vertebrates lack them, but have spindle-shaped cells named *thrombocytes*.

These seem to be generally similar in function.

2. *Size and shape.*

Platelets are tiny disks, averaging 3 μ in diameter.

Viewed on the flat, the shape is round to oval (often stellate when fixed).

In edge view the shape is like a spindle or rod.

3. *Number.*

The normal range is 250,000 to 350,000 per cu. mm.

Platelets are difficult to count accurately, partly because of their fragility.

Also they tend to clump in drawn blood and stick to anything they touch.

4. Structure.

Blood dyes demonstrate two regions interior to the plasma membrane of the platelet.
Centrally the protoplasm is granular and deeply basophilic (the *granulomere*).
Peripherally the protoplasm is pale and homogeneous (the *hyalomere*).

5. Origin and fate.

Platelets arise by fragmentation of the cytoplasm of the giant cells of bone marrow.
Their life-span has been determined to be about nine days.
Their disposal is presumably by the phagocytic activity of macrophages.
This is held to occur in the liver, spleen and bone marrow.

6. Appearance in sections.

Occasionally platelets show within vessels, when preserved and stained properly.
They are tiny protoplasmic fragments with a basophilic staining preference.

7. Functional correlations.

Platelets of circulating blood agglutinate and adhere to injured regions of vessels.
Such a *white thrombus* plugs leaks and covers injured spots.
Agglutinated platelets are associated with clotting, both inside and outside of vessels.
A plasma protein (*fibrinogen*), under enzymic influence, becomes threads of *fibrin*.
This meshwork entangles the blood cells and a jelly-like *clot* results.
Evidence associates the cytoplasmic granules with the clot-promoting factor.
A fibrin clot soon becomes smaller, firmer and stronger.
Knots of platelets throughout the mesh cause fibrin threads to twist and bend.
This clot-retraction is an important factor in stopping bleeding.
Disintegrating platelets liberate *serotonin,* an agent that constricts small blood vessels.

D. BLOOD PLASMA:

1. Composition.

Plasma constitutes 55 per cent of blood; cellular elements total 45 per cent.
It is isotonic with an 0.85 per cent solution of sodium chloride.
Many substances are contained in the slightly alkaline plasma.
These include: gases; proteins; carbohydrates; lipids; inorganic salts; organic substances, such as enzymes and hormones.
Certain suspended particles are demonstrable by phase or dark-field microscopy.
Chylomicrons are minute fat globules, more numerous after a fatty meal.
Hemoconia, or blood dust, probably represent cellular debris.

2. Appearance in sections.

Acidophilic fibrin-threads and plasma show at times within vessels.
The *fibrin* occurs as delicate to coarse interlacing filaments, minutely cross-banded.
The plasma is commonly a finely granular, but otherwise structureless, mass.

3. Functional correlations.

Plasma activities are related to respiration, coagulation, temperature regulation, buffer mechanisms and fluid balance.
Plasma also transports hormones, antibodies, foodstuffs and excretory wastes.
Fibrin forms and blood coagulates when the circulation ceases or when blood escapes.
Plasma, defibrinated by clotting or whipping, is known as blood *serum.*
It is a clear, yellowish fluid, no longer capable of clotting.
This is because fibrin and cellular elements largely entangle in the clot.

II. THE LYMPH

Lymph is a fluid, collected from the tissues and returned to the blood stream.

Its origin is from the fluid that occupies the tissue spaces of the body.

The *tissue fluid* is material that has escaped through the wall of blood capillaries.

But the endothelium is a semipermeable membrane; hence the larger molecules of plasma, such as colloids and fats, are mostly retained by capillaries.

The dialyzed fluid loses nutrients and oxygen to the extravascular tissues.

The tissue fluid also acquires the waste end-products from tissue metabolism.

Hence it becomes quite different from the original dialysate.

Some tissue fluid is absorbed by blood capillaries (those tributary to venules).

The remainder is taken up by lymphatic capillaries, whereupon it is called *lymph*.

Lymphatic endothelium allows colloids to enter; most blood endothelium does not.

Lymph from the small intestine (*chyle*) is milky because of fat globules taken up.

Lymph from the liver is unusually rich in proteins.

The smallest lymphatic vessels carry a practically noncellular lymph.

On reaching the lymph nodes, cells (mostly small lymphocytes) are added; erythrocytes lack.

Lymph coagulates, but the process advances slowly and the clot is soft.

Chapter VII

The Development of Blood

Blood cells are short-lived, and are constantly being destroyed and replaced.

The process by which blood cells are formed is named *hemopoiesis*.

In the embryo and fetus, total blood is formed successively in these places: the yolk sac; mesenchyme and blood vessels; liver; spleen, thymus and lymph nodes; bone marrow.

In the late fetus, and thereafter, blood is formed in the marrow and lymphoid tissues.

Under certain pathological conditions the liver, spleen and lymph nodes can regain hemopoietic functions like those of the bone marrow.

A. RIVAL INTERPRETATIONS:

Hemopoiesis is the area of greatest controversy in the entire field of histology.

Maximow and Sabin were the major proponents of rival, contesting schools of thought.

The chief points of disagreement involve the following things:

    1. The identification of the mother cell(s) of the several lines of differentiation.

        Terminology differences, related to divergent opinions concerning cell characteristics
and relationships.

        The concept of all blood cells belonging to a single family group versus that of the
existence of separate, distinct families of cells.

    2. The development of all blood cells outside the vascular channels versus the devel-
opment of leucocytes outside such channels and erythrocytes inside.

The theories of hemopoiesis can be summarized as follows:

    1. *Unitarian (or Monophyletic) Theory.*

        It derives all blood elements from a common mother cell.

    2. *Dualistic (or Diphyletic) Theory.*

        It derives nongranular leucocytes from one stem cell and granular leucocytes and
erythrocytes from a different stem cell.

        (Some have used this term to designate a concept that assigns red cells to one
developmental line and white cells to another line.)

    3. *Trialistic (Tri- or Polyphyletic) Theory.*

        It derives blood cells from three distinct stem cells.

          These give rise to: lymphocytes; monocytes; granulocytes and erythrocytes.

Probably the best total evidence favors the unitarian theory.

Also, this theory enjoys the support of a majority of hematologists.

Hence it will be simplest to base the following account on this interpretation.

Only minor parenthetical comments will indicate the alternative views of Sabin.

It should be emphasized, however, that the controversies over primal origins of blood cells do
not affect factual descriptions of developmental stages in the several lines.

From this standpoint the disputed aspects of hemopoiesis are largely academic.

B. HEMOPOIETIC TISSUES:

In normal, postnatal life, blood formation is less widespread than in the fetus.

After birth it is restricted to the lymphoid organs and red bone marrow.

    These two different sources are implied when the terms *lymphoid* (for nongranular leuco-
cytes) and *myeloid* (for granulocytes and red corpuscles) are used.

    But this convenient distinction is not realized at all times.

    In early fetal stages such separate specialized sites do not exist.

In adults the separateness may again be lost under abnormal conditions.
This occurs in *myeloid metaplasia*, in which lymphoid organs imitate red marrow.

1. Lymphoid hemopoietic tissue.

The chief lymphoid organs engaged in hemopoiesis are the spleen and lymph nodes.
Less important are the thymus, tonsils, scattered nodules and diffuse masses.
The lymphoid organs are the chief source of lymphocytes and monocytes.
Only a small number (about 5 per cent) of such cells arise in bone marrow.
For this reason, these derivatives of lymphoid organs are called *lymphoid elements.*
The basic tissue in these organs is a reticulum harboring lymphocytes.

2. Myeloid hemopoietic tissue.

In the fetus and child, *red bone marrow* occurs in all the bones.
At about the time of puberty it begins to be replaced in some regions by fat.
This fatty marrow is then termed *yellow bone marrow.*
In adults red marrow is restricted to the spongy regions of certain bones.
These are: vertebrae; ribs; sternum; cranium; clavicles; scapulae; pelvis.
Sites in the limbs are limited to the proximal ends of the humerus and femur.
The total marrow (red and yellow) accounts for nearly 5 per cent of body weight.
This is astonishing, since it weighs twice as much as the liver.
Yellow bone marrow typically is mostly fat; it does contain some crowded marrow tissue.
Actually all intergrades between yellow and red marrow can occur.
Normally there is no evidence of hemopoietic activity in ordinary yellow marrow.
Nevertheless, this power is dormant and can be revived under stress.
Example: red marrow replaces yellow after hemorrhages or in anemias.
Red bone marrow consists of a supporting framework, vascular channels and free cells.
The framework is a typical reticulum, with reticular cells stretched along it.
Ordinary blood vessels connect with sinusoids lined with fixed macrophages.
This lining is a type of the so-called *reticulo-endothelium.*
The distinctive marrow tissue is a pulpy mass of cells, both immature and mature.
These marrow cells collectively are called *myeloid elements.*
Interspersed are a varying number of fat cells, plasma cells and lymphocytes.
The chief characteristic components of myeloid tissue are the several stages in the
development of red blood corpuscles and granular leucocytes.
Giant cells (megakaryocytes) and blood platelets are further components.

C. THE STEM CELL:

It is plain that all blood cells trace their descent from mesenchymal progenitors.
It is equally clear that, sooner or later, various descendants acquire differences.
These specializations are not only structural but also in potentialities.
The main controversy hinges on whether the formative cells seen in lymphoid and myeloid
tissue are identical and interchangeable, or whether they are different in structure and
capacities. If identical, the type of specialization depends on the local environment.
Maximow, the chief advocate of the unitarian view, believed that the stem cell is a multipotent
element that can be called a *hemocytoblast.*
It is present both in the lymphoid organs and in the bone marrow.
It is a large ameboid cell, identical with a medium-sized and large lymphocyte.
The cytoplasm is fairly abundant and is noticeably basophilic.
The nucleus is large, open-structured and contains one or more irregularly shaped
nucleoli; it is a relatively primitive, spheroidal nucleus.
The hemocytoblast, in turn, is derived from a primitive reticular cell.
This is essentially a fixed, undifferentiated, nonphagocytic mesenchymal cell.
Maximow maintained that the small lymphocytes in blood-forming organs can grow larger.
In its usual state it can be considered an inactive form of hemocytoblast.
On becoming a medium-sized lymphocyte it is a potential hemocytoblast.

D. DEVELOPMENT OF LYMPHOID ELEMENTS:

Nongranular leucocytes arise in lymphoid tissues, and to some degree in red marrow as well.
  Lymphocytes arise chiefly in lymphoid tissue that is organized into nodules.
    Chief sites are the lymph nodes and spleen.
    Minor production in the thymus gives rise to a short-lived type (p. 62).
  Monocytes are sister cells of lymphocytes, but modify in a phagocytic direction.
    They develop in splenic sinuses, and also in hepatic and marrow sinusoids.
According to Maximow, nongranular leucocytes differentiate from mitotic *hemocytoblasts*.
  The intermediate stages of differentiation are not particularly distinctive.
  Neither the nucleus nor cytoplasm undergoes marked changes.
The daughter *lymphocytes* become the ordinary small-sized ones encountered so abundantly.
  The chromatin network is denser than in the mother cell, hiding the single nucleolus.
  A few azurophil granules may develop in the cytoplasm.
Typical *monocytes* acquire a horseshoe-shaped nucleus; nucleoli are usually not visible.
  The cytoplasm remains basophilic, but stains a grayish blue.
  It also may acquire many fine, pale-staining azurophil granules.
Many monocytes and lymphocytes pass into lymphatic channels and so reach the blood stream.
(According to Sabin, a 'primitive white blood cell' becomes a *lymphoblast* or a *monoblast*, depending on its environment; the lymphocyte, on the contrary, is an end-product, incapable of differentiating into anything else.)
Some further information on these matters will be found on p. 143.

E. DEVELOPMENT OF MYELOID ELEMENTS:

A minor activity of the red marrow is the production of lymphocytes and monocytes.
  Also present are some plasma cells.
But the development of myeloid elements is the distinctive feature of this tissue.
  These elements comprise the red-cell series, the granulocyte series and the giant cells of
    bone marrow (megakaryocytes).
According to Maximow, the stem cell of all three series is the *hemocytoblast*.
New hemocytoblasts arise chiefly by their own mitotic divisions.
  Some can differentiate from reticular cells that round up and detach.
  Hemocytoblasts average not more than 3 per cent of all marrow cells.

1. Erythrocytes.

  Stages are characterized by a reduction in cell size, an increasing content of hemoglobin
      and a shrinking, progressively darker-staining nucleus (finally discarded).
    Cell division continues into the metarubricyte (normoblast) period.
    The course of erythrocyte development is believed to take three days.
  A. PRORUBRICYTES (BASOPHILIC ERYTHROBLASTS).
    This stage is smaller than the stem-cell (hemocytoblast).
      Its nuclear network is slightly coarser; the cytoplasm is deeply basophilic.
      The basophilia is due to an increased presence of ribonucleic acid.
  B. RUBRICYTES (POLYCHROMATOPHILIC ERYTHROBLASTS).
    Mitosis in the preceding stage has halved the size of the cells.
    The nucleus is checkered with coarse chromatin masses; nucleoli are now obscured.
    The cytoplasm is losing its ribonucleic acid and is acquiring hemoglobin.
      Hence it colors variably with both the acid and basic components of the stain.
      The result (purplish; lilac; gray) explains the name 'polychromatophilic.'
  C. METARUBRICYTES (NORMOBLASTS).
    Mitosis in the preceding stage (and in this one) again halves the size of the cell.
    The nucleus becomes increasingly shrunken and pycnotic; mitosis ceases.
    The cytoplasmic hemoglobin stains strongly acidophilic (almost maximally).
  D. ERYTHROCYTES.
    The nuclei of normoblasts have been lost by extrusion; organelles have disintegrated.
    Red blood corpuscle is another term for this enucleated cell.

Immature stages still contain some residual ribonucleoprotein.

This becomes demonstrable by supravital staining or phase microscopy.

Because of the net-like pattern the cells are called *reticulocytes*.

Red corpuscles enter the sinusoids, possibly through growth pressure from behind.

(According to Sabin, the stem cell of the erythrocyte series is a specific cell type, the *megaloblast*, derived from reticular cells that line the marrow sinusoids.)

2. *Granulocytes.*

According to Maximow, the common stem cell is a typical *hemocytoblast*.

The general name for various stages of differentiating daughter cells is *myelocyte*.

These cells are characterized by a progressive (but moderate) reduction in size, an increasing darkening and lobation of the nucleus and a progressive accumulation of specific cytoplasmic granules.

As a group, these are the most numerous cells inhabiting the marrow.

A. PROGRANULOCYTES.

The earliest type that is easily distinguishable is the *progranulocyte*.

This large cell is ameboid and mitotic; it comprises about 4 per cent of all marrow cells.

Nonspecific granules begin to appear in the basophilic cytoplasm.

B. MYELOCYTES.

Three times as abundant are daughter cells known as *myelocytes*.

They proliferate repeatedly, but eventually become smaller and cease dividing.

Cytoplasmic basophilia decreases; specific granules appear in large numbers.

The specific kind of granule foreshadows an *eosinophil*, *basophil* or *neutrophil*.

Nuclei indent and assume a horseshoe shape; chromatin increases in density.

C. METAMYELOCYTES.

The most numerous cells (emerging from the final mitoses) are called *metamyelocytes*.

These are juvenile types of leucocytes, with characteristic granular content.

Neutrophils far outnumber the other two granulocyte types.

The nucleus, at first horseshoe-shaped, gradually acquires its typical lobation.

D. MATURE GRANULOCYTES.

The terminal stage is that of the definitive granulocytes of the blood.

These mature cells enter the sinusoids and thus reach the blood stream.

Nonmotile forms are forced through the sinusoidal wall by tissue pressure.

(According to Sabin, the 'primitive white blood cell' produces a *myeloblast* which is the progenitor of the several granulocytes.)

3. *Megakaryocytes.*

According to Maximow, this giant cell takes origin from the *hemocytoblast*.

The nucleus enlarges and undergoes a peculiar multiple nuclear division.

The daughter nuclei merge and the same type of mitosis is repeated.

Concomitant cytoplasmic growth produces a giant cell, some $100\,\mu$ in diameter.

The nucleus is complexly lobed; the lobes may connect by thin strands.

The cytoplasm is finely granular, but has a clear ectoplasm at the periphery.

Multiple fragmentation of the cytoplasm produces the *blood platelets*.

Megakaryocytes do not live long, and their cytoplasm disintegrates.

The shrunken nuclei are often carried to the lungs, lodging in capillaries.

(Sabin derives these cells from reticular cells that line the marrow sinusoids.)

F. NUMERICAL RELATIONS:

The red marrow controls the proportions of cell-types present in the blood.

The relative numbers of the different kinds of these cells vary but little normally.

This is true of both the marrow and the circulating blood.

Pathologically, however, these ratios may become altered.

Example: in local infections neutrophils increase; in typhoid fever they decrease.

Correlated with the increase in cell numbers, by mitosis, goes a decrease in cell size.

In other words, individual volumes are inversely related to numbers.

Example: progranulocytes (large cells) comprise 4 per cent of nucleated marrow cells; metamyelocytes (smaller cells) comprise 22 per cent.

Yet the volume of all metamyelocytes scarcely surpasses that of progranulocytes.

The total number of cells at each stage of a series remains at a quite constant level.

This is owing to advancing stages being offset by steady losses to the blood stream.

About 1.5 per cent of the cells of normal marrow are in mitosis at any given time.

Under normal conditions the replacement-demands are largely met by mitoses of immature forms rather than by the stem cells themselves.

That is, hemocytoblasts are relatively dormant and add few cells to the total yield.

This, however, is adequate to maintain pools of dividing daughter cells.

Under stress, on the other hand, hemocytoblasts become active.

This is because the ordinary manner of supply is then inadequate.

The ratio of leucocytic forms to nucleated red cells is about 3:1.

This is correlated with their longer stay in the marrow and shorter life when mature.

The hemopoietic tissues are not depleted during the production of mature cells.

Not all daughter cells go on at once to succeeding stages.

Some remain at the same stage as their mother cell and divide again.

G. Marrow as an Organ:

A general account of bone marrow, apart from its hemopoietic activities, will be found in a subsequent chapter (p. 84).

Chapter VIII

Cartilage

Cartilage, the 'gristle' of the body, is a specialized type of supporting tissue.
  It is a fairly firm substance that will bear weight and give some rigidity.
  Like connective tissue, it consists of *cells, fibers* and *ground substance.*
      The ground substance and fibers, together, constitute the *matrix* of cartilage.
Mature cartilage occurs in three subtypes:
  1. *Hyaline;* this is the fundamental and commonest kind.
  2. *Elastic;* this type specializes by adding elastic fibers to the matrix.
  3. *Fibrous;* this type specializes by increasing the collagenous fibers in its matrix.

A. HYALINE CARTILAGE:

1. *Occurrence.*

Ribs (ventral ends); long bones (articular ends).
Nose; larynx; trachea; bronchi.
External acoustic meatus.
Fetal skeleton (cartilages of adults are remnants of this).

2. *Macroscopic appearance.*

Cartilage occurs in plates, columns or irregular masses.
It is solid, but somewhat flexible and elastic.
  It is easily cut with a knife.
Hyaline cartilage is translucent, with a bluish to pearly tint.
  Hyaline means 'glassy'; this quality is a property of its matrix.
It is enclosed within a fibrous envelope, except on articular surfaces.

3. *Microscopic structure.*

A thin total slice shows *cells* embedded in a clear, stainable *matrix.*
The whole cartilage-slice is bordered by a fibrous strip, the *perichondrium.*
  A. PERICHONDRIUM.
      It is composed of coarse, firm connective tissue.
          This is densely interwoven and consists mostly of collagenous fibers.
      Next to the cartilage the perichondrium tends to be more cellular.
          This specialized layer is not obvious after cartilage growth ceases.
      At the inner surface, its cells and fibers grade insensibly into cartilage tissue.
  B. CELLS.
      These *chondrocytes* are large (up to 40 μ), and tend toward a spherical shape.
          Yet mutual pressure, resulting from mitotic cell clusters, often distorts them.
      Near the perichondrium the cells are relatively young and flattened.
          Here they gradate into the fibroblasts of the perichondrium.
      Under the free surface of a joint they also become flattened.
      The basophilic cytoplasm contains fat droplets and glycogen.
          On fixation it usually suffers marked shrinkage, vacuolation and distortion.
  C. CELL GROUPS.
      In young cartilage, before internal growth begins, cells occur singly.
          Also near the perichondrium or a joint surface they remain single permanently.
      In somewhat older cartilage the cells usually occur in groups (*cell nests*).

They then are arranged in rounded groups or in rows.

Between the compressed cells there may be a thin layer of matrix.

Such groupings are due to mitoses and internal growth (p. 74).

D. MATRIX.

It appears to be homogeneous (but actually is not), and is basophilic.

Spaces in it, occupied by cartilage cells, are named *lacunae.*

In life a cartilage cell (or resulting daughter cells) fills its lacunae fully.

Lacunae are revealed when cartilage cells shrink in routinely prepared sections.

Each shows as a smooth-walled cavity containing a shrunken chondrocyte.

1. *Physical Structure.*

The matrix appears to the eye to be amorphous and homogeneous.

Actually it is a stiff, gelatinous ground substance, permeated by a feltwork of fine collagenous fibrils (43 per cent of dry weight).

The fibrils are not visible in fresh preparations, because their refractive index is the same as that of the ground substance.

Yet the polarizing microscope will reveal these fibrils in thin sections.

Fibrils do not show the typical banding and do not group in bundles.

Thus the matrix contains basophilic ground substance, masking acidophilic fibrils.

The gelatinous ground substance can be removed by tryptic digestion.

When this is done, the fibrillar framework is made plain.

2. *Chemical Composition.*

The composition of cartilage matrix is complex.

One component is the collagen belonging to the collagenous fibers.

The principal component of the ground substance is *chondro-mucoprotein.*

This is mucoprotein plus *chondroitin sulfates* A and C, which are acid.

There is a high content of water (70 per cent).

Matrix dissolves in boiling water, forming *chondrin* or cartilage-glue.

Chondrin consists of gelatin and chondro-mucoprotein.

The distribution of the several chemical substances throughout the matrix can be shown by differential staining reactions.

These specializations are correlated with growth and aging of the matrix.

Nearest a cell is a refractile zone, the so-called *cartilage capsule.*

It is merely the youngest and most basophilic part of the matrix.

The deep staining is due to a high concentration of acidic chondroitin sulfates and to fewer fibrils in this local region of the matrix.

Another zone is sometimes seen outside a single capsule, or surrounding a group of capsules belonging to a cell cluster.

This *territory,* or *chondrin ball,* is less basophilic than the capsules.

In it occur less chondroitin sulfates and more fibrils.

The *general matrix,* between territories, may take an acid stain, as does matrix beneath the perichondrium.

This is because there the collagenous fibrils are not masked by the usual concentration of the chondroitin sulfates.

4. *Nutrition.*

In general, cartilage matrix lacks intrinsic blood vessels, lymphatics and nerves.

Vessels that occasionally become enclosed are coursing to another destination.

Only in large cartilages are there blind channels containing blood vessels.

These occur, for example, in the epiphyses of the fetus and adult.

Moreover, there are no canaliculi in the matrix along which fluids might pass.

Hence nutrients, oxygen and cell wastes must seep through the matrix.

This diffusion is adequate, since the requirements of cartilage are not high.

Actual experiments show that dyes quickly permeate living cartilage.

Capillaries in the perichondrium both supply and receive metabolic materials.

Articular cartilage derives its nutrition from the synovial fluid that bathes it.

5. *Development and growth.*

Mesenchymal cells enlarge into crowded spheroidal cells, bathed by a mucinoid fluid.

This preliminary tissue is named *precartilage*.

Somewhat similar is the *notochordal tissue* of the embryo.

This is the forerunner of the *pulpy nuclei* of later intervertebral discs.

Thin plates of matrix, deposited by the cells, enclose and separate them.

These cells, now *chondrocytes*, thereby become embedded in cartilage matrix.

Mesenchyme, surrounding the enlarging primordial mass of cartilage, is compressed.

The resulting envelope becomes the fibrous *perichondrium*.

Continued growth of the cartilage is by two methods: (1) *interstitial;* (2) *appositional.*

A. INTERSTITIAL GROWTH.

Cells that are well buried undergo mitosis and form groups of two to several cells.

The deposition of matrix progressively separates the daughter cells and produces the so-called *capsules* about them.

Continued laying down of matrix, by the cells, separates cells still further.

The 'capsule' proves to be merely a zone containing newly formed matrix.

Hence the earliest capsule loses its identity as newer matrix crowds it away.

That is, the earlier capsules merge and become a *territory*.

Still later the substance of a territory is, in turn, crowded away.

It then loses its identity as it blends with the more remote matrix.

This method of growth occurs in relatively young, expansile cartilage.

The cell groups seen in old cartilage indicate the condition that existed when interstitial growth finally came to an end.

B. APPOSITIONAL GROWTH.

This chief type of growth is from the perichondrium, as a tree grows from its bark.

The innermost cells of the perichondrium specialize into *chondroblasts*.

These deposit matrix about them; in turn, they become overlaid by still newer cells and matrix, added from the perichondrium.

As young cartilage cells get buried deeper in matrix they enlarge into spheroids.

These cells may then participate in interstitial growth, as described above.

6. *Regressive changes.*

In the developing fetus *calcified cartilage* appears as a temporary strengthening expedient during the replacement of cartilage by developing bone (pp. 91, 93).

Such impregnation of cartilage matrix interferes with the diffusion of nutrients.

The effect on cartilage cells can be death and dissolution.

As cartilage ages there is cell loss and a decline in the basophilia of its matrix.

Decreased basophilia is due particularly to a decrease in chondroitin sulphate A.

In old age the calcification of some cartilages is a characteristic phenomenon.

The matrix then becomes opaque, hard and brittle through lime deposits.

A rarer secondary change is the formation of so-called *asbestos fibers*.

Silky, lustrous, parallel fibers are deposited.

They do not have the properties of collagenous fibers.

Tissue softening, or even cavity formation, may result.

B. ELASTIC CARTILAGE:

1. *Occurrence.*

This type occurs in locations where support with flexibility is required, as follows:

External ear (auricle); auditory tube, in part.

Epiglottis.

Larynx (corniculate, cuneiform and arytenoid cartilages).

2. *Macroscopic appearance.*

It is yellow (because of elastic fibers), and more opaque than hyaline cartilage.

It is also more flexible and elastic.

An ensheathing perichondrium is present.

3. Microscopic structure.

Elastic cartilage is fundamentally like the hyaline type.

The *cells*, singly and in groups, and their capsules are similar.

The general matrix also contains *ground substance* and masked *collagenous fibrils*.

But, in addition, it contains a meshwork of branching, *elastic fibrils*.

The elastic fibers vary in thickness and abundance in different cartilages.

They also are thicker and more closely packed in the interior of a cartilage.

They may be so abundant locally as to obscure the ordinary matrix.

Growth occurs in the same ways as in hyaline cartilage.

C. FIBROCARTILAGE:

1. Occurrence.

This type occurs in locations where a tough support or tensile strength is desirable:

Intervertebral disks; articular disks.

Pubic symphysis; some articular cartilages; rims of some sockets.

Lining of tendon grooves.

Insertions of some tendons and ligaments.

(Fibrocartilage never occurs wholly alone, but merges insensibly with neighboring hyaline cartilage or with fibrous tissue.)

2. Macroscopic appearance.

This tissue has an opaque appearance and a firm, fibrous texture.

A perichondrium is lacking.

3. Microscopic structure.

The *cartilage cells* are of the ordinary type, but are relatively sparse.

They occur as single cells, groups and rows.

Visible matrix is limited to the near vicinity of cartilage cells.

It may be scarcely noticeable, but may even show deep staining *capsules*.

Preponderant in the tissue are the massed, coarse *collagenous fibers*.

These fiber-bundles usually take a common direction, yet they may interweave.

In development, such bundles largely displace the ground substance.

D. REGENERATIVE ABILITY:

Injuries are not repaired by the cartilage tissue itself.

This is because adult cells are imprisoned in matrix and probably never divide.

Tissue from the perichondrium and adjacent fascia proliferates and fills in the defect or gap.

In young, growing animals certain cells convert into chondroblasts.

These cells deposit new matrix and become chondrocytes.

A fracture of a mature cartilage usually becomes united by dense fibrous tissue.

Some of this fibrous tissue, however, may be replaced by bone.

Homografts of cartilage, brought into a suitable nutrient bed, persist.

The naturally imprisoned cells are protected from antibodies and lymphocytes.

E. APPEARANCE IN SECTIONS:

Large cells (singly, in groups or in rows) occur in an abundant basophilic matrix.

Single cells are rounded when deeply located.

Near the cartilage surface they are flattened and adjoin a fibrous sheet.

The occurrence of cell groups in the interior is common and characteristic.

Mutually apposed surfaces are flattened.

The cartilage cells are shrunken and vacuolate, owing to loss of water and fat.

They often drop out of their opened matrix cavities (lacunae).

The matrix is basophilic and often stains more deeply in the vicinity of cells.

It varies in appearance in the three cartilage types.

In *hyaline cartilage* it is abundant and seemingly structureless.

In *elastic cartilage* it contains varying numbers of elastic fibers.
> These are usually not well shown unless stained differentially.

In *fibrocartilage* the ground substance is largely replaced by collagenous fibers.
> Ordinary matrix is seen only in the near vicinity of cells.

A fibrous, perichondral sheath envelops hyaline and elastic cartilage alone.

F. Functional Correlations:

Hyaline cartilage provides support that combines resiliency with fair rigidity.
> In joints it withstands compressing forces, produced by weights sustained.
>> The smooth free-surface makes possible nearly frictionless movement.

Other types specialize in the directions of flexibility, and toughness (against shear).

Cartilage is a skeletal tissue that can grow rapidly enough to keep pace with the growth of a fetus, infant and child. (Bone grows too slowly to maintain the pace.)

Cartilage produces provisional models of most of the future bones.
> Within and around these models the replacing, definitive bones develop.

It also plays the leading role in the elongation of many bones.
> Such growth centers (actually disks) add bone progressively to parts already formed.

The orientation of fibers in cartilage is related to the direction of external forces.

S^{35}, injected as sodium sulfate, is detected first in cartilage cells and then in matrix.
> In growing cartilage this indicates the source and deposit of new ground substance.
> In adult cartilage it suggests a normal, continuous turnover of matrix material.

Similarly the route of matrix-collagen can be followed by administering tritiated proline.
> It is traced from endoplasmic reticulum to the Golgi complex and into the matrix.

Chapter IX

Bone, Bone Marrow and Joints

I. BONE

Bone, or *osseous tissue*, represents the highest differentiation among supporting tissues.
It is a rigid tissue that constitutes most of the skeleton of higher vertebrates.
    A 'bone,' as a total skeletal unit, is a true organ.
Like other supporting tissues, bone consists of *cells*, *fibers* and a *ground substance*.
    But a distinguishing feature is the presence in the ground substance of inorganic salts.

A. GENERAL FEATURES:

1. Macroscopic appearance.

    Bone consists of both compact and spongy regions of hard-matter.
        It is hard and tough, but somewhat elastic.
    The color in life is a pinkish blue.
    Externally it is covered with a fibrous *periosteum*.
    Internally its cavities are filled with *marrow tissue*.
        A thin condensed layer, next to the bone, is the ill-defined *endosteum*.

2. Chemical composition.

    Earthy (inorganic) and animal (organic) components are intermixed in bone.
        The inorganic components give hardness and rigidity.
        The organic components give tenacity, elasticity and resilience.
    The pure inorganic component can be obtained by *calcination*.
        When burned, bone first turns black as the organic component carbonizes.
        Then it turns white as the organic matter becomes totally consumed.
            The residue is chalky and brittle; the loss by weight is 38 per cent.
        The general shape and internal arrangement are retained.
        Analysis proves the earthy residue (62%) to consist of the following:
            calcium phosphate (85%); calcium carbonate (10%); others (5%).
    The pure organic component may be obtained by steeping a bone in dilute acid.
        This treatment dissolves out the lime salts; it is called *decalcification*.
        A tough, flexible substance remains that retains the form of the bone.
            It is easily cut or bent; a slender bone can even be tied in a knot.
        This residue retains faithfully most of the structural details.
            For this reason decalcification is a preliminary step in preparing sections.
        Decalcified bone consists almost wholly of collagenous fibers.
            This bone collagen has sometimes been called *ossein*.
            It yields gelatin on boiling; this is a source of commercial gelatin.
    Also retained is the amorphous ground substance named *osseomucoid*.

3. Compact and spongy bone.

    Differences in the texture of bony regions are plain to the unaided eye.
    Compact bone is external in position, whereas *spongy bone* is more internal.

Compact bone is solid, except for microscopic canals.

Spongy bone, also called *cancellous bone* or *trabecular bone*, is a lattice-work.

It is composed of short bars, plates, tubes and globular shells.

The two types differ chiefly in their degree of porosity.

A long bone (*e.g.*, femur), sawed lengthwise, shows these relations well.

The two ends of the bone consist mostly of tissue that is obviously spongy.

Its irregular spaces continue into the main marrow cavity of the shaft.

All such cavities, large and small, lodge bone marrow.

By contrast, the 'shaft' is a hollow cylinder whose compact wall seems imporous.

Most bones of the body have their entire interior filled with spongy bone.

4. Classification of bones.

Every bone of the body contains both compact and spongy tissue.

The amounts of these and their local distributions vary.

There are several groups of bones, based on shape, as follows:

A. SHORT BONES.

These are roughly cuboidal in shape.

Example: bones of the wrist and ankle.

They consist of spongy bone enclosed within a shell of compact bone.

B. FLAT BONES.

Actually they are characterized by being relatively thin, rather than truly flat.

Example: ribs; shoulder blade; bones of the cranial vault.

Two plates of compact bone enclose a middle layer of spongy bone.

In the cranium the flat plates are named *tables;* the spongy layer is the *diploe.*

C. LONG BONES.

This category includes bones of a somewhat cylindrical shape.

Example: most of the limb bones.

The main tubular shaft (*i.e.*, *diaphysis*) is chiefly compact bone.

Each end-region of the bone (including the *epiphysis*) is chiefly spongy bone.

D. IRREGULAR BONES.

These are of irregular and varied shapes, not belonging in the previous categories.

Example: vertebrae; many bones of the skull.

Like short bones, they consist of a compact exterior and a spongy interior.

The compact bone is usually in the form of a thin shell.

B. STRUCTURAL ELEMENTS:

1. Bone cells.

These faintly basophilic *osteocytes* are specialized connective-tissue cells.

For a time, during bone development, they acted as formative cells (*osteoblasts*).

A little later they became imprisoned as matrix was progressively deposited.

Their size varies; they are approximately $10 \times 35 \ \mu$, in flat view.

Their outline is irregularly oval (on the flat) or biconvex (on edge).

In life, bone cells fill little cavities (*lacunae*) in the bone matrix.

Fine cytoplasmic processes enter the angular bays of a lacuna.

In developing bone the processes of bone cells extend even farther.

That is, they occupy capillary tubes (*canaliculi*) radiating from the lacunae.

In this way bone cells come into contact by fine cytoplasmic processes.

In mature bone of mammals the processes apparently have been largely withdrawn.

2. Bone matrix.

Although apparently homogeneous, matrix really has a double structure.

The condition is something like that of a heavily starched cloth.

There are both a fibrous fabric and substances that stiffen and mask it.

One component is organic (*fibers*); the others, inorganic (*lime*) and organic (*cement*).

A. ORGANIC COMPONENTS.

The major component in bulk is collagenous fibrils of the ordinary banded kind.

The fibrils are fine, but are gathered in bundles 3 to 5 μ thick.

Such bundles are named *osteocollagenous fibers.*

The fibers are united by a special cementing substance (see beyond).

B. INORGANIC SALTS.

The mineral salts of bone tissue are located on the fibers and within them.

They total 62 per cent of the dry weight of a bone.

Calcium phosphate comprises 85 per cent of this inorganic deposit (p. 77).

The bone salts have the structure of an apatite mineral (with needlelike crystals).

They are deposited in a regular, orderly manner with respect to the fibers.

This arrangement is in relation to the cross banding of collagen.

C. CEMENT.

There is a *cementing substance* that unites individual fibers of bone.

This is the primary ground substance of the matrix.

It is a viscid substance—a mucopolysaccharide containing chondroitin sulfate.

Also, adjacent lamellae are united, as are adjacent sets of lamellae.

Adjacent sets include Haversian systems and interstitial lamellae.

All such sets are delimited by a distinct *cement membrane.*

The membrane is a refractile layer of dark-staining binding substance.

A layer of cement marks a pause between minor phases of local construction.

It also marks beginning reconstruction following a wave of local destruction.

D. LACUNAR CAPSULES.

Lacunae and canaliculi are bordered by a layer of special organic cement.

This forms a thin *lacunar capsule*, similar structurally to cement membranes.

It is homogeneous and the index of refraction is high.

In unstained sections the lacunar capsule appears as a shining ring.

Silver treatment blackens the capsule; basic dyes stain it also.

It is resistant to chemical attack, such as strong acids or hot alkali.

3. Woven bone.

The prenatal type of spongy bone has its fibers irregularly interwoven.

Woven bone is characteristic of rapid bone development.

The irregular fiber-pattern is isotropic with polarized light.

4. Lamellae.

Postnatal bone development is carried out at a slower pace than the fetal rate.

Such bone matrix is arranged in layers (*lamellae*) 3 to 7 μ thick.

Lamellae occur in parallel series, either flat or curved (concentric).

This results from the rhythmical manner in which matrix is deposited.

Lamellae are the most characteristic structural feature of adult bone.

The fiber components of each lamella run in roughly parallel courses.

Their spiralling direction agrees with the long axes of lacunae in that lamella.

Adjacent lamellae of any series alternate in fiber direction.

That is, the fibers of one lamella course at a considerable angle to those of adjoining lamellae on either side of it.

It explains why lamellae appear to be so distinct, one from another, in sections.

This alternation gives maximum rigidity and strength.

Lamellae are arranged in sets (*Haversian systems; periosteal lamellae;* etc.).

Even the *trabeculae* (*i.e.*, beams) of postnatal spongy bone consist of lamellae.

5. Lacunae.

A *lacuna* is shaped like a melon seed; its size averages $35 \times 10 \times 6$ μ.

In prenatal, woven bone the orientation of lacunae is random.

In lamellar bone the arrangement of lacunae (and their canaliculi) is orderly.

The flat surface of a lacuna lies parallel to the lamellae.

But a lacuna may actually lie within a lamella, or largely between two lamellae.
The long axis agrees with the direction of fibers in its containing lamella.
Tiny tubes, or *canaliculi*, project from all surfaces of a lacuna; many are long.
Some bend, and all pass in a perpendicular direction through the lamellae.
Canaliculi branch and anastomose freely with those of other lacunae.
Canaliculi, next to periosteal and endosteal surfaces, open freely onto them.
Others, adjacent to Haversian or Volkmann's canals, open into those canals.

C. BONE ARCHITECTURE:

1. Periosteum.
A. RELATIONS.
This fibrous sheath envelops bone except on articular surfaces, sesamoid bones, and
insertions of tendons and ligaments.
Its union with the underlying bone varies in strength.
It is firm on short bones, at epiphyses and where some tendons insert.
The bolting-down is accomplished by *Sharpey's fibers* (see beyond).
B. STRUCTURE.
Two layers are described, but they are not sharply demarcated.
The outer layer is dense, fibrous and vascular.
It consists mostly of collagenous fibers.
The inner layer is looser, more elastic and more cellular.
It appears clearest, as a distinct zone, only when bone is developing.
At this time bone-forming cells (*osteoblasts*) are characteristic of it.
In the normal adult this layer does not contain osteoblasts, as such.
Yet, on stimulation (*e.g.*, by fracture) it becomes reactivated.
Osteoblasts then reappear and the layer again becomes plain.
Vessels and nerves, from the external layer, pass through to the bone.
C. SHARPEY'S FIBERS.
These are coarse collagenous fibers (or bundles of fibers).
They turn inward from the inner periosteum and enter the bone matrix.
Here they pass through the periosteal lamellae, like spikes.
They are sometimes called *perforating fibers*.
Their general course is perpendicular to lamellae.
By embedding in matrix, Sharpey's fibers serve to bolt periosteum to bone.
They also continue from tendons, fastening them into periosteal bone.
Sharpey's fibers also occur in some sets of interstitial lamellae.
These sets represent buried fragments of earlier periosteal lamellae.
They never occur in Haversian systems or endosteal lamellae.

2. Compact bone.
This type consists of lamellae, in orderly arrangements, and of minute canals.
Layered bone is almost exclusively the product of postnatal osteogenesis.
A. PERIOSTEAL AND ENDOSTEAL LAMELLAE.
These are series of parallel lamellae lying next to the periosteum or endosteum.
In tubular bones they have a concentric, cylindrical arrangement.
They are traversed, either vertically or at an angle, by *Volkmann's canals*.
Such canals contain blood vessels, lymphatics, nerves and osteogenic cells.
In one direction they communicate with the periosteum or marrow cavity.
In the opposite direction they connect with *Haversian canals* (see beyond).
B. HAVERSIAN CANALS.
Compact bone is really quite vascular, although microscopically so.
Haversian canals conduct blood vessels, lymphatics and nerves through bone.
They are lined with cells possessing osteoblastic potentialities.
They are abundant in compact bone, acting as the axes of Haversian systems.
Any canal surrounded by concentric lamellae is an Haversian canal.
The largest canals are 0.1 mm. in diameter; most are less than half this size.
Their general course follows the main axis of a long bone.

They branch and anastomose; in this manner they become continuous with the Volk-
mann's canals of the periosteal and endosteal lamellae.
Some cross connections between Haversian canals are Volkmann's canals.
These are canals that actually pierce the lamellae of two Haversian systems.
By definition a Volkmann's canal is one that pierces through lamellae.
c. HAVERSIAN SYSTEMS.
These are cylindrical branching tubes, present only in compact bone.
Each *Haversian system*, or *osteon*, is arranged about an Haversian canal.
Its wall is relatively thick, whereas its lumen (Haversian canal) is narrow.
An Haversian system consists of concentric tubular layers; its diameter is 300 $\mu \pm$.
Each bony layer, 3 to 7 μ thick, is known as an *Haversian lamella*.
The total number of lamellae in a system varies between 4 and 20.
Bone cells lie, in roughly concentric circles, between or within lamellae.
Those canaliculi that border an Haversian canal communicate with its cavity.
Those located at the periphery of a system almost always loop back.
Only rarely do they end blindly or join canaliculi of another system.
d. INTERSTITIAL SYSTEMS.
These sets of lamellae fill-in the spaces between Haversian systems.
They are irregular in size and in shape.
The orientation of the component lamellae varies greatly.
Some sets are parallel to the surface of the bone and curve but little.
These are surviving remnants of earlier periosteal lamellae.
Others are distinctly curved remnants of Haversian systems.
They survived destruction during a wave of bone remodeling.

3. Spongy bone.

This type is simpler and less regularly organized than compact bone.
A. ARRANGEMENT.
The total bony mass is enclosed within a variably thick layer of compact bone.
The spongy mass is composed of trabeculae, plates, tubules and globular shells.
All the interspaces are filled with vascular marrow.
B. STRUCTURE.
Prenatal bone is spongy and of the irregularly woven type.
The fundamental composition of postnatal, spongy bone is lamellar.
The pattern is variable and Haversian systems are lacking.
Some cylindrical cavities occur, bounded by concentric lamellae.
These simulate Haversian systems, as do sections cut through globular shells.
Spongy and compact bone blend in structure where they become continuous.

4. Endosteum.

This delicate layer lines the marrow cavities, covers the irregular surfaces of spongy bone
and extends, as a lining, into the canal system of compact bone.
In adult bone it consists merely of condensed connective tissue of the bone marrow.
Endosteum is analogous to the thick periosteum in its formative powers only.
During the period of bone development it contains active osteoblasts.
In the adult these cells are not identifiable as such.
Yet, like periosteum, it retains the latent capacity to form and dissolve bone.

5. Bone Marrow.

This tissue will be described in a separate topic (p. 84).

D. VESSELS AND NERVES:

In bones, in general, *arterioles* enter from the periosteum at many points.
They course within systems of the Volkmann and Haversian canals.
After supplying the bone they reach the marrow.
Some *venules* from the marrow retrace the arterial course in reverse.

These 'arterioles' and 'venules' are essentially capillary-like in actual structure.

In long bones one or more larger arteries also enter about midway of the shaft.

These *nutrient arteries* course in a prominent, oblique canal directly to the marrow.

Here they branch into proximal and distal divisions.

Nutrient veins are represented; they retrace the arterial course in reverse.

Nevertheless, most of the blood in the marrow leaves by another route.

Numerous veins find exits at the extremities of the bone.

Lymphatic vessels exist in the marrow, in the various canals and in the periosteum.

Many sensory *nerves* occur in the periosteum.

Other nerves, presumably vasomotor, accompany the arterial vessels.

E. METABOLIC PATHWAYS:

Bone is rich in small vessels, yet no capillary mesh exists within bone matrix itself.

In compact bone, vessels are restricted to its surfaces and conducting canals.

In spongy bone the vessels course mostly in the marrow spaces, between bony masses.

In bone the dense matrix does not permit adequate diffusion of nutrients, gases and wastes.

Instead, canaliculi establish communications between lacunae and neighboring canals, and between lacunae and the adjacent periosteum and marrow.

More precisely, the canaliculi open into tissue that is provided with capillaries.

Diffusion within this continuous, communicating system provides for interchanges.

Oxygen and nutrients leave the capillaries and enter the tissue fluid outside.

Diffusion carries them through the fluid-filled canaliculi to lacunae.

Here bone cells take up what is needed and pass the remainder on to other cells.

Catabolic wastes leave the cells and spread by diffusion in a reverse course.

This method of transmission and interchange is relatively slow, but adequate.

A saving factor is the modest requirements of the relatively inactive bone cells.

Moreover, the farthest bone cells are usually less than 0.1 mm. from a capillary.

About 0.2 mm. is the farthest from a capillary that a bone cell can survive.

In spongy bone completely solid trabeculae are not more than about 0.2 mm. thick.

Thicker trabeculae are supplied with canals and blood vessels.

F. REGENERATIVE ABILITY:

This topic is discussed on p. 96.

G. APPEARANCE IN SECTIONS:

1. Osseous tissue.

Adult bone is lamellated; its layered arrangement is distinctive.

The appearance in sections depends on how the component fibers are cut.

A lamella cut 'with the grain' shows longitudinal fibrillations.

A lamella cut 'across the grain' shows granular dots.

Decalcified bone usually suffers from a marked blurring of details.

This is due to swelling of osteocollagenous fibers by the reagents used.

The decalcified matrix takes an acidophilic stain, like any collagenous fibers.

Bone cells are shrunken, and canaliculi are more or less obscured.

Ground sections of dry bone present a picture of lifeless matrix.

The details of matrix structure, however, are shown at their best.

Bone cells have disappeared and their lacunae contain air.

By direct light, lacunae are bright; by transmitted light, dark.

This is because of the low refractive index of air.

Lacunae differ in shape, depending on the plane of section.

Cut parallel with lamellae, the lacunae are oval.

Cut vertical to lamellae, either a long or short oval is seen.

This depends on whether the long or short cell-axis is cut across.

Canaliculi, like lacunae, are dark by transmitted light.

They appear either as hair-lines or as dots, depending on the plane of section.

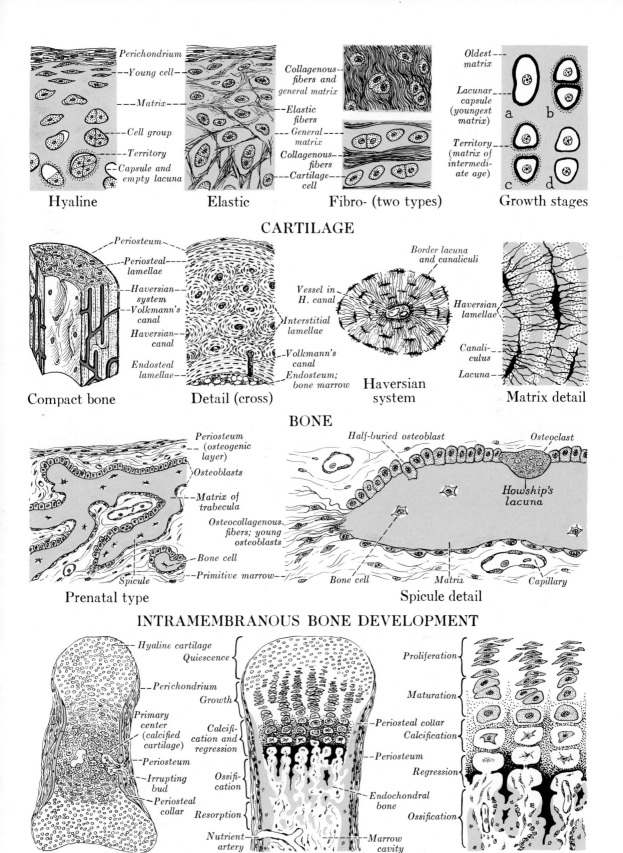

Hyaline   Elastic   Fibro- (two types)   Growth stages

Perichondrium
Young cell
Matrix
Cell group
Territory
Capsule and empty lacuna

Collagenous fibers and general matrix
Elastic fibers
General matrix
Collagenous fibers
Cartilage cell

Oldest matrix
Lacunar capsule (youngest matrix)
Territory (matrix of intermediate age)

CARTILAGE

Compact bone   Detail (cross)   Haversian system   Matrix detail

Periosteum
Periosteal lamellae
Haversian system
Volkmann's canal
Haversian canal
Endosteal lamellae

Interstitial lamellae
Volkmann's canal
Endosteum; bone marrow

Border lacuna and canaliculi
Vessel in H. canal

Haversian lamellae
Canaliculus
Lacuna

BONE

Prenatal type   Spicule detail

Periosteum (osteogenic layer)
Osteoblasts
Matrix of trabecula
Osteocollagenous fibers; young osteoblasts
Bone cell
Primitive marrow
Spicule

Half-buried osteoblast
Osteoclast
Howship's lacuna
Bone cell
Matrix
Capillary

INTRAMEMBRANOUS BONE DEVELOPMENT

Beginning stage   Later stage   Ossification detail

Hyaline cartilage
Perichondrium
Primary center (calcified cartilage)
Periosteum
Irrupting bud
Periosteal collar

Quiescence
Growth
Calcification and regression
Ossification
Resorption
Nutrient artery

Periosteal collar
Periosteum
Endochondral bone
Marrow cavity

Proliferation
Maturation
Calcification
Regression
Ossification

INTRACARTILAGINOUS BONE DEVELOPMENT

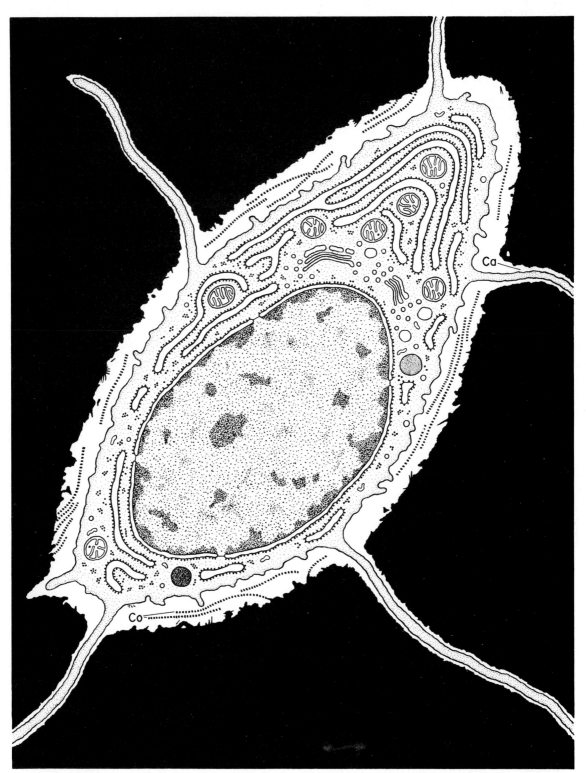

OSTEOCYTE. The dense bone matrix imprisons a bone cell. Its cytoplasm is poorer in organelles than that of active osteoblasts, yet rough endoplasmic reticulum, free ribosomes, Golgi stacks, mitochondria and lysosomes occur. In a space between osteocyte and matrix lie some collagen fibrils (Co), while cell processes extend into communicating canaliculi (Ca). The double-layered nuclear membrane is typically interrupted by 'pores' and bears ribosomes externally.

2. *Transverse section through shaft of a long bone.*

Periosteal and endosteal lamellae occur in slightly curving, parallel series.
Haversian systems form sets of concentric rings about central canals.
> Each resembles a tree-trunk, with rings and a hollow center.

Interstitial lamellae have irregular locations between Haversian systems.
Bone cells, within lacunae, occur in fairly regular rows in adult bone.
> However, they may be situated between lamellae or in them.

Sections, cut through the main shaft, show a central marrow cavity free (or nearly free) of spongy bone and filled with bone marrow.
Sections, cut near the ends, show marrow interspersed with much spongy bone.

3. *Longitudinal section through shaft of a long bone.*

Periosteal and endosteal lamellae appear much as in transverse sections.
The changed appearance of Haversian systems is striking.
> They are less conspicuous because the ringed arrangement is lost.
> Parallel lamellae, flanking an elongate canal-space, are seen.
> Branching and anastomosis between systems occur here and there.
> Canals are not seen nearly so abundantly as are the bony walls of the systems.

Cement membranes may furnish the only clue to the boundary between systems.

4. *Vertical section of a flat bone.*

Next to the free surface, above and below, is compact bone bordered by periosteum.
> This upper and lower layer may be thick (*e.g.*, tables), or extremely thin.
> Each layer consists of a series of parallel lamellae.
> Haversian systems occur, but they are not abundant.

Connecting the compact layers is a varying amount of spongy bone (*e.g.*, the diploë).
> Marrow tissue occupies the spaces of the spongy bone.

5. *Vertical section of short and irregular bones.*

Beneath the periosteum there is a varying amount of compact bone.
> Whether thin or thick, it is always lamellated.

The interior consists of spongy bone and marrow.

H. FUNCTIONAL CORRELATIONS:

Bones provide skeletal support to the body.
> Lamellar architecture is directly related to the functional stresses encountered.
> Maximum support is furnished with the least material and weight.
> Bone resists a bending force of 35,000 lbs./sq. in. before fracturing.
> In tensile strength it approximates cast iron—and at one-third the weight.

Protection is afforded to vital organs in the head, chest and pelvis.
Leverage action is effected through muscles acting upon bones.
> Movement is accomplished by the presence of joints at the ends of bones.
> Locomotion and movements of parts of the body are thus made possible.

A lodging place is provided for bone marrow.
Bone is not an inert tissue, even though it has a low metabolic rate.
> It is plastic, and remodeling can take place to accommodate changed stresses.
> This occurs after a badly set fracture, or following disuse or increased use.

Bones store most of the body calcium, but this deposit is labile (especially in young osteons).
> There is a normal, physiological turnover of the calcium salts, under hormone control (p. 175).
> > Much of the skeleton replaces its mineral salts over a period of months.
> > Also the calcium store is a reserve that can be drawn on rapidly.
> > > This occurs in meeting needs in other tissues; it may be excessive in pregnancy.

Bone cells are relatively dormant in mature bone; they are incapable of mitosis.
> Yet they are responsible for the well-being and maintenance of the matrix.
> Also they seem to aid in the physiological release of mineral salts.

Periosteum helps to anchor some tendons and ligaments.
> It conducts blood vessels and nerves to the bone.

The periosteum plays an important part in bone development.
It is also actively concerned in the repair of injuries to bone matrix.

II. THE BONE MARROW

The cylindrical cavity of bone shafts and the irregular spaces of spongy bone are filled with soft,
vascular marrow tissue; as a whole, it weighs twice as much as the liver.
The total bone marrow of the body can be regarded as an organ.
Until middle childhood all marrow is of the hemopoietic type (*i.e., red bone marrow*).
By the end of adolescence most of the red marrow has been replaced by fat cells.
This inactivated tissue is called *yellow bone marrow.*
Under stress, however, it can return to active hemopoiesis.
In the normal adult, red marrow occurs chiefly in the sternum, ribs, vertebrae and cranium.
It consists of a supporting framework, sinuses and free cells occupying the interspaces.
There is no need for the amount of red marrow that would fill a total adult skeleton.
In aged or emaciated persons the yellow bone marrow undergoes changes.
The fat cells lose their oil content and the tissue acquires a reddish tint.
Because of a jelly-like consistency the tissue is then called *gelatinous bone marrow.*
The following details on framework, vessels and cells apply to red bone marrow only.

A. FRAMEWORK:

Reticular fibers make a rather loose latticework or spongework.
Lying along these fibers are primitive and phagocytic reticular cells.
Fat cells, usually single, also are scattered about in this stroma.

B. VASCULAR RELATIONS:

Large, tortuous sinusoids occur abundantly, supported by the reticular framework.
These channels are lined by flattened, phagocytic reticulo-endothelial cells.
Another name given to these reticular cells is *fixed macrophages.*
Such cells may detach and become free in the sinusoidal blood.
The sinusoidal wall permits newly formed blood cells to slip through.
Thus gaining the lumen, they are added to the blood stream.
Nutrient marrow-arterioles reduce to capillaries which, in turn, empty into sinusoids.
Sinusoids then converge into venules which leave the marrow by several routes.
Lymphatic vessels have not been demonstrated in bone marrow.

C. FREE CELLS:

Most of the cells lying free in the meshes of the reticulum are blood cells.
Represented are all stages in the maturation of red and white elements (p. 69).

D. APPEARANCE IN SECTIONS:

In decalcified bone the topographical relation of marrow to bone is characteristic.
Spongy bone shows irregular bony plates embedded in red or yellow bone marrow.
A shaft of a long bone shows compact bone enclosing a central mass of yellow marrow.
Typical yellow bone marrow is not easily distinguished from adipose tissue.
For the most part, the crowded residue of marrow tissue is wholly inconspicuous.
In some instances, however, little clusters of marrow cells occur among the fat cells.
Red bone marrow is notable for its cellularity and (usually) scattered fat cells.
Megakaryocytes and stages in the maturation of blood cells are uniquely diagnostic.
Among the stages seen, basophilic myelocytes are usually notably absent.
This is because their granules dissolve in aqueous fixatives.

E. FUNCTIONAL CORRELATIONS:

Yellow marrow in the adult is a dormant tissue hemopoietically.

The potentiality of returning to the functional state, however, is not lost.
Red marrow is the chief hemopoietic center of the adult, releasing cells to the circulation.
It is the normal site where red corpuscles and granular leucocytes differentiate.
Also aged or damaged corpuscles are phagocytosed and destroyed.
Macrophages function like those elsewhere in the reticulo-endothelial system (p. 47).
The marrow participates in immunologic functions.

III. THE JOINTS

Bones are connected by *articulations;* this region of union is also called a *joint.*
By means of these connections the individual bones co-operate in forming a skeleton.

A. SYNARTHROSES:

In general, these are immovable joints.
Some that are slightly movable are named *amphiarthroses.*

1. Syndesmosis.

The union between bones is by dense fibrous tissue (collagenous or elastic).
Example: the sutures of the skull are collagenous tissue; the ligamenta flava, uniting
vertebral arches, are dense elastic tissue.
In a cranial *suture* the fibers are largely continuous with periosteal fibers.

2. Synchondrosis.

The connection is by cartilage (hyaline or fibrocartilage).
Example: union of growing epiphysis and diaphysis (hyaline); pubic symphysis (fibrocartilage); intervertebral disk (mostly fibro-, but some hyaline).

3. Synostosis.

Originally separate bones begin to be united by osseous tissue at 30 years.
These bones were earlier joined by cartilage or by fibrous tissue.
Example: union of mature epiphysis and diaphysis; aging sutures of the skull.
The zone of union of an epiphysis and diaphysis is sometimes called the *metaphysis.*

B. DIARTHROSES:

These are freely movable joints, with a *joint cavity* interposed between the two parts.
Articular cartilages cover the ends of the bones; they are bare disks, 0.5 to 6.0 mm. thick.
They are usually hyaline cartilage, spared from the general ossification.
Superficial cells are flat; deeper cells tend to be arranged in vertical columns.
The deepest layer, adjoining bone, is calcified and fixed firmly to the bone.
The *joint capsule* envelops the articulation, like a collar.
Its outer layer, continuous with the periosteum, is densely fibrous.
The inner layer, the *synovial membrane,* lines the joint cavity (except for cartilages).
This is a looser vascular layer, surfaced discontinuously with fibroblasts.
The surface layer is sometimes called a 'false epithelium' (p. 34).
The membrane may be thrown into folds or processes (*synovial villi*).
Glairy, lubricating *synovial fluid* originates from the membrane.
It arises largely as a dialysate of the blood plasma and lymph.
Chemically it is a muco-polysaccharide and protein complex.
An *articular disk, articular meniscus* or a ligament may project into the joint cavity.
It lies within an intruding, wedge-shaped portion of the synovial membrane.
The disks are mostly fibrous, but may convert into fibrocartilage.
Synovial membrane is lacking in regions of the disk where rubbing occurs.
Blood vessels and lymphatics supply the capsule, and especially the synovial membrane.
Nerves and nerve endings occur chiefly in the outer, fibrous layer of the capsule.

C. Regenerative Ability:

The capsule, capsular ligaments and synovial membrane repair injuries perfectly.

Injuries to articular cartilages remain unhealed, except when near synovial membranes.

A removed meniscus may be replaced by growth inward from the fibrous capsule.

D. Functional Correlations:

Articulations connect the individual bones into a functional skeletal system.

A wide range of movement is made possible, depending on local requirements.

Nevertheless, movement is not an essential characteristic of joints in general.

Some joints are as immobile as the bones they connect.

Synchondroses provide an opportunity for long bones to grow in length near their ends.

In doing this, the epiphyseal growth zone is unhampered by pressure and contact.

Flat and irregular bones expand by growth in connective tissue at articular margins.

Chapter X

The Development and Growth of Bones

A. SOME UNIQUE QUALITIES OF BONE:

As bone evolved, several new features appeared, not found in cartilage.
Nature had experimented with stiffening cartilage by calcifying its matrix.
>This tissue was not a success because it could not metabolize properly.
>The very deposit of lime salts presented a barrier to diffusive interchanges.
Bone solved the problem of rigid support and introduced four distinctive features.

1. A canalicular system.

Tiny tubules within the matrix provide a means for carrying out metabolism.
At the boundaries of bone, the tubules open into tissue spaces.
>In this way the tissue fluid in these spaces becomes continuous with fluid within the entire canalicular system and makes possible diffusive interchanges.

2. Internal vascularity.

The canalicular system can operate effectively only through very short distances.
>Bone cells cannot survive when farther than 0.2 mm. from a capillary.
Hence bone acquired a vascular supply within its matrix.
>These internal vessels are carried in special canals (Haversian and Volkmann).
The co-operative action stated in (1) and (2) permits bone to live indefinitely.

3. A new type of appositional growth.

Interstitial growth, as in cartilage, became impossible for bone.
>This is because the amorphous ground substance becomes stiff with lime.
>>The lime deposits promptly after the formation of ground substance.
Growth in thickness follows the general appositional plan used by cartilage.
>This is by the addition of matrix directly beneath a fibrous periosteum.
By contrast, a new type of appositional growth was perfected to care for elongation.
>The new method employs a special plate of cartilage, the *epiphyseal disk*.
>>This disk grows progressively near its outer surface.
>>Its inner surface is correspondingly destroyed and replaced by bone.

4. Reconstruction.

Fetal (mostly spongy) bone is destroyed locally and reformed, again and again.
After birth, newly formed matrix is deposited in layers (*lamellae*).
>This bone is also eroded and reconstructed repeatedly.
>During the reconstructions Haversian systems are fashioned in some bones.
>Finally parallel systems of lamellae (periosteal; endosteal) are laid down.

B. OSSIFICATION FUNDAMENTALS:

The histogenesis of bone, or *osteogenesis*, is the same wherever it occurs.
>Two types (*intramembranous* and *intracartilaginous*) are traditionally described.

These merely refer to particular environments in which bone happens to develop.
For this reason some generalities concerning the process of ossification can be presented at the outset as fundamental concepts.
Afterward, certain special problems confronting developing bones can be considered.
These pertain to development in membrane and cartilage, and to continuing growth.

1. *Distinctive specialized cells.*

Two cell types, distinctive for osseous tissue, make their appearance.

A. OSTEOBLASTS.

These specialized bone-formers presumably differentiate from mesenchyme.
Such recruitment continues, since mature osteoblasts do not divide.
Osteoblasts are medium-sized cells, each with an eccentric nucleus.
They come to lie on the surface of growing bone, forming an 'epithelioid' layer.
When functionally active, this sheet resembles a simple cuboidal epithelium.
There is, however, a wide range in cell shape at different locations.
Apparently the flatter, paler cells are inactive (and depleted?) elements.
Osteoblasts have delicate processes; many touch those of adjacent cells.
The cytoplasm facing the site of bone deposit contains most of the organelles.
There is much endoplasmic reticulum, rich in ribosomes.
The RNA is responsible for the cytoplasm staining deeply basophilic.
There are specific granules that stain with PAS, as does organic matrix of bone.
Both kinds of granules are causally related to the deposition of *osteoid*.
This tissue is ground substance embedding collagenous fibers.
These fibers of bone are named *osteocollagenous fibers*.
The cytoplasm contains much *alkaline phosphatase* during bone deposition.
As bone deposition proceeds, many osteoblasts become imprisoned in the matrix.
These become bone cells (*osteocytes*), located within individual lacunae.
The retention of cytoplasmic processes during cell-entombment accounts for the establishment of interconnecting canaliculi in bone matrix.
After an osteoblast becomes a bone cell, its matrix-forming activities cease.
Except, apparently, for the deposition of a *lacunar capsule* about it.

B. OSTEOCLASTS.

These elements are also known as the *giant cells of bone development.*
They are large multinucleate cells, with pale to acidophilic, foamy cytoplasm.
The cell may measure up to 100 μ; nuclei number from several to dozens.
Osteoclasts are commonly seen in regions where bone is being resorbed.
In regions of calcified cartilage they are often called *chondroclasts*.
They sometimes occupy shallow pits in bone known as *Howship's lacunae*.
The cytoplasm may form a fringe next to the bone matrix.
The osteoclast ('bone breaker') was so named because it was supposed to be directly responsible for the dissolution of bone matrix.
Except for their common presence in resorbing regions, convincing evidence fails.
Some doubts can be cast on any active role in the resorptive process.
Osteoclasts are not mechanically erosive or helpfully phagocytic.
At best, phagocytosis cannot explain how debris is produced.
Evidence is lacking for enzyme production (organic matrix digestion) or for creating an acid environment (bone mineral dissolution).
Bone resorption sometimes proceeds in their complete absence.
The origin of the osteoclast is multiple, and may vary with circumstances.
It is the product of cell fusions, not of repeated nuclear division.
Mesenchymal cells of the marrow stroma produce some osteoclasts.
Inactive osteoblasts also merge to form such giant cells.
Bone cells, becoming free by bone dissolution, are added as well.
Thus the osteoclast may result from bone resorption, rather than causing it.

2. Tissue participants.

A. PRIMITIVE MARROW.

In a region where a so-called membrane bone will develop there is mesenchyme.

This tissue provides both osteoblasts and vessels for development.

Presently, as *primitive marrow,* it becomes active in the formation of spongy bone.

At a site for a 'cartilage bone,' local mesenchyme first forms a cartilage model.

The perichondrium then sends one or more buds of vascularized tissue into the cartilaginous model of a future bone.

(Such perichondrium is called *periosteum* as soon as it overlies bone.)

Cartilage melts away before this advancing *irruptive tissue.*

This tissue differentiates into *primitive marrow*, including osteoblasts.

It at once engages in the formation of spongy bone in the newly excavated cavities of the cartilage.

B. PERIOSTEUM.

The inner layer of the periosteum of every developing bone becomes osteogenic.

This general activity supplements the earlier furnishing of local irruptive buds at the start of cartilage-bone development.

On its internal surface a sheet of osteoblasts arises and deposits bone there.

Fetal *periosteal bone* is spongy; postnatally it is deposited in compact layers.

C. ENDOSTEUM.

The peripheral layer of marrow tissue is also osteogenic (*i.e.,* bone-producing).

It contributes bone; notable are the late, definitive, *endosteal lamellae.*

But an endosteal surface is also a site of earlier bone resorption.

By it, spongy bone is removed and the marrow cavity of a long bone enlarged.

D. CARTILAGE.

Cartilage is well adapted to serve as a provisional model for future bones.

It is sufficiently rigid to act as a temporary fetal skeleton.

Unlike bone, it develops rapidly and can keep up with the growth of the fetus.

Cartilage also provides the unique *epiphyseal disks* in many bones.

Such plates occur in long bones, and in some flat and irregular bones.

At these disks continued cartilage proliferation, followed by destruction and bone deposition, accomplishes growth in length.

3. Osteogenesis.

A. SPICULAR BONE.

Early bone, almost everywhere, makes its appearance in the form of *spicules.*

These 'little spikes' arise at multiple points.

Osteoblasts, differentiating at local sites, make a start on matrix formation.

At first, the matrix is essentially like that of ordinary connective tissue.

Here *osteocollagenous fibers* intermingle with amorphous *ground substance.*

Both materials are products of protein synthesis on the part of osteoblasts.

Such provisional matrix is soft; it is sometimes called *osteoid tissue.*

Directly following, there is a deposition of lime salts in the osteoid mass.

This stiffening substance completes the definitive *matrix.*

The mechanism of the deposit of calcareous crystals is not well understood.

The process, however, is wholly separate from syntheses by osteoblasts.

These crystals first appear as little islands deposited in the osteoid substance.

They occur earliest on the surface of fibrils, and later within them.

Their alignment is orderly, and in relation to collagen banding.

As a spicule becomes of appreciable size, osteoblasts clothe it on all sides.

Spicules become thicker by the continued formation of new matrix.

This occurs beneath the snugly fitting epithelioid layer of osteoblasts.

Laggard osteoblasts are trapped and imprisoned as bone cells.

Osteoblastic replacements come from differentiating mesenchymal cells.

The deposition of matrix fails wherever bone cells occur.
This failure leaves a space (*lacuna*) about each cell body.
Similarly, a tubular *canaliculus* surrounds each cell process.
Spicules increase in length by adding matrix at the growing tip.
Here osteoblasts and differentiating fibers often fan out like a brush.

B. SPONGY BONE.
Elongation and branching lead to unions between previously separate spicules.
In this way, *spongy bone* arises and takes form.
Continued deposition makes the *trabeculae* (beams) of the bony spongework thicker and the whole system increasingly compact.
Such early bone is not laid down in layers, but is of the woven type.
That is, its fibers run in random, interlacing directions.

C. LAMELLAR BONE.
After birth the woven, spongy bone of the fetal skeleton is replaced.
Previously this matrix had undergone repeated erosions and replacements.
By contrast, the definitive type of bone is lamellated (*lamellar bone*).
This is true both of compact and of spongy bone.
Only to a slight extent does lamellar bone begin to appear before birth.

C. INTRAMEMBRANOUS DEVELOPMENT OF BONE:

The details of osteogenesis will not be described again in the remaining topics.
Instead, only the development of bone into an organ (organogenesis) will be discussed.
Still to be considered are two specific problems confronting a developing bone.
One is the way osteogenesis adapts to the particular environment encountered; that is, within a membranous or cartilaginous forerunner of the future bone.
The other is the development of an architectural form, adapted to local needs.
This involves remodeling to meet both mechanical and metabolic requirements.
The present account will deal only with the general organogenesis of membrane bones.
In later topics the remodeling in response to functional demands will be described.
The products of intramembranous ossification are often called *membrane bones*.
The name merely implies that the bone arose in mature mesenchyme.
Such tissue constitutes a cellular and fibrillar plate or 'membrane.'

1. Occurrence of membrane bones.
A. PURE MEMBRANE BONES.
Flat bones of cranial vault; irregular bones of the face.
B. MIXED MEMBRANE AND CARTILAGE BONES.
Occipital; temporal; sphenoid.
(In addition, it should be emphasized that every cartilage bone ends its development by becoming largely membrane bone, through secondary periosteal replacements.)

2. Early development.
The site of a future bone is a plate of primitive connective tissue (old mesenchyme).
Each bone starts its development at one or more points (*ossification centers*).
The earliest centers begin to appear in the eighth week of fetal life.
A center becomes richly vascularized and actively proliferative.
Spicules of bone arise in a center and soon expand in a radiating manner.
Continued spreading produces a wheel-like pattern, within the membranous model.
Branching and anastomosis soon make this a spongy meshwork of trabeculae.
Thickness is subordinated to rapid, centrifugal (*i.e.*, spreading) growth.
Hence the preponderant growth parallels the flat surfaces of the membrane.
By birth the cranial bones have met along most of their margins.
They are surrounded by connective tissue which organized early as a *periosteum*.
On its inner surface, osteoblasts have helped to thicken the total bony mass.
Thickening of trabeculae has reduced greatly the earlier interspaces.
These contain vessels and marrow, but the bone is a fairly compact plate.

3. *Later development.*

For some time after birth the cranial bones are simple, bony plates—wholly spongy.

Gradually the periosteum begins to lay down parallel lamellae.

Thus in childhood are produced the characteristic *tables* made of compact bone.

Thinning of the thick, central trabeculae produces the widely spaced *diploë.*

As the brain enlarges, the calvarium has to make additional room for it.

Also the calvarium acquires a progressively more gentle curvature.

During these readjustments appositional growth is largely on one surface of each table, whereas resorption occurs mostly on the other surface.

During the period of continued growth and reconstruction some *Haversian systems* are created in the compact bone of the tables.

Their manner of formation, in general, will be described on p. 94.

The method of marginal growth of a membrane bone is disputed.

Some think that new matrix is formed progressively in the region of the suture.

Others hold that expansion occurs by periosteal deposits of increasing area.

With this goes a resorption of the earlier bone at a deeper level.

D. Intracartilaginous Development of Bone:

Most of the bones of the skeleton are preceded by cartilaginous models.

Thus there is an intermediate stage not encountered in developing membrane bones.

This cartilage is, however, a provisional tissue that is eroded and replaced by bone.

It is this feature that gives additional complexity to the history of these bones.

During the replacement of cartilage, ossification occurs within the eroded regions.

This fact explains why the terms *intracartilaginous* or *endochondral* are used.

Yet, as the bone continues to grow and becomes reconstructed, the final osseous tissue in a mature bone is almost wholly a direct deposition by periosteum.

The simplest events characterize short bones, since these have no epiphyses.

The most complex history is found among the irregular bones.

These may have multiple centers of ossification, both primary and secondary.

A typical long bone of the forearm or leg shows all the essential features simplest.

There is one primary center for the shaft (*diaphysis*) of a long bone, and one secondary center for each end (*epiphysis*).

Hence this type of bone will serve as a basis for the descriptions in subtopics 1-6.

Primary ossification centers appear early in some cartilages of the primitive skeleton.

The earliest organize in the second fetal month.

The latest primary centers (wrist; ankle) do not arise until childhood.

A few *secondary (epiphyseal) centers* are present in cartilages before birth.

The great majority, however, do not appear until childhood or adolescence.

1. *Early history of cartilaginous model.*

The site of a future bone is indicated by a condensed mass of mesenchyme.

This differentiates into precartilage and then into typical hyaline cartilage.

At the periphery is a fibrous sheath, the *perichondrium.*

Such a cartilage serves as a provisional model for the bone.

Increase in length comes from interstitial growth, chiefly near the ends.

Increased thickness is partly interstitial, but mostly appositional (perichondral).

A. Primary Center.

The site of the first ossification center is indicated by changes in cartilage cells.

These are located internally, midway of the shaft of a long bone.

Hence this center is also called the *diaphyseal center.*

These cells enlarge and the intervening matrix is correspondingly thinned.

Such large, mature cells are able to secrete alkaline phosphatase.

At the same time, lime salts are deposited in the adjacent cartilage matrix.

This *calcified cartilage* stains intensely with basic dyes.

The enlarged cartilage cells soon die because they have walled themselves off from nutrients diffusing through the matrix.

When they die the calcified matrix becomes unstable and begins to dissolve.

This leaves irregular cavities within the matrix.

Intermingled with the cavities are undissolved calcified spicules and disintegrating cartilage cells.

B. PERIOSTEAL COLLAR.

Meanwhile the inner, cellular layer of the perichondrium is becoming active.

Some cells differentiate into osteoblasts and produce an *osteogenic layer*.

A thin, cylindrical *collar* of spongy bone is deposited about the cartilage.

This early collar encloses approximately the middle third of the cartilage model.

Henceforth the overlying, former perichondrium must be called *periosteum*.

The bone, forming in a typically intramembranous manner, is *periosteal bone*.

It acts as a splint to compensate for strength lost by cartilage dissolution.

C. IRRUPTIVE PERIOSTEAL BUDS.

Vascular connective tissue from the periosteum pushes through one or more gaps in the bony collar; each is known as an *irruptive periosteal bud*.

It soon encounters the altered cartilage about the primary center.

As a bud advances, the thinned partitions between cartilage cells dissolve.

The cartilage cells perish by the time their distended lacunae open up.

Arriving at the center, the tissues of the bud proliferate rapidly.

This tissue-mass progressively occupies the spaces made available by the destruction of cartilage cells and matrix.

Some of the mesenchymal cells differentiate into osteoblasts.

This vascular, invading tissue is now called *primary marrow*.

D. EARLY ENDOCHONDRAL BONE.

Osteoblasts gather on the undestroyed remnants of the calcified cartilage, using these as a scaffolding on which to work.

They straightway proceed to encrust them with bone.

Since the surviving calcified cartilage was in the form of an irregular meshwork, the encrusting bone is spongy as well.

Its trabeculae are characterized by having cores of calcified cartilage.

The osseous mass, thus established, is the *primary ossification center*.

Located midway of the shaft, it is also known as the *diaphyseal center*.

2. *Growth in length.*

A. ADVANCE OF OSSIFICATION FROM PRIMARY CENTER.

As endochondral ossification spreads toward the ends of the cartilage, the events are similar to those in establishing the primary center.

But the stages are more clearly segregated in a series of transverse zones.

Of course, each zone changes character as ossification advances on it.

That is, the same cells forming zones 1, 2, 3 (as listed below) soon comprise 2, 3, 4 and still later 3, 4, 5, etc.

Passing from the ends of a cartilage toward the primary center, a series of gradual stages can be recognized that illustrates the sequence of events.

1. *Quiescent (or Reserve) Zone.*

Nearest the ends is primitive hyaline cartilage, showing slight, slow growth.

At first this zone is relatively extensive, but it shortens progressively as steadily advancing ossification encroaches on it.

2. *Proliferative Zone.*

Next centralward in the cartilage is an active, mitotic zone.

A cell divides and the daughter cells repeat, forming conspicuous columns.

These rows are arranged parallel with the long axis of the cartilage.

A row grows chiefly by adding cells near the quiescent zone.

The cells of a row are crowded, flattened and separated by little matrix.

There is, necessarily, much more matrix between adjacent total rows.

Such columns of young cells, oriented in the long axis of the cartilage, tend to add length rather than breadth to the cartilage-mass.

3. *Maturation Zone.*
> Here mitoses cease, but the cells and lacunae enlarge to a 'cuboidal' shape.
>> This increases still further the length of cell rows and their matrix.
>> All such growth is interstitial, expanding growth.
> The maturing cells produce increasing amounts of phosphatase and glycogen.

4. *Calcification Zone.*
> Deeply basophilic, calcified matrix features this relatively narrow zone.
> The cells of this level have reached the peak in their life cycle.

5. *Regressive Zone.*
> Here the cartilage cells are dying or undergoing actual dissolution.
> The matrix between successive cells is dissolving, thus opening up lacunae.
>> These spaces add to tubular channels already produced in the matrix.
> The thicker plates of cartilage between cell rows (*i.e.,* the walls of the tubular channels) are not eroded significantly.
>> Their calcified matrix offsets weakenings in eroded cell columns near by.
> Vascular primary marrow is extending into the newly opened spaces.
> Osteoblasts differentiate from mesenchymal cells of the marrow tissue.

6. *Ossification Zone.*
> Osteoblasts gather on the exposed plates of calcified cartilage.
>> They promptly clothe them with an encrustation of bone.
> This addition extends significantly the spongy bone already present.

7. *Osseous Zone.*
> At first a zone of endochrondral bone extends from the region undergoing ossification all the way to the primary center.
> It might seem that this zone would continuously increase in length.
>> Actually this is not the case, as the next stage will explain.

8. *Resorptive Zone.*
> The advance of ossification toward the ends of the cartilages is offset by a compensatory resorption of bone nearer the midpoint of the diaphysis.
> Resorption is chiefly at the oldest (or central) ends of the bony mass.
>> This keeps the internal masses of spongy bone nearly constant in length.
> It also progressively lengthens the marrow cavity.

B. DEFINITIVE MARROW CAVITY.
> The clearing away of endochondral bone leaves an increasingly large 'cavity.'
>> Actually this common central space fills with differentiating tissue.
>> This tissue is the *secondary marrow* (or definitive red marrow).
> The progressive removal of bone is matched with periosteal activity.
>> The bony, periosteal collar not only thickens but also extends at each end.
>> These new deposits compensate for the loss of endochondral bone.
> Henceforth, at any level that has lost its endochondral bone, the periosteal collar must provide all the required strength and support.

C. OSSIFICATION IN SECONDARY CENTERS.
> After birth, *secondary ossification centers* arise in the cartilage remaining at the ends.
>> A center organizes within the cartilage at each end of a typical long bone.
>> These two secondary centers are also called *epiphyseal centers.*
>>> They will produce the permanent bony *epiphyses.*
> The sequence of changes follows that already described for the shaft.
>> But the proliferating cartilage cells form irregular clusters, not rows.
> Buds of vascular osteogenic tissue irrupt from the perichondrium (and marrow?).
>> They reach the center of an organizing epiphysis, and here osteoblasts lay down bone on the exposed remnants of calcified cartilage.
>> Ossification then spreads peripherally in all directions.
> Not all the cartilage is replaced by spongy bone, and this is important.
>> About the free end enough is spared to constitute the *articular cartilage.*
>> Also a plate is left between the epiphyseal and diaphyseal bone.
>>> This transverse plate is known as the *epiphyseal disk.*
>>> It is a temporary synchondrosis; *metaphysis* is a name given this region.

D. GROWTH FROM EPIPHYSEAL DISKS.

All late elongation of a long bone emanates from the two epiphyseal disks.

Except at the start, when the epiphysis is still establishing itself, bone is not added from the distal (epiphyseal) surface of the disk.

Active growth does continue at the proximal surface, facing the diaphysis.

Hence the disk proliferates cartilage steadily near its distal surface, and its older cartilage is replaced by bone deposited at its proximal surface.

The formation of axial rows of cells, the calcification of cartilage and the deposit of bone on these calcified plates continues, as earlier in the shaft.

Cartilage growth and bony replacement just balance each other in the disk.

As a result, the thickness of the epiphyseal disk remains constant.

When final growth is attained, proliferation in the disk ends.

Its cartilage is then wholly replaced by bone.

Diaphysis and epiphysis finally unite by a bony union; it is a *synostosis*.

This plane is marked permanently by the so-called *epiphyseal line*.

Henceforth, any further elongation is impossible.

The lengthening of long bones at the disks is wholly practical.

It permits elongation, without interference with functioning joints just distal.

3. *Growth in thickness, or diameter.*

Long bones increase in diameter by the deposition of new periosteal bone.

This is *appositional growth*, carried out by membranous osteogenic tissue.

The periosteum retreats outward, like the bark of a growing tree.

If this process continued indefinitely, bones would be too thick-walled and heavy.

Also the marrow cavity would be no wider than in a young fetus.

This result is avoided by new bone being added progressively outside while a somewhat less amount is being resorbed from the oldest bone (facing the marrow) on the inside.

In this way the bony wall thickens, but in a controlled manner.

An accompanying benefit is an increase in the diameter of the marrow cavity.

A cylindrical *marrow cavity* first arose as the endochondral bone was removed.

The definitive marrow cavity is much more voluminous.

It contains extensive additions gained from the erosion of periosteal bone.

Toward the epiphyses spongy bone is retained as a permanent feature.

The marrow cavity, as such, does not extend into these regions.

4. *Gross remodeling.*

Bone is a plastic tissue that can adapt its external shape and internal architecture so as to meet new requirements advantageously.

Changed stresses result from accidents, disease, use and disuse.

They also may derive from planned, clinical intervention.

Even in fetal life, bones modify the shape of earlier roughly modeled stages.

Also it is plain that, as a long bone lengthens, its thick ends recently lay at levels where now there is a slender shaft.

These problems are solved by extensive remodeling programs.

But remodeling is not accomplished as a sculptor might push and reshape clay.

It can result only from resorptions in some regions and depositions elsewhere.

5. *Formation of Haversian systems.*

Important in postnatal osteogenesis is the production of *Haversian systems*.

These serve to distribute vessels advantageously throughout compact bone.

Haversian systems always course lengthwise in the shaft of a long bone.

They have several different sources of origin.

Some earlier ones form in the longitudinal tunnels produced from the peripheral regions of the advancing epiphyseal disks.

These are called *primitive Haversian systems*.

Others are made possible by the filling-in of cylindrical canals that are secondarily dissolved out of the compact bone of the shaft.

Still others are preceded by longitudinal grooves just beneath the periosteum.

Such grooves are closed-over and buried by later-formed bone.

The tunnels, arising in this way, are then converted into Haversian systems.

Regardless of the source of their tunnel, all Haversian systems develop alike.

At the outset, the tunnel that precedes any future system is lined with osteoblasts.

It also contains at least one blood vessel. A new system can form in a few weeks.

First, a cement membrane is laid down at the periphery of the tunnel.

Next, successive layers of bone are deposited, beginning at the tunnel's periphery.

This is the only direction possible — from the outside toward the center.

Finally the spacious tunnel is reduced to a slender canal about the vessel.

6. Other internal reorganization.

Gross changes, necessitated by growth and new requirements, lead to compensatory internal reorganization of the bone substance.

These alterations are brought about by bone destruction and new deposition.

The alterations are carried out in an experimental, indecisive manner.

Alternate waves of construction and destruction repeat in the same region.

In this way over-deposits and over-resorptions are gradually corrected.

A fundamental reorganization accompanies the maturing of a bone.

Until the end of fetal life nearly all osseous tissue is spongy and nonlamellar.

Thereafter, periosteal bone is laid down in compact, distinct layers *(lamellae)*.

As a bone thickens, periosteal blood vessels are left behind in radial canals (Volkmann's) that interconnect Haversian systems and also traverse periosteal lamellae.

In a similar manner collagenous fibers *(Sharpey's)* of the periosteum become buried by the continuing deposit of bone matrix.

Processes of construction and destruction alternate as long as bones grow.

These occur spasmodically in local regions, and not in general synchrony.

Former Haversian systems are destroyed and rebuilt repeatedly.

In doing this, parts may escape destruction and become *interstitial lamellae*.

As such they are odd-shaped masses filling-in between new systems.

Other interstitial series represent fragments of former periosteal lamellae.

As bone growth nears completion, definitive *periosteal* and *endosteal lamellae* are laid down that persist, undisturbed, as complete concentric layers.

The periosteum is predominantly concerned with deposition and the endosteum with resorption, but these roles can be reversed.

This happens notably where the shaft swells into the end of a bone.

As the bone elongates further, this region has to reduce to a slender shaft.

The internal rebuilding of bone continues, at a slower rate, throughout life (p. 83).

As a result, the internal pattern becomes more and more complex.

It is a mosaic made of a steadily increasing number of bony pieces.

The deposit of lamellar bone adds a thickness of about one micron per day.

7. Short and irregular bones.

The foregoing descriptions were based on conditions in a typical long bone.

Only a few comments need to be added about other types of cartilage bones.

A. SHORT BONES.

From a center of ossification, spongy-bone formation spreads in all directions.

At the periphery a thin layer of cartilage is spared.

This serves as a proliferative zone, beneath which ossification takes place.

It results in the bone expanding progressively in all directions.

When this phase of internal growth is completed, the external shell of proliferative cartilage is replaced by bone.

The fibrous envelope, now periosteum, first deposits additional spongy bone.

This layer varies in thickness in different short bones.

Later its spongy structure becomes compact.

B. IRREGULAR BONES.

The variety of shapes and component parts can be suggested by two examples.

A *vertebra*, modeled in cartilage, exhibits several centers.

The body develops much like a short bone from a single center.
But there are also an epiphyseal center and disk at each end.
Each vertebral arch has a center from which bone grows out.
This growth also spreads into its several protuberant 'processes.'
In addition, there are three secondary centers with disks.
The *scapula* is mostly a flat bone that develops from two centers.
But, in addition, there are seven secondary centers.

E. REGENERATIVE ABILITY:

Osseous tissue (bone cells and matrix) is not able to repair losses directly.
It cannot, of itself, heal local injuries or gross fractures.
But from associated tissues the repair can be accomplished.
At the time of a *fracture* there is hemorrhage from torn vessels, and clotting.
Proliferating fibroblasts and budding capillaries invade the clot.
The clot becomes organized by this *granulation tissue.*
The resulting *procallus* consolidates, and cartilage develops within it.
This product is the *temporary callus;* it unites the fractured bones strongly.
Cartilage invasion is accompanied by calcification and erosion.
The process repeats the steps seen in fetal endochondral ossification.
Osteoblasts appear in the deep layer of the periosteum and also in the endosteum.
Spongy bone is laid down which progressively replaces the callus.
Bony union is restored, after which the *bony callus* becomes compact.
Internal reorganization then takes place and bony excesses are resorbed.
Bone *grafts* are commonly used to bridge gross defects or for plastic reconstructions.
This bone does not persist, and its periosteum is only a minor contributor to repair.
Osteogenic tissue of the host is the significant reparative agency.
New bone spreads over the dead ends of the host bone and over the transplant.
Eventually both the dead ends and the transplant are replaced by new bone.
Hence the transplant serves merely as a temporary bridge and pathway.

F. CONTROLLING FACTORS:

The genetic constitution is a basic factor in osteogenesis and morphogenesis.
Genes control the occurrence of osteogenesis and the presence or absence of cartilage.
They also determine the normal timing and order in which ossification centers appear.
They likewise superintend the fusion of epiphyses and the cessation of growth.
Functional use, however, adds final refinements to the architecture of bone.
Vitamins play important roles in conditioning normal ossification.
D-deficiency is accompanied by faulty absorption of calcium from foods.
This leads to *rickets*, in which the cartilage cells hypertrophy and persist.
It causes the epiphyseal disks to become thick and irregular.
Also neither the cartilage matrix nor the osteoid tissue calcifies to any degree.
C-deficiency leads to the condition known as *scurvy.*
This is marked by an impaired production or maintenance of collagenous fibers.
Calcification is also affected because of reduced phosphatase production.
A-deficiency interferes chiefly with the remodeling of growing bones.
They become thick through lack of compensatory resorption.
Hormones are participants in the growth and maintenance of bone.
The hypophyseal growth-promoting hormone is essential to normal bone growth.
But this is only one phase of its general influence on body growth.
Oversecretion and undersecretion lead to *gigantism* and *dwarfism*, respectively.
Thyroid hormone has a nonspecific influence on the growth of bone.
The effect is probably due to its controlling role on the general metabolic rate.
In precocious sexual development, either sex hormone accelerates skeletal maturation.
This closes epiphyses prematurely and results in stunted growth.
The gonadal hormone of each sex has important relations to the growth rate.
The appearance of centers, rate of maturation and closing of epiphyses are correlated
with the normal or abnormal developmental rate of the gonads.

Parathyroid and thyroid (calcitonin) hormones regulate the life-long resorption of bone, mostly from incompletely ossified young osteons (p. 95).

This resorption releases calcium to the blood, whose calcium-level normally remains constant through a balance maintained between release and deposit.

Excess hormone production is accompanied by pathological osseous resorption.

Parathyroid activity is controlled by another hormone, *calcitonin* (p. 173).

G. APPEARANCE IN SECTIONS:

A developing bone is characterized by spongy bone, bone marrow and periosteum.

The cut surfaces of spongy bone appear as branching trabeculae.

In active regions osteoblasts occur in rows along trabeculae.

The marrow tissue is variable in appearance, depending on its age.

It may be primitive and simply organized, or congested and specialized as red marrow.

At the periphery of the bony mass the periosteum occurs as a condensed, fibrous zone.

Compact bone, layered bone and Haversian systems are late (postnatal) features.

A membrane bone is notable for its lack of cartilage.

A cartilage bone is distinguished by cartilage and stages in its replacement.

Cartilage cells are multiplying, enlarging and disintegrating.

Cartilage matrix, in the vicinity of enlarged cells, is calcifying.

This is made evident by increased basophilic staining there.

Cartilage erosion, leaving spike-like remnants, is a feature.

Bone deposition in this region is upon such calcified remnants.

Secondary (epiphyseal) centers are late (mostly postnatal) features.

Chapter XI

The Muscular Tissues

Muscle comprises the 'flesh' of the body, and much of the walls of hollow organs.
It is a tissue through which movements of the body and its parts are made possible.
    To this end, cells have specialized in the protoplasmic property of contractility.
    These cells also are rather efficient in the protoplasmic property of conductivity.
Muscle cells are elongate elements, and contraction operates in this long axis.
    Thread-like shape and functional polarity make contraction maximally effective.
The unit of muscle tissue is a cell that is usually called a *muscle fiber*.
    This usage (*i.e.*, an entire cell is a 'fiber') is unique for muscle.
    By contrast, a connective-tissue fiber is noncellular; a nerve fiber is a cell process.
The protoplasm of a muscle cell is given a special name, *sarcoplasm*.
    This term is applied especially to the unspecialized (*i.e.*, nonfibrillar) cytoplasm.
The contractile elements are the minute thread-like *myofilaments* within the fiber.
    These, grouped as *myofibrils*, are cytoplasmic specializations, distinctive of muscle.
Muscle is classified on both a functional and a structural basis.
    Functionally it is either *involuntary* or *voluntary*.
        The distinction depends on whether or not its action is controlled by the will.
    Structurally it is either *striated* (cross-striped) or *smooth* (unstriped).
        The distinction rests upon the presence or absence of serial banding of the fiber.
    The two classifications can be combined, as follows:
        1. Smooth involuntary muscle; this is *smooth muscle*, mostly present in hollow organs.
        2. Striated involuntary muscle; this is *cardiac muscle* of the heart wall.
        3. Striated voluntary muscle; this is *skeletal muscle*, attached to the various bones.
Muscular tissue enters into the composition of many organs as building material.
    But a skeletal muscle, considered as a structural and functional unit, is an organ.

I. SMOOTH MUSCLE

This type is also called plain, nonstriated, unstriped and involuntary.
It has the simplest structure among the three kinds of muscle.

    1. Occurrence.

        Walls of hollow viscera (except heart), of ducts and vessels.
        Skin; spleen; eye; penis; broad ligament; visceral pleura.

    2. Shape.

        The individual fibers are elongate, tapering spindles.
            In some special locations, forked or star-shaped fibers occur.
        Sections almost never include the full length of a fiber.
            Maceration loosens and isolates fibers, and so demonstrates their true length.

    3. Size.

        There is marked variation in the length of fibers (18 to 200 μ) in different regions.
        The greatest diameter is also variable (3 to 8 μ).

4. *Structure.*

A. NUCLEUS.

The shape is elongate (ovoid to cigar-shape), depending on fiber length.
The pale nucleus lies midway of its fiber, where the fiber is broadest.
It is almost centrally located, and extends in the long axis of the fiber.
The nucleus shortens when the muscle cell contracts.
  It then tends to wrinkle or twist by passive distortion.

B. CYTOPLASM (SARCOPLASM).

The *plasma membrane* is delicate, and not visible with the light microscope.
  It is far thinner (0.015 μ) than the total sheath of a striated muscle fiber.
The cytoplasm appears homogeneous when fresh, and usually after fixation.
  Yet the electron microscope reveals *myofilaments* 0.003 and 0.008 μ thick.
These organelles are unstriped threads coursing lengthwise in the fiber.
  They are the contractile elements, more solid than the general sarcoplasm.
  Their relations to the two contractile proteins (*actin* and *myosin*) are unknown.
Clusters of myofilaments about 0.3 μ thick may appear after fixation or maceration.
  These *myofibrils* are said to be artifacts, produced by clumping.
The general cytoplasm (*sarcoplasm*) embeds the vast number of myofilaments.
  It exists, but is not noticeable between the closely packed myofibrils.
  It is visible about the nucleus, and especially extending beyond its ends.
  The various *organelles* are grouped inconspicuously near the nucleus.

5. *Grouping of fibers.*

Some solitary fibers or loose networks occur (*e.g.,* in certain regions of the skin).
However, the common, functional unit is a *fascicle* (*i.e,* bundle) of fibers.
  Its fibers pack together in an arrangement that is economical of space.
  Thick middle regions and thinner ends are staggered in adjacent fibers.

A. ISOLATED BUNDLE.

Example: erector muscles of hairs.

B. AGGREGATED BUNDLES.

An irregular spongework exists, as in the penis and prostate gland.
A layer is well defined when its component bundles orient similarly.
  Example: intestine; ductus deferens.
A layer is ill-defined when its bundles interlace or take different directions.
  Example: stomach; bladder; uterus.

6. *Inter-relation of fibers and bundles.*

Adjacent fibers make intimate contact at numerous points on their surfaces.
  Here plasma membranes fuse in the manner of epithelial 'tight junctions' (p. 41).
Each fiber is invested with material much like that of a basal lamina (p. 41).
  It is also surrounded by a network of reticular fibers.
  Here there may also be some fine collagenous fibers and elastic nets.
Bundles and sheets of muscle fibers are separated by ordinary areolar tissue.
In these ways the smooth muscle of a structural unit is united into a functional unit.
  The pull of one fiber is transmitted to another, and of one fascicle to another.
  The result is a unified action rather than localized twitches of individual fibers.

7. *Stretching and contraction.*

When a hollow organ dilates, the passive stretching thins the layers considerably.
  The multiple fusions do not permit the cells to 'glide,' as once taught.
Muscle contraction is slow, sustained and resistant to fatigue.
  The whole fiber may contract as a unit, or local waves may pass along it.
    The latter produce swollen, dark-staining *contraction nodes*.
    These prominent bands tend to align, wave-like, across a sheet of muscle.

Contraction may maintain a constant muscular tension (*i.e.*, *tone*) in an organ.
At times it also may exert a more vigorous, propulsive force.

8. *Vessels and nerves.*

Smooth muscle is only moderately well supplied with *blood vessels*.
Capillaries course in the connective tissue that surrounds bundles of fibers.
But they do not invade bundles and supply individual fibers.
The capillary mesh is elongate, in agreement with general fiber direction.
Autonomic *nerve fibers* branch and end on some muscle cells of a bundle.
Each ends by one or more terminal knobs in contact with the plasma membrane.
Yet relatively few of all the fibers of a muscle receive a terminal nerve twig.
Exceptionally (*e.g.*, ductus deferens) fibers receive individual innervation.
The mechanism of excitation-spread to uninnervated fibers is not surely known.
It presumably depends on intimate contact between muscle fibers. (p. 101).
Loss of nerve supply does not lead to the degeneration of muscle fibers.

9. *Regenerative ability.*

Fibers can enlarge considerably through functional stress.
Extraordinary is the increase in length (70 to 500 μ) in the pregnant uterus.
Adult fibers sometimes show evidence of proliferation after injury or loss.
Also, reserve mesenchymal cells can apparently differentiate into smooth-muscle fibers.
For the most part, however, these activities and capacities are limited.
Large injuries are filled-in by connective tissue that becomes a scar.

10. *Appearance in sections.*

A. LONGITUDINAL SECTION.
The fibers appear like parallel bands, which taper toward the ends.
Adjacent fibers tend to overlap in a staggered fashion.
Their full length is never demonstrable in a single section.
The length of a fiber, as seen, depends upon several factors:
The actual length of the particular fibers examined.
The plane of section with respect to the axis of the fiber.
The straightness of the fiber with respect to the plane of section.
No distinct fibrils are discernible within well preserved fibers.
Dark-staining, crosswise bands sometimes show in a muscle or on individual fibers.
These are prominent regions of local contraction, 'set' by fixation.
The nucleus is moderately to highly elongate.
It lies midway of the fiber length.

B. TRANSVERSE SECTION.
The fibers show as circular or polygonal disks of variable size.
These sizes range from the full fiber breadth to mere dots.
This depends on the level of section through each fiber.
Only some of the largest disks include a nucleus.
The nucleus is located at or near the center of the disk.
The cytoplasm appears homogeneous in well preserved tissue.
No distinct stippling (*i.e.*, sections of cut myofibrils) is seen.
The sparse connective tissue between fibers is inconspicuous.
Bundles or sheets of fibers are separated by areolar tissue.

C. DIFFERENTIATION OF SMOOTH MUSCLE FROM CONNECTIVE TISSUE.
Muscle fibers are protoplasmic and commonly stain darker with eosin.
Nuclei lie inside muscle fibers, but occur between connective-tissue fibers.
In longitudinal sections, muscle nuclei are longer and often wrinkle.
No other kinds of cells occur between the muscle fibers within a bundle or sheet.
In other words, such smooth muscle is notably a 'pure culture.'
Some stains differentiate smooth muscle from connective tissue sharply.
These stains are especially valuable where intermingling occurs.

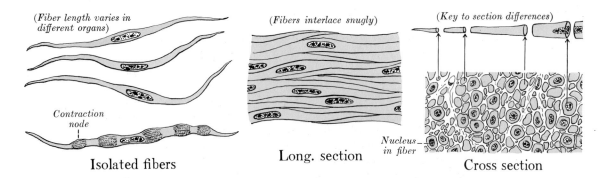

(Fiber length varies in different organs)

(Fibers interlace snugly)

(Key to section differences)

Contraction node

Nucleus in fiber

Isolated fibers

Long. section

Cross section

SMOOTH MUSCLE

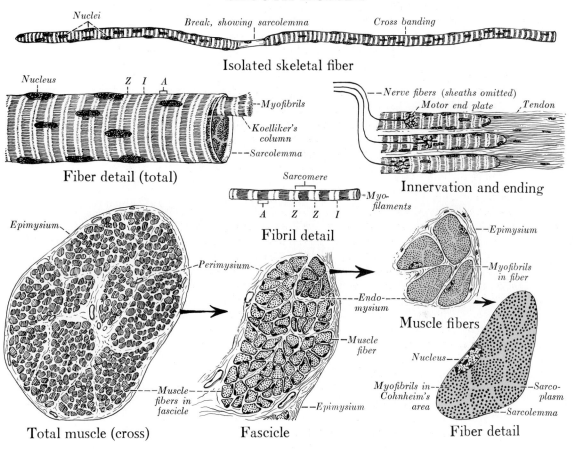

Nuclei

Break, showing sarcolemma

Cross banding

Isolated skeletal fiber

Nucleus   Z I A

Myofibrils

Koelliker's column

Sarcolemma

Fiber detail (total)

Nerve fibers (sheaths omitted)
Motor end plate   *Tendon*

Innervation and ending

Sarcomere

Myo-filaments

A Z Z I

Fibril detail

Epimysium

Perimysium

Endo-mysium

Muscle fiber

Muscle fibers in fascicle

Epimysium

Epimysium

Myofibrils in fiber

Muscle fibers

Nucleus

Myofibrils in Cohnheim's area

Sarco-plasm

Sarcolemma

Total muscle (cross)

Fascicle

Fiber detail

SKELETAL MUSCLE

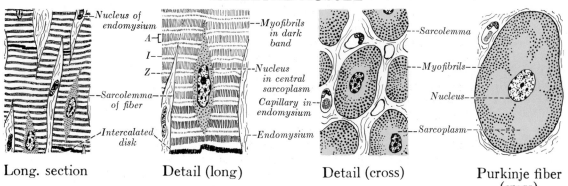

Nucleus of endomysium

A

I

Z

Sarcolemma of fiber

Intercalated disk

Myofibrils in dark band

Nucleus in central sarcoplasm

Capillary in endomysium

Endomysium

Sarcolemma

Myofibrils

Nucleus

Sarcoplasm

Long. section

Detail (long)

Detail (cross)

Purkinje fiber (cross)

CARDIAC MUSCLE

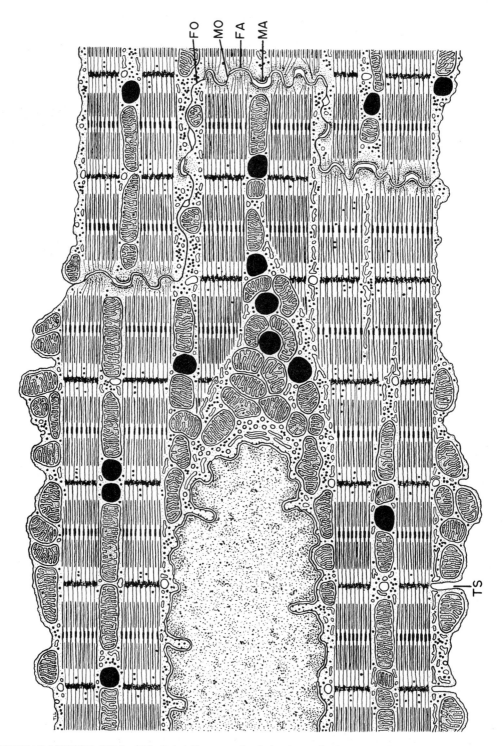

CARDIAC MUSCLE CELL. Fibril details are as in skeletal muscle, but sarcoplasm and mitochondria are more abundant. A transverse tubule (TS) enters at the level of a Z line and points to a triad in the sarcoplasmic reticulum between two myofibrils. A typical sinuous junction of two cells has dense material adhering to the abutting plasma membranes, thereby producing an intercalated disk. Desmosomal conditions (FA, MA) occur, as well as tight junctions (FO, MO) where plasma membranes fuse.

The Mallory stain colors collagenous fibers a bright blue.

Smooth muscle is stained feebly pinkish.

The Milligan stain colors smooth muscle a magenta hue and collagenous fibers in sharply contrasted blue or emerald green.

11. *Functional correlations.*

The elongate fiber, with myofilaments oriented similarly, enhances contractile efficiency.

Arrangements of fibers in layers, oriented differently, permit antagonistic action.

The lack of two kinds of associated filaments correlates with the lack of cross-striping.

The slow response of smooth muscle relates to its lack of individual fiber innervation.

Also its myofilaments respond less vigorously than do cross-striated ones.

Excitation spreads from innervated to uninnervated fibers.

The presence of tight junctions between fibers aids in this transmission.

Involuntary, autonomic control characterizes all so-called vegetative organs.

This and slow, sustained, fatigue-resisting response are suitable adaptations.

Circular muscle in hollow organs (*e.g.*, artery) controls tonus and the size of lumen.

In other organs (*e.g.*, gut) circular and longitudinal layers co-operate in propulsion.

II. SKELETAL MUSCLE

Skeletal muscle is a voluntary, cross-striated type of muscle.

It comprises the 'flesh' attached to the vertebrate skeleton.

But only in mammals does it have a deep red color.

The unit of structure is the *skeletal muscle fiber,* a multinucleate cell, produced by cell fusions.

1. *General features.*

A *muscle fiber* is an extremely long, and fairly thick, multinucleate cell.

The thickest of these thread-like elements are just visible to the naked eye.

A single living fiber is yellowish; muscle is red only when its fibers are massed.

The fiber is contained within a tough, structureless sheath.

This is a specialized membrane, known as the *sarcolemma.*

The numerous *nuclei* are arranged about the periphery of a mammalian fiber.

The fiber contains dozens to hundred of *myofibrils.*

Each is prominently cross-banded (alternating dark bands and light bands).

Between the myofibrils there is less specialized cytoplasm (*sarcoplasm*).

2. *Shape.*

Each fiber is a single, long, protoplasmic thread.

Its general shape is cylindrical (or prismatic through pressure).

Toward the extreme ends there is gradual tapering.

In some instances the ends bifurcate or branch.

Example: tongue; skin of face.

3. *Size.*

A. LENGTH.

An individual muscle fiber is usually said to be between 1 and 40 mm. long.

The total length of human fibers would then be tens of thousands of miles.

It is claimed that much longer fibers occur in nontapering muscles (*e.g.*, sartorius).

B. DIAMETER.

The ordinary limits lie between 10 and 40 μ.

The thickness varies with the type of muscle, and even within the same muscle.

Example: the gluteus has coarse fibers; the ocular muscles, fine fibers.

The diameter of fibers increases with age, exercise and male-hormone influence.

An adult fiber may be as much as ten times its diameter at birth.

Even in old age fibers are thicker, though less numerous, than earlier.

Exercise will increase fiber thickness by 25 per cent.

The augmented muscularity of adolescent boys is attributable to testosterone.

The diameter of fibers decreases in a period of emaciation or disuse.

4. *Nuclei.*

These are numerous (about 35 per mm.), the total number depending on fiber length.

The nucleus is ovoid to fairly elongate and is oriented lengthwise of the fiber.

In mammals its characteristic position is peripheral, close beneath the sarcolemma.

Yet in many 'red fibers' (see beyond) the nuclei are scattered, taking any position.

5. *Sarcolemma.*

Each fiber is enclosed by a close-fitting, tubular sheath — compound in structure.

It stains poorly and is best seen where a fiber is crushed, torn or shrunken.

It is structureless, transparent, elastic and tough; its total thickness is 0.1 μ.

The inherent elasticity makes it conform to changing fiber shape.

The sarcolemma proper is a plasma membrane nearly 0.01 μ thick.

Outside is a basal lamina, ten times thicker, composed of mucopolysaccharide.

Supporting this amorphous sheath (and partly embedded) are reticular fibers.

6. *Myofibrils.*

These are unbranched, parallel threads that extend the length of a fiber.

Their average thickness ranges between 1 and 2 μ; the thinnest are 0.2 μ.

The fibrils often are seen in bundles, called *Koelliker's columns,* probably artifacts.

Such bundles are separated from each other by relatively abundant sarcoplasm.

A Koelliker's column in cross-section is called a *Cohnheim's area.*

Electron micrographs demonstrate that each myofibril is a compound thread.

It contains fundamental units, the *myofilaments,* of two sizes and lengths.

Each consists of chains of long protein molecules of *actin* or of *myosin.*

The thicker filaments (myosin) are restricted to the extent of the dark band.

Each is about 1.5 μ long, 0.01 μ thick, and studded with evenly spaced spines.

The thin filaments (composed of actin) extend throughout the light band.

They also continue for a distance into the adjacent dark band.

Its length in the half light-band is about 1.0 μ; its diameter is 0.005 μ.

Where thick and thin filaments overlap, their arrangement is geometrically regular.

Six thin filaments mark off an hexagonal area about each thick filament.

Three thick filaments mark off a triangular area about each thin filament.

There is an intricate system of projections from thick filaments at regular intervals.

Presumably these can hook onto the thin fibers and pull, ratchet-wise.

7. *Myofibrillar banding.*

Each fibril bears alternate *dark* and *light bands,* about 300 to each millimeter.

These bands are not surface markings but involve the total fibril thickness.

The corresponding bands on all fibrils in a fiber align usually at the same levels.

This generally correct register accounts for the total pattern of cross-striping.

It can be compared to the rows of knuckles and phalanges across the fingers.

Hence the total appearance of a fiber is that of a long riband (actually a rod) crossed
by alternating dark and light stripes (actually disklike regions).

It is notable that the sarcoplasm does not participate in this obvious banding.

A. DARK BAND.

It is also called the *anisotropic band* (abbreviated to *A band*).

This band is strongly refractile and dark in the living fibril, with ordinary light.

It is doubly refractive (anisotropic) to polarized light, showing as a bright region.

The birefringence is a property of the myosin of the thick myofilaments.

These filaments are restricted to the extent of the A band.

The middle region of the A band at times appears paler than the rest.

It is seen only in a relaxed fiber and is named the *H band.*

It represents a region into which actin myofilaments do not extend.

The A band consists of a more concentrated substance that resists stretching.

This portion of the fibril stains well with dyes.

B. LIGHT BAND.

It is also called the *isotropic band* (abbreviated to *I band*).

This band is poorly refractile, pale in the living fibril and is bisected by a Z line.

It is singly refractive (isotropic) to polarized light.

Only the thin myofilaments (actin) occur in this band; they insert on the Z line.

Their free ends extend into the A region for a variable distance.

This distance depends on the degree of contraction in the fibril.

The light band contains more water than the dark band, and stretches easily.

It does not stain with ordinary dyes.

C. ADDITIONAL MARKINGS.

A thin *Z line* bisects each I band transversely.

It is a dense zone in which each actin filament joins a group of special filaments.

It is limited to the fibrils, and hence does not cross the sarcoplasm between fibrils.

Such a relation keeps the filament in register with others.

Electron microscopy has demonstrated the presence of two still feebler stripes.

The *M line* bisects the H band; it represents connections between myosin filaments.

These lateral interconnections keep myosin filaments in register.

The *N line* crosses the I band, between Z and A; its nature is uncertain.

In relaxed muscle, the A, H, I and Z bands are plainly visible.

The entire muscle fiber bears these markings, repeated in identical sequence.

During contraction the appearance of these parts undergoes change (p. 104).

8. *The sarcomere.*

In practice, it is customary to consider the fiber as a series of fundamental units.

Each of these structural units is a *sarcomere*, about 2.5 μ long.

A sarcomere is any segment of the fiber included between successive Z bands.

It contains all of an A band and the half of each I band that borders on A.

Mild trypsin digestion destroys the Z lines.

The fiber then fractures into sarcomere segments.

A sarcomere is a unit of histological structure and physiological action in a fiber.

A finer unit of structure and function is the myofibril within a sarcomere.

9. *Sarcoplasm.*

This comprises the less specialized cytoplasm between myofibrils and about nuclei.

It is clear and less refractile than any region of the myofibrils.

The amount of sarcoplasm varies considerably in different fibers.

Some are rich in sarcoplasm; these have coarse fibrils, weakly cross-striped.

Others are poor in sarcoplasm; these have thinner fibrils, with well defined striping.

In some animals (*e.g.,* cat, rabbit) the various muscles fall into two color-categories.

Red muscles (or 'dark' muscles) have most of their fibers rich in sarcoplasm.

White muscles (or 'light' muscles) have most of their fibers poor in sarcoplasm.

In most mammals, both kinds of fibers (and intermediates) mingle in the same muscle.

One or the other tends to predominate, but no muscle is actually pale.

Sarcoplasm is fundamentally a clear protoplasm, but it contains various specializations:

Mitochondria; Golgi network; sarcoplasmic reticulum.

Pigment: myoglobin is much like hemoglobin and gives color to the fiber.

Nonliving inclusions are glycogen 'granules' and lipid droplets.

Sarcoplasmic reticulum is a system of specialized, smooth endoplasmic reticulum.

Membrane-lined tubules surround each myofibril in regular arrangements.

A set of such tubules courses lengthwise throughout a definite, periodic interval.

At each end of a set there is a transverse expansion into a terminal *cisterna.*

The cisternae of adjoining sets associate with a slender *transverse tubule.*

This combined *triad* encircles a fibril at the level of the A-I junction.

The tubule is an invagination of the basal lamina and plasma membrane.

10. *Structural changes during contraction.*

Active contractility resides in the myofibrils.

Contraction can shorten a relaxed fiber up to two-thirds, or more, of its former length.

The fiber then thickens and the sarcomeres shorten.

In contraction, as followed in stained sections, the following events are noted:

The distance between the Z bands lessens progressively.

The length of the I bands diminishes progressively (and can obliterate).

This brings the Z bands progressively nearer the A bands.

The length of the A band remains constant, as the polarizing microscope proves.

If the shortening is extreme, a so-called reversal of striping occurs.

The ends of each A band, then crowded by the Z bands, become denser.

This region is then a zone that stains darker than the rest of the sarcomere.

The electron microscope indicates that only one active shift takes place.

This is done by the thin (actin) myofilaments.

They slide along the thick (myosin) myofilaments of the A disk.

The action is presumably the result of a rachet-like series of hook-ups.

As the two actin sets approach, the H band shortens progressively and may disappear.

Actin attachment to the two Z bands draws the latter in tow passively.

Thus the entire sarcomere becomes shorter; also I bands shorten and may disappear.

11. *Muscle as an organ.*

A. STRUCTURAL PLAN.

Muscle fibers are aggregated into functional groups known as *muscles*.

The number of fibers in a muscle depends chiefly on its size.

Example: biceps, 260,000 fibers; stapedius, 1500 fibers.

The muscle fibers are grouped into bundles, called *fascicles*.

Some muscles have large fascicles, and thus show a coarse grain.

Example: gluteus maximus; deltoid.

Others, such as the ocular muscles, have a very fine grain.

In many muscles no fascicle extends the full length of the muscle.

Connective tissue embeds fibers, surrounds fascicles, and encloses the muscle.

(The toughness of meat depends mostly on the amount of this tissue present.)

The delicate connective tissue between the muscle fibers is called *endomysium*.

Collagenous, elastic and reticular fibers occur there.

The fibrous sheath around each fascicle is the *perimysium*.

Portions carrying larger vessels are thicker and often produce radial septa.

The fibrous sheath around the whole muscle is the *epimysium*.

B. ARRANGEMENT OF MUSCLE FIBERS.

Some fibers extend the entire length of a fascicle and attach at each end of it.

Some fibers attach at one end of a fascicle and terminate freely within it.

Some fibers lie wholly within the fascicle, attaching to neither end.

It is commonly said that most fascicles longer than 5 cm. contain no fibers that extend through their entire length.

C. UNION OF MUSCLE WITH TENDON.

The connective tissue of a muscle makes a continuous system of fibrous tissue.

That is, epi-, peri-, and endomysium are local portions of a sheath-system.

This 'harness' merges with the fibrous tissue that anchors a muscle in place.

Such attachments, on which a pull is exerted, are tendons and aponeuroses.

In addition, the ends of muscle fibers themselves become firmly anchored.

The manner of union of muscle with tendon has been debated for many years.

Electron micrographs show that there is no direct continuity of these fibers.

Instead, tendon fibrils continue as the reticular fibers of the sarcolemma.

12. *Vessels and nerves.*

Blood vessels follow the connective tissue into muscle.

In the endomysium a rich, elongated network of capillaries surrounds each fiber.

Actually, each capillary serves two or more fibers that abut upon it.
Lymphatics occur in the epimysium and in the perimysial septa only.
Muscle sensibility is mediated exclusively through sensory *muscle spindles* (p. 294).
　　They occur only in muscles required for the maintenance of posture.
Motor activity is mediated through specialized *motor end-plates.*
　　Motor nerve fibers that supply a muscle branch repeatedly within the muscle.
　　　　A terminal twig from such branching comes to an end about midway along a
　　　　　　muscle fiber, making a slightly elevated plaque there.
　　　　It then loses its myelin sheath and its neurolemma in part.
　　　　The axonal-twig ends in a 'crow-foot' or other pattern directly on the sarcolemma.
　　　　Its bulbous termination contains numerous mitochondria and vesicles.
　　At the site of junction the sarcolemma is depressed and folded into troughs.
　　　　The underlying sarcoplasm is massed here, producing the *sole plate.*
　　　　　　It contains more than the ordinary number of muscle nuclei.
Every muscle fiber receives one of these specialized motor endings.
　　In most instances a single branching nerve fiber innervates many muscle fibers.
　　　　This set of muscle fibers is arranged in a compact group, often a fascicle.
　　　　It constitutes a separate functional contractile unit (up to 160 fibers or more).
　　In muscles with delicate precise movements, individual nerve fibers branch less.
　　　　In one of the ocular muscles each nerve fiber innervates a single fiber only.
Neurons exert a trophic influence which maintains muscle fibers in good condition.
　　Motor-nerve injury leads to muscle atrophy (as in infantile paralysis).

13. *Growth and regenerative ability.*

Growing muscles lengthen by fibers adding new sarcomeres at muscle-tendon junctions.
Growing muscles thicken by first synthesizing new filaments; the enlarged fibrils then split.
Nucleated remnants of injured muscle fibers can regenerate to a certain extent.
Large injuries to a muscle are usually filled-in and healed by a connective-tissue scar.

14. *Appearance in sections.*
　A. LONGITUDINAL SECTION.
　　Fibers are solitary acidophilic bands, both long and relatively broad.
　　　　The fibers of any given muscle are fairly uniform in size.
　　Cross-striping is bold and conspicuous under moderately high magnification.
　　　　But locally, or under certain conditions, striations may show poorly (if at all).
　　A longitudinal, fibrillar arrangement may or may not be apparent within a fiber.
　　Nuclei may appear to occupy any position with respect to fiber breadth.
　　　　But more are seen at the sides; all actually occupy border regions of a fiber.
　B. TRANSVERSE SECTION.
　　Fibers show as more or less rounded polygons, prominent and fairly equal in size.
　　Fibrils are cut across and appear as distinct dots.
　　　　These dots may be grouped in clusters (Cohnheim's areas).
　　The sarcolemma is a thin, limiting line.
　　Nuclei lie close beneath the sarcolemma; an interior position is exceptional.
　　Delicate connective tissue (endomysium) separates the fibers.
　　　　Coarser connective tissue encloses bundles of fibers (fascicles).

15. *Functional correlations.*

Skeletal muscle contracts faster than does smooth muscle.
　　But it fatigues easier and its action is less sustained.
　　It is set off by a smaller stimulus, yet consumes more energy.
Muscles that are most constantly active have more red fibers, rich in sarcoplasm.
　　These contract slower, have a longer twitch and withstand fatigue better.
　　Example: ocular; respiratory; masticatory.
Muscles capable of quicker and more powerful contraction have more white fibers.

These fibers are rich in myofibrils, but exhaustion occurs sooner in them.

In fast moving muscles the sarcomeres are shorter (more contractile units per mm.).

Example: digital muscles; biceps.

The size increase of exercised muscles is due to an increased amount of sarcoplasm.

The gain in volume of a fiber through such cell hypertrophy can be twofold.

The total mechanism of muscular contraction is understood but partially.

Discovery of the shift of actin filaments has aided understanding greatly.

Yet the way of making new side linkages between filaments is obscure.

Energy for contraction is liberated through a series of known oxidizing reactions.

In this, adenotriphosphate is changed to the diphosphate.

The free phosphate ions, thus released, constitute the store of energy.

This energy-store is converted into kinetic energy without significant heat.

How the protein filaments accomplish this has not been explained.

The diphosphate is rephosphorylated into the triphosphate before another contraction.

The efficiency of muscle in converting energy to work is 25 per cent.

(Steam engine, 9 to 14 per cent; diesel engine, 29 to 35 per cent.)

Transverse tubules are a system specialized for spreading the contraction-impulse fast.

They are extensions of the plasma membrane and share its properties.

Sarcoplasmic reticulum perhaps triggers contraction by releasing calcium ions.

Mitochondria are located between myofibrils, and in relation to their banding.

This is correlated with the high energy required for muscle contraction.

That is, the mitochondria are a source of adenotriphosphate.

Lipid droplets are usually associated with mitochondria, indicating a source of energy.

This is supported by a content of enzymes suitable for fatty-acid oxidation.

The vesicles in the axonal endings in the motor end-plate contain *acetylcholine*.

This substance is released on the arrival of the nerve impulse.

It serves as the chemical mediator that induces contraction of the muscle fiber.

III. CARDIAC MUSCLE

This involuntary, cross-striated muscle is peculiar to the myocardium of the heart.

It also extends onto the roots of the large vessels joining the heart.

Cardiac muscle is much like skeletal muscle in structure.

But in development, innervation and function it resembles smooth muscle.

1. General features.

Cardiac muscle consists of short columns, united into a close meshwork.

The meshwork simulates a syncytium because cell junctions are not easily seen.

The main columns of the mesh in any local region extend in a common direction.

These are connected by slenderer, slanting branches.

Formerly a 'muscle fiber' referred to any column in a presumed syncytial mesh.

Although columns are now known to be cellular, the term 'fiber' is still used.

Connective tissue fills-in the slit-like interstices of the meshwork.

This *endomysium* is well pronounced in mammals alone.

A cell contains *sarcoplasm* and *myofibrils*, like skeletal muscle, but only one nucleus.

2. Shape and size.

Each cell is an elongate prism, whose cross-sectional shape is quite variable.

The diameter of cardiac cells varies between 9 and 22 μ.

The thickest are not much larger than the thinnest skeletal fibers of an adult.

3. Cell boundaries.

Each column of the cardiac meshwork consists of a single row of several cells.

The plasma membranes, where cells abut, are resolved only with the electron microscope.

Their junctions tend to follow sinuous, interlocking planes.
Maceration with potassium hydroxide isolates the component cells of a column.

4. Nuclei.

The shape is ovoid and the orientation agrees with the long axis of the cell.
A nucleus retains a central position, midway within its cell, as in embryonic stages.

5. Sarcolemma.

This thin sheath encapsulates the cell, as in a skeletal muscle fiber.
Structurally the two are alike (*cf.,* p. 102); the cardiac type is thinner and more adherent.

6. Sarcoplasm.

This is rather abundant; it is correlated with the heart's capacity to withstand fatigue.
(The heart does enough work daily to lift itself a distance of 35 miles.)
The amount of sarcoplasm and the central nucleus simulate a 'red' skeletal fiber.
Sarcoplasm embeds the nucleus and extends beyond it in a spindle-shaped axial mass.
This axial mass lacks myofibrils, but a Golgi complex and some pigment occur here.
Elsewhere sarcoplasm embeds myofibrils and the abundant mitochondria.
Large *transverse tubules,* associated with myofibrils, are located over the Z bands.
These are invaginations of the plasma membrane and its basal lamina.
Sarcoplasmic reticulum is a network, associated with T-tubules, but not as triads (p. 103).

7. Myofibrils.

The *myofibrils* are distinct, but less robust than those of skeletal muscle.
Their extent is restricted to each individual cell in a column.
The actual endings, however, like the limits of a cell, are not easily seen.
Fibrillar striping is like that in skeletal muscle (p. 102), but closer and fainter.
During contraction a similar sequence of events occurs (p. 104).
The myofibrils sometimes are seen gathered into *Koelliker's columns,* as in skeletal muscle.
Transverse sections of these artifacts show as *Cohnheim's areas.*

8. Intercalated disks.

Prominent markings pass across columns of cardiac cells at irregular intervals.
They may not transect the entire fiber, and may take a stepped or zig-zag course.
Such *intercalated disks* are blackened by silver nitrate and stained by some dyes.
Disks occur only where delicate plasma membranes demark contiguous cells.
Dense substance, next to the irregular transverse boundaries, stains deeply.
This reinforcing substance resembles Z lines and lies at their position.
The total arrangement at a disk corresponds to a desmosome in epithelium.
Also at some places along the disks, where cells adjoin, there are tight junctions.
Only the electron microscope demonstrates all these details correctly.
The number of disks seen increases with age, and especially in overworked hearts.

9. Purkinje fibers.

Despite its cellularity, cardiac muscle is a good conductor of excitation impulses.
The heart also has an *impulse-conduction system* made of specialized muscle cells.
It constitutes a cellular network at the junction of endocardium and myocardium.
Its 'Purkinje fibers' are composed of large cells with much central sarcoplasm.
Their fibrils are few and occupy a peripheral position in the cells.
The most prominent part of the system is the *atrio-ventricular bundle.*

10. Gross arrangement of muscle.

The meshwork of cell columns is partially segregated by thicker connective tissue.
This partial isolation produces bundles and plates of muscle.
Many of these continue so as to interconnect the right and left halves of the heart.
The cell columns of any such system take a common lengthwise direction.

In general, layers located at different levels in the wall course in different directions.
Hence any slice through the heart shows fiber groups cut in various planes.

11. *Vessels and nerves.*

Blood capillaries form plexuses in the endomysial connective tissue about fibers.
This supply is about twice as rich as in skeletal muscle.
Lymphatic capillaries are also present especially in the endomysium.
Autonomic *nerves* end in knobbed brushes on cardiac muscle 'fibers.'
They belong both to the sympathetic and parasympathetic nerve divisions.

12. *Regenerative ability.*

Cardiac muscle is more resistant to injuries than other types of muscle.
Regeneration after tissue injury is scarcely evident.
Healing is almost wholly by fibrous invasion, producing scar tissue.
The response to increased work is by cell hypertrophy; new fibers are not formed.

13. *Appearance in sections.*

A. LONGITUDINAL.
There is a system of branching strands, bearing fine cross-striations.
This banding may show poorly, or not at all, in local regions.
There is considerable variation in the width of fibers seen in any region.
Intercalated disks are diagnostic features, but may lack proper staining.
Nuclei occur in the axis of the band, not marginally.
Endomysial connective tissue is rather plentiful.

B. TRANSVERSE.
Irregularly shaped areas are separated by considerable connective tissue.
These areas are variable in size, but smaller than ordinary skeletal fibers.
The nucleus, when included, is central and relatively large.
Some sections of fibers, lacking a nucleus, show a central mass of sarcoplasm.
Cohnheim's areas often are arranged like radiating wedges.

14. *Functional correlations.*

Branching of cardiac muscle provides an effective spread of contraction throughout.
Purkinje fibers conduct stimuli that co-ordinate the atrial and ventricular beats.
Tight junctions permit the rapid spread of electrical excitation from cell to cell.
The abundance of mitochondria and lipids correlates with the high energy requirements.
Intercalated disks and sinuous end-to-end cell junctions are mechanically useful.
They bind cells together and withstand the lengthwise pull of contraction.
Sarcoplasmic pigment accumulation, with aging, results from metabolic 'wear and tear.'

15. *Comparison of the three muscle types.*

A. LONGITUDINAL SECTION.
Smooth-muscle fibers are relatively small spindles; cardiac fibers, a coarsely branching network; skeletal fibers, very large solitary bands.
Smooth muscle is unstriped; cardiac, weakly striped; skeletal, strongly striped.
Smooth-muscle nuclei are slenderer and more elongate than the other two.

B. TRANSVERSE SECTION.
Smooth-muscle fibers are much smaller than the other two.
Skeletal fibers are larger than cardiac.
Smooth-muscle fibers show wide size variation; cardiac fibers, moderate variation; skeletal fibers, fair uniformity in any given muscle.
Smooth-muscle fibers lack any evident stippling (myofibrils); cardiac and skeletal fibers show fibrils as plainly visible dots.
Smooth- and cardiac fibers have central nuclei; skeletal fibers, peripheral nuclei.
Smooth-muscle nuclei are largest, relative to fiber diameter; skeletal are smallest.
Cardiac and skeletal muscle are embedded in connective tissue (endomysium).
Smooth muscle packs tightly; there is no obvious tissue between fibers.

Chapter XII

The Nervous Tissues

Irritability and conductivity are inherent properties of protoplasm.

> *Irritability* is sensitivity to stimuli, with the setting up of an impulse response.
> *Conductivity* is the transmission of such a wave of excitation.
> These qualities reach their highest expression in the nervous tissue.

Most nerve cells are massed in, or near, the *central nervous system* (brain; spinal cord).

Nerve-cell processes are capable of transmitting impulses over long distances.

> Some lie wholly within the central nervous system.
> Others extend beyond the brain and cord, or lie largely or wholly outside of them.
> > They constitute the *peripheral nervous system.*

I. THE NEURON CONCEPT

A. NEURON:

A *neuron* is a nerve cell, consisting of a cell body and all its processes.

> It arises from a single embryonic cell, the *neuroblast.*
> It retains its physical independence and connects with other neurons by contact only.
> It is the structural and functional unit of the nervous system.

Many years elapsed before these facts were established and cell-chain concepts disproved.

> It had seemed improbable that cell processes could extend for inches or even feet.

Nevertheless, established custom has retained some of the old terminology.

> The main cell-body of a neuron is commonly called the *nerve cell.*
> The thread-like cell processes are called *nerve fibers.*
> (Originally these terms referred to separate things, as in connective tissue.)

B. SYNAPSE:

Neurons come into intimate contact (but not continuity) with other neurons.

> This specialized region of physiological junction is named a *synapse.*
> Here the neuron-units are still separated by intact plasma membranes (p. 118).

II. THE CELL BODY

The main portion of a total neuron that looks like an ordinary cell is the *cell body,* or 'nerve cell.'

> A technical name for the cytoplasm alone is *perikaryon* (*i.e.,* the region about the nucleus).

A. GENERAL FEATURES:

1. Size.

> Nerve cells are mostly large in comparison with other body-cells.
> In man the extremes in diameter are 4 and 135 μ.
> Cell size is roughly correlated with the length of the main process, or *axon.*

2. Shape.

> Cell shape is dependent on the number and arrangement of cell processes.

A. UNIPOLAR CELL. A nearly globular cell, with a slender stem that bifurcates.
Example: cells in the ganglia alongside the brain and spinal cord.
B. BIPOLAR CELL. A spindle-shaped cell with a process at each end.
Example: cells of acoustic ganglia; some retinal neurons; olfactory neurons.
C. MULTIPOLAR CELL. A cell with several to many processes; the commonest type.
Variant shapes are illustrated by stellate-, pyramidal- and pear-shaped cells.
Example: cells in the autonomic ganglia and central nervous system.

3. *Numbers.*

A computation has been made of the total number of nerve cells in one region.
In the cerebral cortex of the brain alone this number is given as 9,200,000,000.

4. *Nucleus.*

Usually there is but one *nucleus,* located more or less centrally.
It is large and spherical, with a distinct nuclear membrane.
There is one (rarely more) prominent *nucleolus,* centrally located.
Chromatin makes a scanty network; the *ground substance* is clear and abundant.
Much of the chromatin is in the unseen, uncoiled, active state.

5. *Cytoplasm (or perikaryon).*

A. PLASMA MEMBRANE.
There is a limiting border to the general cytoplasm of a neuron.
This typical *plasma membrane* is the seat of impulse conduction.
B. NEUROPLASM.
This name denotes the general cytoplasm, containing organelles and inclusions.
Living *neuroplasm* usually appears homogeneous with the light microscope.
Dark-field or phase microscopy reveals the presence of granules.
Staining proves it to be basophilic and demonstrates other constituents.
C. ORGANELLES.
Mitochondria, a diffuse *Golgi complex, lysosomes* and *microtubules* occur.
The problematical microtubules of nerve are specifically named *neurotubules.*
A *centrosome* is present in neuroblasts, but is inconspicuous in mature cells.
This change is correlated with the inability of the mature neuron to divide.
Unbranching *neurofibrils* exist in both the cell body and cell processes.
They are firm protoplasmic threads, embedded in the neuroplasm.
Each fibril is composed of a bundle of much finer (0.008μ) threads.
Only the electron microscope resolves these tubular *neurofilaments.*
Neurofibrils have apparently been observed in some living cells.
They are clearly demonstrated by special silver techniques.
The utility of neurofibrils to the neuron still remains undetermined.
Nissl bodies are a flaky material, ranging from fine to coarse in different neurons.
Phase microscopy demonstrates them as discrete clumps in living cells.
Electron microscopy reveals concentrations of granular endoplasmic reticulum.
The arrangement is one of stacks of flat sacs bearing clusters of ribosomes.
Other ribosomes lie in the general neuroplasm, free of the membranes.
Nissl bodies are present in the cell body and branching dendrons.
They are absent from most axons and their conical base (axon hillock).
Basic aniline dyes stain the Nissl bodies strongly.
This is owing to the concentration of ribonucleoprotein in their ribosomes.
Ribosomes are sites of continuous synthesis, replacing used-up neuroplasm.
Such protein material flows into and down the cell processes.
After an injury to a neuron, the Nissl bodies undergo *chromatolysis.*
This involves: swelling of the cell body; peripheral displacement of the
nucleus; disruption and dispersal of the Golgi complex.
Some of the Nissl bodies collect near the periphery of the cell.
More centrally they break down to fine particles, but do not disappear.

Much of the neuroplasm then stains palely with basic aniline dyes.
On recovery of the neuron, Nissl bodies reorganize as before the injury.
    D. INCLUSIONS.
Granules, lipid droplets and packets of vesicles occur in the neuroplasm.
Pigment granules are of widespread occurrence in man.
Brownish black, coarse granules (*melanin*) occur in primates, in general.
They are present only in certain cells of definite regions.
Example: substantia nigra of the midbrain; some ganglion cells.
Yellow to brownish granules occur mainly in the larger nerve cells of man.
They are fine and tend to aggregate as they become numerous.
They represent a *lipochrome pigment* of a special fatty nature.
Such pigment increases with age, and probably represents metabolic slag.
Secretory products (hormones) are elaborated by some nerve cells of the brain.

6. Appearance in sections.

Nerve cells are mostly large; they are usually cut into several slices.
Hence the nucleus or nucleolus is not included in every section observed.
The most common cell shape is rounded or irregularly angular.
The cytoplasm is basophilic and granular.
Often there is some indication of the flaky Nissl substance.
The nucleus is large and round; it contains scanty chromatin.
There is a prominent, rounded, basophilic nucleolus.

B. NERVE CELLS OF CENTRAL SYSTEM:

These cell bodies are multipolar, but vary in size and shape.
The anterior-column cells (stellate) of the spinal cord, Purkinje cells (pear-shaped) of the cerebellum, and pyramidal cells of the motor cortex illustrate the range in form.
Cells, similar in type and function, tend to aggregate in local groups, called *nuclei*.
Their naked cell bodies are embedded in nerve fibers and neuroglial tissue.

C. NERVE CELLS OF PERIPHERAL SYSTEM:

These cell bodies are associated in groups that are known as *ganglia*.
Since ganglia are major features of the nervous system and consist of more than bare nerve cells, they will be described in the following, separate topic.

III. THE GANGLIA

The distinctive component of a ganglion is a group of cell bodies belonging to neurons.
These are located outside the central system, although interconnected by nerve fibers.
They are associated with either the cranio-spinal or the autonomic system.

A. GENERAL FEATURES:

A *ganglion* is supported and surrounded by connective tissue.
Nerve fibers are present, many or all of which belong to the ganglion cell bodies.
Other fibers enter some ganglia and synapse with its neurons.
Still others may merely pass through, seeking other destinations.
The larger ganglia are prominent swellings that contain up to 50,000 *ganglion cells*.
By contrast, the smallest consist of but few cells.
A cell-body is enveloped by a thin cellular capsule, consisting of *satellite cells*.
These cells make a single-layered envelope, supported by a basement membrane.
Their mother cell in the neural crest was similar to that of the ganglion cell.
The daughter cells of each merely took different lines of specialization.
Satellite cells are continuous with the neurolemma sheath of the cell process.
In life only a thin film of tissue fluid separates satellites from ganglion cell.
The cellular capsule is reinforced externally by a delicate connective-tissue sheath.
This blends with the general vascular stroma, which embeds nerve fibers as well.
It is continous with the endoneurial sheath (of Henle), enclosing the axon.

B. Cranio-Spinal Ganglia:

Some make nodular enlargements on the dorsal (posterior) roots of the spinal nerves.
>   Others occur on the sensory roots of certain cranial nerves.
All the cell bodies belong to sensory (afferent) neurons.

1. Cell shape.

The so-called unipolar cells are globular or pear-shaped.
>   Actually they are pseudo-unipolar; the common stalk is a portion of the perikaryon.
The acoustic ganglia are exceptional in retaining bipolar, embryonic-type cells.
>   In addition, these cells lack a capsule composed of satellite cells.

2. Cell size.

The cells fall into two groups, small and large.
Small cells range between 15 and 25 μ; they have unmyelinated fiber-processes.
Large cells range up to 100 μ; their associated nerve fibers are myelinated.

3. Neuron details.

The cell body exhibits no unusual features; Nissl bodies, however, are fine granules.
There is a single stem-process which presently bifurcates T- or Y-fashion.
>   Both of these branches have the structure of an efferent process (*i.e.*, an axon).
>   If the stem is cut, impulse conduction and synaptic transmission are undisturbed.
Nevertheless, the thicker peripheral process is functionally afferent (*i.e.*, a dendron).
>   It enters a peripheral nerve and terminates as a sensory receptor.
>   The thinner, central process is an axon; it passes into the spinal cord or brain.
>   No fibers of other neurons traverse the ganglion; hence no synapses occur here.
The main process of large cells may wander within the capsular space before emerging.
>   It occasionally arises by more than one root, or gives off short collaterals.

C. Autonomic Ganglia:

Some make a series of enlargements along the sympathetic trunks.
>   Others occur on the more peripheral plexuses and within the walls of visceral organs.
All the cell bodies belong to motor (efferent) neurons.

1. Cell shape.

Typical *autonomic ganglion cells* are multipolar; the general shape is stellate.
>   A few bipolar and unipolar cells are said to occur also.

2. Cell size.

They are smaller (15 to 45 μ) than the larger representatives of the cranio-spinal series.

3. Neuron details.

The cell body has the general structure of typical nerve cells.
>   Its cytoplasm often contains prominent masses of pigment, especially with aging.
>   Nuclei tend to be eccentric in position and two (or more) sometimes occur.
The several cell processes usually pierce the capsule.
>   But sometimes short dendrons ramify and remain inside the capsule.
Sometimes, but not always, the axons and dendrons are distinguishable.
>   The axon (called a *postganglionic fiber*) lacks a myelin sheath.
>   It usually arises from a dendron-stem, not independently from the cell-body.
In the outlying ganglia, typical capsules may be lacking about the cell body.
>   Instead, the ganglion cells are enmeshed in an interlacing system of cells.
>   These spindle-shaped elements are equivalent to satellite cells.
All autonomic ganglion cells are apparently motor in function.
>   Most of them (perhaps all) enter into synapse with a *preganglionic fiber*, whose cell
>   body lies within the central nervous system.

D. **Appearance of Ganglia in Sections:**

Large, encapsulated cells intermingle with nerve fibers and connective tissue.
Connective tissue also envelops the whole ganglion.
The cellular capsule is the distinguishing feature of ganglion cells in general.
Its epithelioid cells have nuclei far smaller than those of a ganglion cell.
A space is frequently seen between capsule and ganglion cell.
In silver preparations this space is greatly exaggerated by shrinkage.
Cranio-spinal ganglion cells show a far greater size range than do autonomic cells.
Cranio-spinal cells are rounded to slightly pear-shape and have one main process.
This process pierces the capsule to gain the outside and become free.
(Naturally most sections miss it by passing in the wrong plane.)
Prominent tracts of nerve fibers course by themselves through the total ganglion.
Autonomic cells are angular in shape (*i.e.*, multipolar).
The cell body commonly contains prominent masses of pigment.
Cell processes are multiple and pierce the capsule at various points.
Only after silver staining is this determinable.
Groups of cells and fibers intermingle confusedly; fiber tracts do not occur.

IV. CELL PROCESSES (NERVE FIBERS)

To provide long conduction paths, cell cytoplasm is drawn out into thread-like processes.
These are variable in number, arrangement and degree of branching.
One to several processes (*dendrons,* or dendrites) conduct impulses toward the cell.
A single process (*axon,* or axis cylinder) conducts impulses away from the cell.
When the receptive and emissive ends are both far away from the cell body, then axon and dendron are structurally alike (*i.e.*, axon-like).
This occurs in the two processes of cranio-spinal ganglion cells.
A cell process may be very long with respect to the size of its cell body.
Example: the length of a fiber from the lower spinal cord to the foot is some 20,000 times the diameter of its cell of origin.
Also cell processes may contain a relatively huge amount of cytoplasm.
Example: an axon can have several hundred times as much cytoplasm as the cell body.
The general cytoplasm of a cell process is *neuroplasm,* as in the cell body.
It contains *neurofibrils* and *neurotubules;* certain processes (dendrons) contain *Nissl bodies.*
Synthesized neuroplasm flows continuously down cell processes, 1 mm. per day.
It replaces neuroplasm catalyzed continuously along the extent of the fiber.
Also replaced are substances, such as acetylcholine, secreted at the synapse.

1. Dendrons.

Multipolar cells, as befits the name, have several to many *dendrons.*
By contrast, a uni- or bipolar cell has but one process that functions as a dendron.
Such a dendron, however, is atypical structurally since it resembles an axon.
A typical dendron is distinguished by its form (dendron means 'tree').
It arises by a broad stem that branches freely in a bush-like manner.
The branches dwindle rapidly in size and end not far from the cell body.
The branches of a dendron are often contorted, varicose and thorny.
The spiny appearance is due to lateral twigs, called *gemmules.*
These are usually swollen or knobbed at their ends.
Dendrons make up much of the felty 'neuropil' of the spinal cord and brain.
They acquire no sheaths (exception, p. 112) and do not build any nerve tracts.
Dendrons are virtually short, branching extensions of the cell body.
Their internal structure is like that of the cell body itself; they lack sheaths.
That is, it is typically fibrillar and granular (including Nissl bodies).

2. Axon.

A neuron has but one *axon*; it is usually longer and slenderer than the dendrons.

Yet in some interconnecting neurons the axon is short and difficult to distinguish.

The axon of a multipolar cell usually begins as an elevation of the cell body.

This conical projection is known as the *axon hillock.*

The larger ones are devoid of Nissl substance, like the axon itself.

The axon does not branch to any degree near its cell of origin.

However, a few branches (*collaterals*) may occur at right angles along its course.

The axon usually ends in twig-like arborizations termed *telodendria.*

The axon has a smooth contour; it is not beset with spines, like a dendron.

It maintains a nearly uniform size until terminal branches arise.

Many axons acquire accessory sheaths along most of their course.

An axon and its sheaths are commonly called a *nerve fiber.*

Nerve fibers tend to run in bundles; these often have a common function.

They are *tracts* in the central system and *nerves* in the peripheral system.

The most important component of a nerve fiber is the *axon* (or *axis cylinder*).

Two kinds of sheaths may enclose this thread-like extension of the cell body.

Externally there is the cellular sheath (of Schwann), the *neurolemma.*

Next to the axon, the neurolemma lays down a fatty *myelin sheath.*

V. CLASSIFICATION OF NERVE FIBERS

The presence or absence of sheaths furnishes a basis for the classification of nerve fibers.

1. Myelinated nerve fibers.
  A. WITH A NEUROLEMMA.
    Such fibers are common in the peripheral nerves of the cranio-spinal series.
    The tubular myelin sheath is interrupted at intervals in regions called *nodes.*
  B. WITHOUT A NEUROLEMMA.
    These fibers occur in the white substance of the brain and spinal cord.
    Here the myelin sheath appears to be an uninterrupted cylinder.
      Actually, nodes and other clefts (incisures) occur, but are not plainly seen.
    Certain neuroglial cells, in association with fibers, take the place of a neurolemma.

2. Unmyelinated nerve fibers.
  A. WITH A NEUROLEMMA.
    All axons of autonomic ganglia are of this type.
    Also included are most of the small fibers of the cranio-spinal nerves.
    Myelinated peripheral fibers, near their terminations, furnish local examples.
      That is, the myelin sheath has been lost already, whereas the neurolemma sheath
        comes to an end somewhat farther on.
  B. WITHOUT A NEUROLEMMA.
    Axons within the gray substance of the brain and cord are naked threads.
    The final terminations of all nerve fibers are devoid of sheaths.
    Some tracts in the brain and spinal cord lack sheaths throughout their entire course.

VI. THE STRUCTURE OF PERIPHERAL NERVES

All the fibers of peripheral nerves are organized as typical axons.

Actually, however, the sensory fibers are functional dendrons.

The following descriptions apply to the main extent of peripheral nerve fibers.

They do not include the terminal simplifications through loss of sheaths.

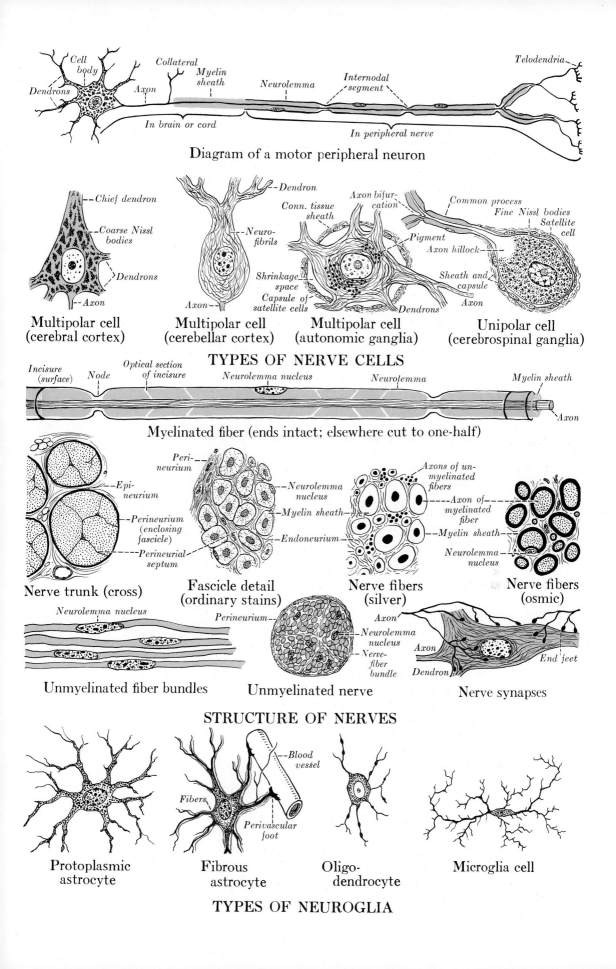

Diagram of a motor peripheral neuron

Cell body
Dendrons
Axon
Collateral
Myelin sheath
Neurolemma
Internodal segment
Telodendria
In brain or cord
In peripheral nerve

TYPES OF NERVE CELLS

Chief dendron
Coarse Nissl bodies
Dendrons
Axon

Multipolar cell
(cerebral cortex)

Dendron
Conn. tissue sheath
Neuro-fibrils
Shrinkage space
Capsule of satellite cells
Axon

Multipolar cell
(cerebellar cortex)

Axon bifur-cation
Pigment
Axon hillock
Dendrons

Multipolar cell
(autonomic ganglia)

Common process
Fine Nissl bodies
Satellite cell
Sheath and capsule
Axon

Unipolar cell
(cerebrospinal ganglia)

Myelinated fiber (ends intact; elsewhere cut to one-half)

Incisure (surface)
Node
Optical section of incisure
Neurolemma nucleus
Neurolemma
Myelin sheath
Axon

STRUCTURE OF NERVES

Epi-neurium
Perineurium (enclosing fascicle)
Perineurial septum

Nerve trunk (cross)

Peri-neurium
Neurolemma nucleus
Myelin sheath
Endoneurium

Fascicle detail
(ordinary stains)

Axons of un-myelinated fibers
Axon of myelinated fiber
Myelin sheath
Neurolemma nucleus

Nerve fibers
(silver)

Nerve fibers
(osmic)

Neurolemma nucleus

Unmyelinated fiber bundles

Perineurium
Neurolemma nucleus
Nerve-fiber bundle

Unmyelinated nerve

Axon
End feet
Dendron

Nerve synapses

TYPES OF NEUROGLIA

Protoplasmic astrocyte

Blood vessel
Fibers
Perivascular foot

Fibrous astrocyte

Oligo-dendrocyte

Microglia cell

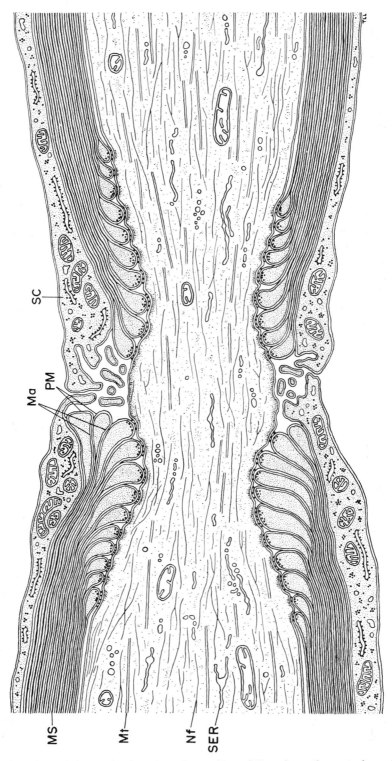

NODE OF RANVIER. A longitudinal section of a myelinated fiber shows the central axoplasm containing microtubules (Mt), neurofilaments (Nf), smooth endoplasmic reticulum (SER), and mitochondria. Two neurolemma cells (SC) abut and interdigitate, but remain separate. At the node the myelin sheath (MS) is lacking; here the individual lamellae separate, each plasma membrane (PM) of a loop containing cytoplasm instead of myelin. The dilated loops (MA) are terminal components of the spirally wrapped and modified sheath.

A. MYELINATED FIBERS:

A fresh *fiber* appears to be a homogeneous, shiny, semitransparent tube.
> Its wall is thick and interrupted at intervals by constrictions, or *nodes.*
> Branching occurs at these nodes, and chiefly at the end of the fiber.
No further details are visible without staining.
> The stained appearance then varies with the technique used.
The thickness of fibers lies between 2 and 20 μ.
> This size-variation depends on the type of nerve and animal examined.
> Large fibers conduct impulses faster, and probably run longer courses.

1. Axon.

In life the *axon* (or *axis cylinder*) is a soft, elastic, homogeneous-appearing jelly.
The unspecialized cytoplasm of an axon (*i.e.,* neuroplasm) is called *axoplasm.*
The semifluid axoplasm embeds the more solid *neurofibrils* and *mitochondria.*
> The neurofibrils (bundled *neurofilaments*) are continuous with those in the cell body.
> There are also *vesicles* (endoplasmic reticulum) and tiny neurotubules.
At the surface of the axoplasm is a plasma membrane, the *axolemma.*
> It is a continuation of the plasma membrane of the cell body.
> It is directly concerned with the transmission of the nerve impulse.
The living axon is several times thicker than the myelin wall which encloses it.
> (Most fixatives have the fault of shrinking the axis cylinder to a thin thread.)

2. Myelin sheath.

The axon is surrounded by a tubular *myelin sheath,* containing fatty *myelin.*
In a fresh fiber the sheath is glistening, white and highly refractive.
> Its presence is responsible for the 'white substance' of the spinal cord and brain.
> Myelin is more fluid than the axoplasm of the axon itself.
> > Postmortem changes quickly break down the labile myelin into droplets.
Myelin is a mixture of complex lipids and protein.
> It is dissolved out by lipid solvents (ether, alcohol, etc.).
> Osmic acid blackens myelin; hematoxylin, after bichromation, also stains it well.
Electron microscopic studies prove that the myelin sheath is modified neurolemma.
> It represents an infolded plasma membrane, fused into a layered spiral wrapping.
> A dense layer and a double, less dense layer alternate throughout the spiral.
> > These layers represent protein and lipid, as in the plasma membrane.
> As many as 50 layers may spiral around the axon, jelly-roll fashion.
The tubular sheath is interrupted at intervals of 0.08 to 0.6 mm.
> This produces constrictions along the fiber, called the *nodes of Ranvier.*
> The total fiber resembles a sausage-chain, whose 'links' are *internodal segments.*
> > Their length is proportional to the length and thickness of a fiber.
Deceptive, false interruptions are the *incisures* or clefts (of Schmidt-Lantermann).
> These oblique, circular clefts subdivide the myelin sheath into *myelin segments.*
> Actually they represent regions where local separations occur between the layers.
> Such slanting segments fit together funnel-fashion; they arise as shearing defects.
A spongy framework is visible in the sheath after myelin extraction during processing.
> This *neurokeratin network* is a precipitated and insoluble protein fraction.
The insulating function of myelin has been inferred; some facts are now known.
> The speed of impulse conduction is correlated with the degree of myelination.

3. Neurolemma.

The *neurolemma* is the toughest and most rigid part of a nerve fiber.
> It dips inward at the nodes and there touches the axon.
> Actually the sheath consists of a series of separate, linked units.
> > Each unit is a single cell that extends the distance between two nodes.
The ordinary microscope shows this neurolemma (or *sheath of Schwann*) as a long, thin
> tube, but this is only a more superficial portion of the whole sheath.

Intervening between it and the axon is that modified portion, the myelin sheath.
The neurolemma is transparent and refractive; it displays little obvious structure.
At the exposed surface there is a plasma membrane, encased by a basal lamina.
Just within the plasma membrane lies a thin, discontinuous layer of cytoplasm.
It is represented best about midway between two nodes.
Here is also located a single nucleus—oval and somewhat flattened.
From this center the cytoplasm radiates in interconnecting strands.
The electron microscope reveals that a developing sheath cell wraps about the axon.
Fusion of directly apposed plasma membranes creates a spiral lamination.
Myelin replaces the cytoplasm except at the two ends *(mesaxons)* of the sheath.
Sheath cells are ectodermal; they originate from primitive neural-crest tissue.
In the central nervous system, oligodendroglia substitute for sheath cells.
They ensheathe the axon and produce a similar spiral of myelin.
The neurolemma is essential to the life and functioning of a peripheral fiber.
Besides being protective and myelin-forming, it may have a nutritive role.
On occasion the cells are proliferative; they are important in nerve regeneration.

4. Appearance in sections.

A. LONGITUDINAL SECTION.

The fibers are pale bands, often of considerable width, grouped in bundles.
(Both smooth muscle and collagenous fibers take ordinary stains better.)
The myelin sheath is pale, but may show a network of neurokeratin.
Neurolemma nuclei are elongate and numerous.
Axons show as axial, well spaced threads when fibers are cut along the center.
They are acidophilic; with silver techniques they are brown to black.
Osmic acid stains the myelin sheath, which shows as parallel, blackened bands.
Within an unstretched fiber-bundle (fascicle) fibers take a zig-zag course.

B. TRANSVERSE SECTION.

The neurolemma shows externally as a sharply defined line about a fiber.
Occasionally a neurolemma nucleus is included, causing a local bulge.
The myelin sheath is a thick, usually unstained (or practically empty) ring.
Osmic acid stains the sheath, which then shows as a blackened ring.
The axon is a small, acidophilic central spot; it is blackened by silver methods.
With osmic preservation the axon is relatively large and the myelin ring thin.
The bundling of fibers to make a circular, ensheathed fascicle is distinctive.
(Neither smooth muscle nor tendon duplicates this arrangement.)
On changing the microscopical focus, a nerve fiber (myelinated or not) maintains its
size and remains in focus; artifacts usually do not.
That is, a fiber extends through the entire thickness of the section.
The images of the fibers often shift position on focusing.
This is because the zig-zagging fibers pass slantingly through the section.

B. UNMYELINATED FIBERS:

These are sometimes called by an older name, *Remak's fibers.*
In fresh, teased preparations they appear to be gray-colored strands, 1 to 2 μ thick.
Ordinary staining shows only plain bands, nucleated at intervals.
Actually each band is a bundle of fine axons, within a common neurolemma sheath.
Apparently every fiber is supplied with some myelin, even though too thin to see or stain.
This view is supported by studies with x-ray diffraction and the polarizing microscope.

1. Axon.

Several axons course together as a compound fiber-cluster.
The group as a whole shares a common neurolemmal ensheathment.
An axon is so slender (0.3 to 1.0 μ) that only the electron microscope reveals details.
Its structure is essentially like that of a myelinated axon (p. 115).

2. *Neurolemma.*

This is a strand made of neural crest cells, arranged in single file.

Each strand contains several to many tiny tubular grooves, opening to the exterior.

Coursing in each channel, and filling it, is an individual axon.

The neck of the channel constitutes a mesentery-like *mesaxon.*

Rarely there is a solitary fiber with an individual sheath.

Encasing the neurolemma cell is a basal lamina.

3. *Appearance in sections.*

Ordinary staining methods color unmyelinated fibers but palely.

Methylene blue or silver techniques demonstrate axons clearly.

A. LONGITUDINAL SECTION.

A compound 'fiber' is a pale band with prominent, elongate nuclei at intervals.

These sheath nuclei seem to occupy the full fiber breadth and interrupt it.

The fibers are grouped in a long bundle (fascicle), paler than connective tissue.

In silver preparations, the axis cylinders are fine, black, crowded threads.

B. TRANSVERSE SECTION.

Individual, compound 'fibers' appear as small, pale, circular areas.

Nuclei, when encountered, are rounded and prominent.

In silver preparations each axon shows as a black dot; these occur in clusters.

The fibers are contained in definite fascicles, ensheathed with connective tissue.

This collagenous tissue colors more deeply with routine stains than do axons.

C. NERVE AS AN ORGAN:

A peripheral nerve, taken as a whole, is an organ (as is a muscle, tendon or bone).

It has, therefore, a distinctive pattern of organization.

Nerves are surpassed only by blood vessels in a wide distribution throughout the body.

1. *Structural plan.*

Individual nerve fibers are separated by fine collagenous fibers.

This interstitial connective tissue comprises the *endoneurium.*

That portion of it closest to each nerve fiber adheres to the neurolemma.

It constitutes a reticulo-gelatinous covering that is named *Henle's sheath.*

Nerve fibers are gathered into distinct *fascicles* (or funiculi), like a wire cable.

A single fascicle may contain up to several thousand nerve fibers.

Each fascicle is enclosed within a dense fibrous sheath, named the *perineurium.*

Wings from the perineurium often invade a fascicle; each is a *perineurial septum.*

These anticipate a separation into smaller fascicles, somewhat distad.

Fascicles are bundled together as a *nerve*, or nerve trunk.

This is accomplished by loose areolar tissue, designated as *epineurium.*

It contains fat cells, blood vessels, lymphatics and some nerve fibers.

Most nerves consist of several to many fascicles; tiny nerves may have but one.

Nerve trunks frequently branch by the divergence and separation of intact fascicles.

Each subgroup then serves as a separate, smaller trunk.

Also fascicles themselves may branch, subdividing into smaller fascicles.

Through the branching and recombination of fascicles, *nerve plexuses* are created.

Most peripheral nerves are mixed, containing both myelinated and unmyelinated fibers.

As a nerve branches progressively, it finally forms twigs, either sensory or motor.

The color of a fresh nerve depends on the nature of its component fibers.

Cranio-spinal nerves appear white because of their dominant myelinated fibers.

Autonomic nerves appear gray because of their unmyelinated fibers.

2. *Vessels and nerves.*

Blood vessels and *lymphatics* course in the epineurial tissue.

Blood vessels pierce the perineurium and form capillary plexuses in the endoneurium.

Nerve twigs in the epineurium supply fibers to the blood vessels related to fascicles.

Such vasomotor fibers are called *nervi nervorum.*

3. *Appearance in sections.*

Except for its smaller branches, a nerve consists of a number of fascicles.

These are embedded in loose connective tissue and spaced well apart.

The fascicles are distinctive because they are regularly cylindrical and firmly ensheathed.

In transverse section they are circular (not angular, as in muscle and tendon).

VII. THE SYNAPSE AND OTHER ENDINGS

The axonal process of many nerve cells ends in relation to another neuron (or neurons).

Such an association constitutes the *synapse,* a local region of impulse transference.

Other axonal terminations are on muscle or glands, where activation is brought about.

Axons (functional dendrons) of ganglion cells serve as receptors of sensory excitation.

Some of these endings are attuned to general sensibility; others serve the special senses.

1. *The synapse.*

This is a specialization for communication between an axon and another neuron.

The contact usually is between an axon and the cell body or its dendrons.

The form of the axonal ending at a synapse exhibits many variations.

Commonly these endings swell into tiny, pear-shaped end-bulbs (or *boutons*).

They usually lack neurofibrils, but contain numerous mitochondria and a multitude of tiny *synaptic vesicles,* located near the region of contact.

Other types are *baskets* or *sprays* that course along a dendron of another cell.

In every instance the association of the two neurons is intimate, but one of contact only.

Actually the junction consists of two thin membranes, only 0.02 μ apart.

These are specialized portions of the plasma membrane of each synapsing neuron.

Some neurons receive only a few terminations; others receive many thousands.

A single axon may supply more than one ending on a second neuron, and on others.

But many neurons may contribute to the total number of synapses on a second neuron.

The possible combinations of communication between neurons are countless.

Nerve impulses pass equally well in either direction along a neuron.

It is the excited synapse that exerts a dynamic polarization.

It acts like a one-way valve, so the impulse continues in one direction only.

This is from an axon to the dendrons or to the cell body of the next neuron.

A chemical agent acts as a mediator in the excitation of a second neuron.

This substance is highly concentrated in the presynaptic end-bulbs.

It is perhaps stored in the innumerable synaptic vesicles located there.

The arrival of a nervous impulse liberates this chemical mediator.

For example, *acetylcholine* is the transmitter that activates skeletal muscle.

Norepinephrine and serotonin are other neurotransmitting agents.

2. *Motor peripheral endings.*

Terminations on all types of muscle have already been discussed (pp. 100, 105, 108).

Endings on glandular epithelium are described on p. 169.

3. *Sensory peripheral endings.*

These receptors occur in relation to epithelium, connective tissue, muscle and tendon.

Some are related to general sensibility and others to the special senses.

They will be treated in Chapter XXV, which deals with sense organs of all kinds.

VIII. AUXILIARY TISSUES OF THE NERVOUS SYSTEM

A. NEUROLEMMA AND CAPSULE CELLS:

These ensheathing elements of peripheral neurons are ectodermal (neural crest) in origin.

They form a continuous layer over ganglion cells and peripheral fibers (pp. 111, 115, 117).

B. EPENDYMA:

The non-nervous, *ependymal cells* are derived from the ectoderm of the neural tube.
They remain, much like an epithelium, lining the cavities of the brain and spinal cord.
Embryonic ependyma is ciliated, and some cells may retain cilia permanently.
At the free end there are *microvilli*; the cytoplasm contains glia-type *fibrils*.
Radiating from the central cavity, the cell tapers and ends within the neural wall.
The tapering end may branch; it becomes a long, thread-like process.
In some regions the cells are specially modified, as in the choroid plexuses (p. 123).

C. NEUROGLIA:

Non-nervous auxiliary cells, of ectodermal origin, occur within the neural wall.
These *neuroglia* substitute for connective tissue, which only follows blood vessels.
There are three main types, demonstrated well only by special selective techniques.

1. Astroglia (or astrocytes).

This group consists of star-shaped cells with branching processes, hence the name.
A. PROTOPLASMIC ASTROCYTE.
It occurs chiefly in the gray substance of the brain and spinal cord.
The cell body bears fairly thick processes which branch repeatedly.
Both cell body and processes contain granular cytoplasm.
Some processes attach to blood vessels by expanded *perivascular feet*.
Some smaller astrocytes act as satellite cells about neuronal cell bodies.
B. FIBROUS ASTROCYTE.
It occurs chiefly between the fiber tracts of the white substance.
The cell bears fewer but longer processes than the protoplasmic type.
They are thinner, straighter and branch but little; some attach to vessels.
Long, unbranched fibrils (bundles of filaments) develop within the cytoplasm.

2. Oligodendroglia (or oligodendrocytes).

These elements are the commonest type of neuroglia.
They are more abundant in the white substance where they ensheath nerve fibers.
In the gray substance they serve as satellites to the cell bodies of neurons.
There is scanty cytoplasm about the nucleus, and but few cell processes.
The processes are small, beaded and not much branched.

3. Microglia.

These cells are invaders of mesenchymal origin (possibly transformed monocytes).
Microglia are more abundant in gray substance than in white.
They occur near nerve cells and blood vessels.
Their nucleus is small; it is elongate or irregular, and stains darkly.
The cytoplasm is scanty, but is drawn out at opposite ends of the cell.
These end-processes branch twistingly and are thorny in appearance.

D. APPEARANCE IN SECTIONS:

After ordinary staining many relatively small nuclei show in the central system.
They lack visible nucleoli, and thus differ from the nuclei of nerve cells.
Astrocytes have the largest, palest, oval nuclei and may show some cytoplasm.
Oligodendroglia have smaller, somewhat darker, rounded nuclei—often in rows.
Microglia have small, irregular to elongate nuclei, the darkest of all.
With the Golgi technique, two types of cell are demonstrated.
Spider cells (astrocytes) have long, branching, radiating processes.
Mossy cells (oligodendroglia; microglia) have short, varicose processes.
With the silver carbonate technique, individual characteristics are revealed faithfully.
The cell types and their diagnostic features are as described above.

E. FUNCTIONAL CORRELATIONS:

Ependyma subserves a supporting role, at least in the fetal brain and cord.
Neuroglia constitute an interstitial, proliferative, auxiliary tissue of the central system.

They are suspected of playing an important role in the metabolic activities of neurons.
They react in definite ways when neurons are affected by a pathological process.

Among others, they proliferate and substitute for destroyed tissue.
Astrocytes are supporting elements, with apparent isolating functions, as well.

Both types have processes in intimate contact with capillaries.

They may aid in the *blood-brain barrier* that regulates exchanges between the two.
Small astrocytes serve as satellites to nerve cells.
Oligodendroglia substitute as sheath cells to the nerve fibers of the brain and cord.
Microglia can become migratory and highly phagocytic elements.

They are the macrophages of the central nervous system.

IX. MICROSCOPIC ANATOMY OF THE BRAIN AND CORD

Aggregations of nerve cells constitute the *gray substance* of the brain and spinal cord.

Nerve cells with a common purpose occur in functional groups, named *nuclei.*
Intermediate regions, rich in nerve fibers, comprise the *white substance.*

Fibers carrying out the same function course in bundles called *tracts.*
The organization of the central system, as to both general architecture and structural details, has
become the specific property of a branch of anatomy known as *neurology.*
Since these topics are treated in special textbooks, no duplication will be attempted here.

X. NERVE STAINS

Ordinary stained sections do not yield satisfactory information on most details.

Neither will any single, special stain serve as an all-purpose method.
Hence individual techniques have been devised to reveal the various neuronal features.

Neurohistology records the composite information gained through their use.

1. Basic dyes.

Dyes, such as *cresyl violet,* stain well the Nissl substance and all nuclei.

Chromatolysis (p. 110), following axon injury, is used to identify cells of origin.

In this way the cells belonging to definite fiber tracts can be traced.
Methylene blue is excellent as a supravital stain for the axon and nerve endings.
Hematoxylin, following mordanting in potassium bichromate, stains myelin.

The myelin sheath colors deep blue; all other tissue elements remain unstained.

2. Silver reduction methods.

A. GOLGI METHODS produce a coarse, black deposit of a silver salt.

The tissue itself is the prime reducing agent, but the response is commonly spotty.
Those neurons that do respond often are delineated in their entirety.

External form, but not internal structure, is made visible in exquisite detail.
Neuroglia also are sometimes demonstrated.
B. CAJAL METHODS utilize photographic developers as reducing agents.

The entire neuron is impregnated with a reduced silver compound.

Cells (including their neurofibrils) and fibers color brown to black.
A modification, by Nauta, colors normal axons brown and degenerating axons black.
C. SILVER CARBONATE REDUCTION, followed by gold toning, is used as a neuroglia stain.

The result is a selective staining of neuroglia and microglia.

3. Osmic acid.

This reagent oxidizes, blackens and renders myelin insoluble.

Combined with potassium bichromate, it blackens the myelin droplets of degenerating
fibers, whereas the myelin of healthy fibers colors yellow.

This method (of *Marchi*) is used in tracing the course of fibers distal to an injury.

XI. PROLIFERATIVE AND REGULATORY ABILITIES

Neuroglia, neurolemma and capsule cells can proliferate throughout the life-span.
By contrast, neuroblasts lose all reproductive power shortly after birth.
   Thereafter neurons are not replaced if destroyed, but can repair a reasonable injury.
      This is especially true of injuries to cell processes in the peripheral nerves.
         A course of degeneration is then followed by gradual restoration (see beyond).
         A corresponding regeneration of nerve fibers does not occur in the central system.
A nerve cell can also regulate derangement of its internal organization.
   Example: recovery from chromatolysis and its related phenomena.
As an adaptive response, a nerve cell can even alter its external form.
   This occurs when its environmental relations change and a readjustment is required.
A *transplant* is made when the ends of a damaged nerve cannot be brought together.
   Neurolemma cells of an autogenous graft seem to survive and proliferate.
   Regeneration then tends to follow the ordinary course of events.
   The main complication is that downgrowing fibers have to pass two sutured regions.

XII. DEGENERATION AND REGENERATION OF PERIPHERAL NERVES

Cutting or crushing a peripheral nerve fiber leads to changes known as *primary degeneration.*
   Both of the ends (central and peripheral), injured by direct trauma, are involved.
   This primary degeneration extends only a short distance from the point of injury.
Within a few days, however, the entire peripheral portion of the fiber is affected.
   This is *secondary degeneration,* or 'Wallerian degeneration.'
   It is a necessary sequel to a trophic separation of an axon from its cell body.
   However, the sheath cells of this portion survive and assist in the regeneration.

1. *Changes in peripheral (disconnected) portion.*

The axons swell, fragment within 3 to 5 days, and largely disappear after 8 to 10 days.
Within a few days after injury, the myelin of fibers fragments into oval portions.
The liquefied remains of axons and myelin are removed by phagocytic ingestion.
   This is carried out by macrophages which invade the neurolemma tubes.
At the end of one week the neurolemma-sheath cells begin to proliferate.
   By the seventeenth day thickened cords (*band fibers*) of sheath-cell result.
      Several may lie within the endoneurial tube that enclosed a former nerve fiber.
   At this time there is little or no degeneration-debris (axonal or myelin) left.

2. *Changes in cell body.*

Most striking is chromatolysis of the Nissl substance (called the *axon reaction*).
   This begins one day after the injury and reaches a maximum in 14 days (p. 110).
   Other features are marked swelling of the cell, peripheral displacement of its nucleus,
      and disruption and dispersal of the Golgi apparatus.
Restitution to normal consumes several months, slowly reversing the alterations incurred.

3. *Changes in central stump.*

Primary degeneration proceeds toward the cell over about two internodal segments.
Within a week after injury, the end of the living axon thickens into a growing tip.
   Many fine branches sprout from such a tip and grow peripherally.
   In man these regenerating axons grow 3 to 4 mm. each day.
Growth across the early scar tissue at the wound-site is guided by sheath cells.
   These cells have proliferated from both cut surfaces of the nerve.
   Some regenerating axons go astray here and never reach the peripheral, degenerated
      portion of the nerve.

4. Restitution of the peripheral portion.

Successful axons enter the endoneurial tubes, following their walls or the surface of the band fiber (or fibers) within each tube.

Later the band fibers enclose them, and again become a neurolemma sheath.

Several to many new axons may enter a single endoneurial tube.

But eventually only one of them persists as the permanent axon.

Some of the axons are inappropriate for the particular termination reached.

For example, a motor axon may attempt to innervate a sensory corpuscle.

Slowly the regenerated axon regains its former diameter.

The total task of cytoplasmic regeneration is formidable.

A single regenerating fiber to the leg may produce axoplasm having a volume 250 times that of the parent cell body.

Myelin sheaths reappear early, but are slow in regaining their former thickness.

5. Additional data.

Unmyelinated fibers of the peripheral system undergo a similar regenerative course.

The only difference is the nonparticipation of a myelin sheath.

In the central nervous system of mammals, regeneration is insignificant.

Sheath cells, as such, are lacking; their guiding role may be a crucial need.

XIII. MEMBRANES AND VESSELS OF THE BRAIN AND SPINAL CORD

A. MENINGES:

The brain and cord are encased within the bony cranium and spinal column.

They are more directly enveloped by fibrous coverings named *meninges*.

The free surfaces of these layers are covered with a simple squamous epithelium.

It is a type that has been called mesenchymal epithelium (p. 34).

1. Dura mater.

This outermost membrane is a separate cylindrical layer about the spinal cord.

In the region of the brain it becomes more or less intimately joined to the internal periosteum of the cranium.

The thick *dura* consists of somewhat vascular, dense fibrous tissue.

The inner surface is covered with a simple squamous epithelium.

It faces upon a thin *subdural space* located between it and the arachnoid.

The outer, free surface (in the extent corresponding to the spinal cord) is also covered with a similar layer of simple squamous epithelium.

It is separated from vertebral periosteum by the *epidural space*.

2. Arachnoid.

This is a thin layer of nonvascular connective tissue, beneath the subdural space.

The *arachnoid* is covered on both surfaces with simple squamous epithelium.

From the main layer, columns extend inward to join the pia mater.

This cobwebby tissue gives the arachnoid (*i.e.*, spider's web) its name.

In the opposite direction stocky *arachnoid villi* project into the dural sinuses.

The local dura, covering this intruding villus, is thin (see beyond).

The labyrinth between the pillar-like columns is the *subarachnoid space*.

3. Pia mater.

The *pia* is a delicate, highly vascular layer of connective tissue.

Its external surface is covered with simple squamous epithelium.

Here also attach the fibrous columns of the arachnoid.

The union is so intimate that the two membranes are often mentioned together.

The single unit is then called the *pia-arachnoid*.

Its internal surface, facing the brain and cord, is bound down by astrocytes.
    Hence it follows all external contours of these parts faithfully.

B. VESSELS AND NERVES:

Arteries pass from the pia mater into the solid substance of the brain and cord.
    Capillary meshworks are denser in the gray substance than in the white.
        Here endothelial cells exhibit tight junctions, thereby preserving a *blood-brain
            barrier.*
            This barrier restricts exchanges between the blood and brain-substance.
Returning *veins* reach the pia, perforate it and open into the *dural sinuses.*
    These are venous collecting channels located within thicker regions of the dura.
There are no *lymphatic vessels* in the central nervous system.
The dura and pia are richly supplied with *nerves.*
    Some are autonomic fibers that innervate blood vessels.
    Others are sensory fibers ending in relation to sensory receptors.

C. CHOROID PLEXUS:

Four regions of the brain have a thin, non-nervous (primitively dorsal) wall.
    These regions are the lateral ventricles and the third and fourth ventricles.
Here the brain wall consists of a single layer of cuboidal ependymal cells.
    This layer conforms to all the characteristics of a simple epithelium.
    Its free surface is supplied with microvilli whose tips are bulbous.
    The basal surface is infolded, as characterizes cells engaged in fluid transport.
Supporting the ependymal sheet is a layer of highly specialized pia mater.
    The combined membrane constitutes a *tela chorioidea.*
The pia sends out capillary loops, pushing the ependymal layer into elevated folds.
    The total vascular complex (tela plus local tufts) is a *choroid plexus.*
The plexuses secrete *cerebro-spinal fluid* into the ventricles.
    From the fourth ventricle the fluid escapes into the subarachnoid spaces.
    Much, at least, passes directly into the dural sinuses through *arachnoid villi.*
        These are stubby projections of the arachnoid membrane into the dural sinuses.
Cerebro-spinal fluid contains proteins (traces), salts and a few leucocytes (mostly
            lymphocytes).
    It fills and surrounds the brain and cord, acting like a shock-absorber for them.

PART III

Special Histology (Organology)

Foreword on the Nature and Origin of Organs

The study of organs is designated as *special histology,* or *organology.*

It is the science that deals with organ architecture and tissue adaptations.

It is clear that both cytology and histology are fundamentally different from organology.

Cytology and *histology* deal with the nature of actual building materials (cells; tissues).

Organology is concerned largely with how the tissues, as structural units, arrange themselves to make associated composites with distinctive architectural patterns.

Yet it also deals with the specialization of tissues for particular work to be done.

Organogenesis describes the developmental courses undergone in the creation of organs.

An *organ* is a somewhat independent portion of the body, performing a specific function.

It is an aggregate of tissues, arranged in a characteristic structural plan.

One tissue is primary in functional importance; others are auxiliary and secondary.

Example: the lining epithelium of the stomach (and the glands outgrown from it) is the primary component; the connective tissue, muscular coat and peritoneal covering are secondary components, or auxiliary features.

In a few organs there is more than one kind of primary functional tissue.

Example: suprarenal cortex and medulla; testis epithelium and interstitial tissue.

A typical organ has a fibrous *framework,* and often an enveloping fibrous *capsule.*

It also has its individual supply of blood, lymph and nerves.

The essential, characteristic, functional cells of an organ are called its *parenchyma.*

By contrast, the internal, auxiliary, supporting tissue is the *stroma.*

Example: the epithelium of a gland is parenchyma; the connective-tissue bed is stroma.

Several types of simple organs have been treated already in the consideration of tissues.

Such are bones, muscles, tendons and nerves.

In general, the functional tissue of organs has a large factor of safety.

Removal of considerable tissue is usually compatible with life.

Example: suprarenal, 90%; pancreas, thyroid, 80%; liver, 75%; kidney, 67%; lungs, 50%.

An *organ system* is a set of organs that collaborate in carrying out related functions.

The component organs sometimes display certain similarities of structure.

Example: nervous system; digestive system; endocrine system.

Naming the germ-layer origin of an organ states the source of the primary tissue only.

Example: the stomach is said to be entodermal because its lining is such; the kidney is said to be mesodermal because its tubules are such.

A few organs are composites, with important parts differing in origin.

Example: suprarenal gland has a mesodermal cortex and ectodermal medulla; teeth have ectodermal enamel, but other parts are mesodermal.

The following table summarizes germ-layer origins for the various organs or organ systems:

DERIVATIVES OF PRIMARY GERM LAYERS

Ectoderm	Mesoderm	Endoderm
Epidermis	Epithelium of:	Epithelium of:
Cutaneous derivatives	Circulatory system	Pharynx
Hairs; nails; glands	Urinary system	Tonsil; adenoid
Epithelium of:	Genital system	Thyroid; thymus
Mouth	Body cavities	Parathyroid
Oral glands; enamel	Connective tissues	Digestive tube
Nasal passages	Blood; bone marrow	Liver; pancreas
Sense organs	Muscular tissues	Respiratory tract
Central nervous system	Skeletal tissues	Larynx; trachea; lung
Peripheral nervous system	Spleen; lymph nodes	Urinary bladder; urethra
Hypophysis; suprarenal medulla	Suprarenal cortex	Vestibule; vagina

Chapter XIII

The Circulatory System

The *circulatory system* includes the heart, blood vessels and lymphatics.
> The heart and blood vessels, alone, comprise the *cardio-vascular system*.
> The major feature, shared by all these parts, is a lining of endothelium.

Blood vessels (and, usually, lymphatics) enter into the composition of all organs.
> Because of this role as building units they are often referred to as *vascular tissue*.
> Actually they are fairly simple organs that invade other organs and nourish them.

In vertebrates the cardio-vascular system is a complete circuit of closed tubes.
> The *heart* is a blood vessel, specialized as a powerful pumping organ.
> *Arteries* conduct blood from the heart to the capillary bed.
>> The quality of blood is not a factor; it may be either rich or poor in oxygen.
> The *capillaries* form a meshwork of the smallest-sized vessels.
> *Veins* return blood from the capillaries to the heart.
>> The blood may be rich in oxygen (pulmonary vein) or deficient (venae cavae).

Lymphatics are vessels that return fluid (lymph) from tissue spaces to the blood stream.
> It is a one-way flow, draining lymphatic networks and blind-end capillaries.

The circulatory system conducts nutrients, oxygen and hormones to all parts of the body.
> It also collects metabolic wastes from the tissues and transports them to the kidneys.
> It is the chief integrator of the various other systems in the body.

The concept of a complete circuit of the blood was enunciated by Harvey (1628).
> Yet the actual demonstration of capillaries came somewhat later (Malpighi, 1661).

I. THE BLOOD VESSELS

The clearest approach is to start with the fundamental and simplest vessel, the capillary.
> Afterward the addition of accessory coats can be traced progressively in larger vessels.

A. CAPILLARIES:

These are bare, endothelial tubes, interconnecting terminal arterioles and venules.
> The name, meaning 'hair-like,' is descriptively appropriate.

Their length in muscle totals some 60,000 miles and presents 1.8 acres of surface.

The total cross-sectional area of the capillary system is 800 times that of the aorta.
> Hence the rate of flow is only 0.4 mm. per second; (aorta, 320 mm. per second).
> A comparison is a fairly stagnant pond and its swift supplying and draining streams.

Structurally capillaries are the fundamental vascular unit, devoid of accessory coats.

1. Size.

The average capillary is about 8μ in diameter.
> This bore will allow red blood corpuscles to pass in single file.

A resting, collapsed capillary is narrower than when blood flows through it.

2. Arrangement.

Capillaries take the form of communicating canals, nearly uniform in caliber.

The pattern may be that of a flattened net or a spongy meshwork.

This is an adaptation to the character of the region supplied.
Commonly the mesh is isodiametric, as in the lung and mesentery.
In elongate structures, like muscle fibers, the mesh is diamond-shaped.
The intensity of metabolism in a region determines the closeness of the mesh.
There is a close network with narrow interspaces in the lung, glands, brain, etc.
There is a sparse network in tendon, nerve, smooth muscle, etc.

3. Structure.

The cells and their nuclei are elongate, and oriented in the long axis of the vessel
Cell margins are usually wavy (*i.e.,* interlocking), and tend to overlap.
Cell boundaries (intercellular cement?) are blackened by silver nitrate.
An endothelial cell is a thin curving plate, bulging in the vicinity of the nucleus.
The cylindrical lining at any level consists of only one to three cells.
The cells are staggered so that their wide and narrow parts alternate.
The cell base rests upon a very thin basal lamina.
The cytoplasm contains tiny closed vesicles; others open on the lumen or exterior.
These are *pinocytotic vesicles;* they apparently transport materials across the cell.
In some body-regions, the cells have extremely thin local areas, or actual pores.
Such locations are notable for participation in fluid transport.
Example: choroid plexus; intestine; endocrines; renal glomerulus.
In other regions the cells lack pores and fit close together; some have tight junctions.
Example: muscle; connective tissue; lung; brain.
Capillaries course through a supporting bed of connective tissue.
Yet this tissue does not furnish any real wall for the capillary.
Only a delicate, reticular network ensheathes the endothelial tube.
Capillaries are accompanied by fixed macrophages and reserve mesenchymal cells.
These *pericytes* are applied to the wall, but do not control the size of the lumen.

4. Diagnostic features.

A capillary is a tiny tube, often collapsed and unnoticed in sections.
Its wall is so thin (less than $1\ \mu$) that it appears as a mere line.
The nuclei, however, make local, bead-like bulges.
They resemble fibroblast nuclei, but lack the prominent nucleolus.
The vessel is embedded in connective tissue, yet this is not a part of the wall.
In longitudinal section a capillary takes the form of two parallel, beaded lines.
The lumen (unlike lymphatic capillaries) maintains a rather uniform bore.
In transverse section a capillary is a thin ring, with or without a nucleus showing.
In most instances the caliber has been reduced somewhat by shrinkage.
It is usually not larger than a red blood corpuscle.
The section resembles, in miniature, a sectioned fat cell.

5. Functional correlations.

Capillaries are functionally the most important of all blood vessels.
They lie in intimate relation to the various tissue elements.
Hence they can deliver nutrients and oxygen, and receive wastes.
They are the vessels at the scene of action of cellular metabolism.
In general, their uptake from the tissue spaces is soluble crystalloids.
Their thin wall and sluggish current are favorable for diffusive interchanges.
Blood pressure and colloid osmotic pressure are important factors.
The endothelium of capillaries seems to lack any power of spontaneous contraction.
Its adaptation to the changing blood-flow is a passive stretch and recovery.
Flow through the capillaries of resting tissues is intermittent.
In active tissues the endothelial area in contact with blood increases greatly.
Capillaries, even when lacking 'pores,' are quite permeable.
Water, gases, salts and some nutrients can pass through cell junctions.
Most colloids and all microscopic particulate matter do not pass normally.

Transport across the cell itself may be accomplished by pinocytotic vesicles.
Permeability varies regionally; under changed conditions it also varies locally.
Blood cells are permitted to pass through endothelium on occasion.
They push a pseudopod between endothelial cells, and the whole cell follows.
Endothelium prevents the coagulation of blood while it is within vessels.
True endothelial cells are not normally phagocytic.
Capillary endothelium can proliferate; it does, for example, in healing wounds.

B. FALSE CAPILLARIES:

Certain other tiny channels resemble capillaries in some general respects.
They possess, however, distinctive features not characteristic of capillaries.

1. Sinusoids.

These passages comprise a special set of channels, set between larger vessels.
Some connect arteriole with venule (spleen; bone marrow).
Others connect venule with venule (liver; hypophysis).
This intermediary relation is similar to the rete mirabile (see below).
Still others interconnect lymphatic vessels (lymph nodes).
Sinusoids have several unique features that specifically characterize them.
They are relatively broad (up to 30 μ), and irregular in caliber.
The lining cells lie in close apposition to the surrounding parenchyma.
A basement membrane is lacking; only a network of reticular fibrils intervenes.
The lining of certain sinusoids (liver; bone marrow) has gaps between some cells.
Cell outlines are not demonstrated with silver, as are those of endothelium (p. 128).
The cells are fixed macrophages, with pronounced phagocytic ability.
They belong to the so-called *reticulo-endothelial* (or *macrophage*) *system* (p. 47).
The lining of other sinusoids (hypophysis; suprarenal) is true endothelium.
Their cells make a complete lining, and they are not phagocytic.
The cells have extremely thin regions that can be mistaken for actual pores.
Perhaps *sinusoidal capillaries* would be a more suitable name for these vessels.

2. Rete mirabile.

This is a capillary-like plexus inserted in the course of an arteriole or venule.
It is a 'marvelous network' because an afferent arteriole (or venule) feeds blood to it and an efferent arteriole (or venule) drains it.
Retia are uncommon in mammals; an arteriolar example is the renal glomerulus.
Analogous vessels are the pituitary sinusoids that interconnect venules.

3. Diagnostic features.

Irregular, broad channels and a close relation to parenchyma suggest sinusoids.
These features, however, are shared by some capillaries (*e.g.*, parathyroid).
The discontinuous macrophages are not easily identifiable as such.
The final proof is physiological—their ability to ingest particulate matter.
A rete mirabile is indistinguishable from ordinary capillaries.

C. PRECAPILLARIES; POSTCAPILLARIES:

These terms designate vessels intermediate between capillaries and arterioles or venules.
They are larger than capillaries and have incomplete accessory coats.

1. Precapillaries.

These vessels are located on the arterial side of the capillary bed.
They are larger than the largest capillaries (12 μ), but less than 40 μ in diameter.
The smallest consist of an endothelial tube and some smooth-muscle fibers.
The muscle fibers encircle the tube, but are scattered.
The largest add connective tissue cells and fibers discontinuously.

2. Postcapillaries.

These vessels are located on the venous side of the capillary bed.
Their maximum diameter is 200 μ.
The smallest consist of endothelium and scattered connective-tissue elements.
Larger tubes also add smooth-muscle fibers discontinuously.

3. Diagnostic features.

Sections that miss the accessory elements resemble oversized, bare capillaries.
Sections that include accessory elements may still fail to show complete coats.
(The presence of complete coats in a tiny vessel signifies arteriole or venule.)

4. Functional correlations.

Pre- and postcapillaries show how blood vessels acquire clearly defined coats.
With the addition of connective tissue, mechanical support is given a vessel.
With the addition of smooth muscle, control of vessel-size becomes possible.
Such *precapillary sphincters* control the flow through capillary beds.
Local beds are even intermittently closed-off in resting tissues.
The main precapillary, feeding a local area, is never completely closed.
It is called a *preferred channel* or a *thoroughfare channel*.
Postcapillaries are more permeable in blood-tissue exchanges than are capillaries.

D. STRUCTURAL PLAN OF BLOOD VESSELS:

All blood vessels, above precapillaries, follow a common plan of organization.
Each specific type of vessel merely shows adaptations for particular purposes.
Certain features of the common plan are emphasized, reduced or omitted.
Certain new features may be introduced to meet local mechanical requirements.
Every typical blood vessel contains three concentric coats (*i.e.*, *tunics*).
1. *Tunica intima* (or interna).
2. *Tunica media.*
3. *Tunica adventitia* (or externa).

1. Tunica intima.

An *endothelium* (simple squamous epithelium) bounds the *lumen*, or central canal.
It rests upon a thin basement membrane of the ordinary sort.
A *subendothelial coat* underlies the endothelium.
This is composed of delicate fibro-elastic tissue, mostly longitudinal.
The *internal elastic membrane* is the outermost component of the intima.
It is typically a fenestrated membrane (*i.e.*, a tube with 'windows').
Sometimes it splits into two or more layers.
On the other hand, the 'membrane' may be reduced to a simple network of fibers.
In an empty or contracted vessel the membrane folds.
These longitudinal wrinkles show as a wavy line in transverse sections.

2. Tunica media.

The primary constituent is smooth muscle, 'circularly arranged.'
Actually the short and often branched fibers make a tight spiral.
Elastic fibers are commonly added, but in variable quantities.
They sometimes occur as fibrous networks, spirally disposed.
The highest development is a series of concentric 'tubes,' perforated with openings.
Networks or tubes alternate with muscle in a layered fashion.
Collagenous fibers occur also in an amorphous, mucopolysaccharide ground substance.

3. Tunica adventitia.

Next to the media, elastic tissue commonly concentrates as an *external elastic layer*.

Closest to the media there may be a definite *external elastic membrane*.
Elsewhere the fibers are often preponderately longitudinal.
The remainder of the adventitial coat is composed of moderately compact fibro-elastic tissue, whose fibers take a predominantly longitudinal (or loose spiral) course.
It acts to restrain the expansile media and interna.
The adventitia grades off into the areolar tissue, nearby.
The latter always accompanies, guys and supports blood vessels.

4. Vasa vasorum.

Blood vessels more than 1 mm. in diameter have nutrient vessels.
These are *vasa vasorum*, which means 'vessels of vessels.'
In arteries they supply the adventitia and are mostly limited to it.
In veins they may penetrate deeper and extend through the media.
This is correlated with the poor quality of blood flowing in veins.
Some claim that the nutrient vessels of veins often drain into the main lumen.
Lymphatics are present in the walls of larger blood vessels.

5. Nerves.

Unmyelinated nerve fibers form networks beneath the adventitia and terminate on the smooth muscle of the media; they are *vasomotor fibers*.
Myelinated *sensory fibers* arborize in the adventitia.

E. ARTERIES:

Arterial blood vessels can be classified into three groups:
1. *Arterioles;* the smallest-sized vessels; predominantly muscular vessels.
2. *Small to medium-sized arteries*; predominantly muscular vessels.
3. *Large arteries*; predominantly elastic vessels.
These divisions are arbitrary and have no sharp limits.
The transition from the elastic to the muscular type is usually gradual.
Intermediate vessels mingle the features, producing a *mixed type* of artery.
Example: external carotid; axillary; common iliac.
On the other hand, the transition may be rather abrupt.
Example: abdominal aorta and its visceral branches.
Furthermore, size and composition are not always typically correlated.
Vessels of smaller caliber may resemble larger arteries.
Example: popliteal; tibial.
Vessels of rather large size may resemble smaller arteries.
Example: radial; celiac; external iliac.

1. Arterioles.

These vessels, as a group, are invisible to the naked eye, or nearly so.
Their diameter lies between about 0.04 mm. and 0.3 mm.
The wall is thicker, relative to the lumen, than in any other blood vessel.
A. TUNICA INTIMA.
This layer is thin; there is no recognizable subendothelial tissue.
The internal elastic membrane is really a network of fibers.
Yet, in sections, it often looks like a true membrane.
B. TUNICA MEDIA.
The media is purely muscular except for a few reticular fibers.
There are 1 to 5 layers of muscle cells; it is the most prominent coat.
C. TUNICA ADVENTITIA.
This fibro-elastic coat is usually thinner than the media.
There is no definite external elastic layer or membrane.

2. *Small and medium-sized arteries.*

This group comprises all arteries belonging to a category called the *muscular type.*
Included are most of the arteries that bear names, and all small unnamed ones.
The smallest are the size of a thin thread.
   A. TUNICA INTIMA.
      A subendothelial layer is represented, but may be very thin.
      The internal elastic membrane is prominent and fenestrated.
         In older individuals it frequently splits locally into two (or more) layers.
   B. TUNICA MEDIA.
      The thick tunica media is predominantly a muscular layer (up to 40 layers).
      The smaller vessels do not have a significant amount of elastic tissue.
      Larger vessels have some elastic tissue arranged in networks.
         In the largest examples of this group, true elastic membranes occur.
         A small amount of thin, collagenous fibers can also be identified.
   C. TUNICA ADVENTITIA.
      Although sometimes thick, it usually only equals the media, or is thinner.
      Bordering on the media there is an elastic layer.
         In arteries not subject to stretching it is weakly represented.
         Nearest the media there is commonly an actual external elastic membrane.
            This is similar in appearance to the internal elastic membrane.
      Outside the elastic layer, the adventitia is chiefly collagenous.

3. *Large arteries.*

This group comprises all arteries that belong to a category called the *elastic type.*
   The elastic tissue is sufficient to color the freshly cut wall yellow.
Included are the aorta and its largest main branches.
      These are the brachio-cephalic, common carotid, subclavian (including its vertebral
         and internal thoracic branches), and common iliac.
The wall is relatively thin in comparison to the large lumen.
   A. TUNICA INTIMA.
      The endothelial cells are polygonal (not elongate, as in smaller vessels).
      The subendothelial layer is thick, with many elastic fibers and some smooth muscle.
      An internal elastic membrane is not a particularly distinctive feature.
         Similar membranes are distributed throughout the media.
   B. TUNICA MEDIA.
      This thickest tunic is composed mainly of elastic and collagenous tissue.
         Hence a large part of these main arteries is nonliving substance.
      In the aorta there are 40 to 60 spiralling elastic membranes, each about 2.5 μ thick.
         Each lamella consists of broad, interwoven bands with prominent gaps.
         Neighboring lamellae frequently connect by slanting bands.
      Interspaces between the concentric membranes contain fibroblasts, an amorphous
         ground substance, fibro-elastic tissue and sparse muscle cells.
   C. TUNICA ADVENTITIA.
      This layer is relatively thin and not highly organized.
      There is no distinctive external elastic layer or membrane.
         The outermost fenestrated membrane could be said to serve this purpose.
      The collagenous fibers take longitudinally spiral courses.
      The adventitia restrains the expansile media and intima from over-distension.

4. *Specialized arteries.*

Some arteries deviate considerably from the generalized plan already described.
      These reflect adaptations to special locations and functional demands.
The intima may contain longitudinal muscle.
      Example: occipital; uterine; palmar.
The media may contain muscle in two layers (inner, longitudinal; outer, circular).
      Example: superior mesenteric; splenic; renal.

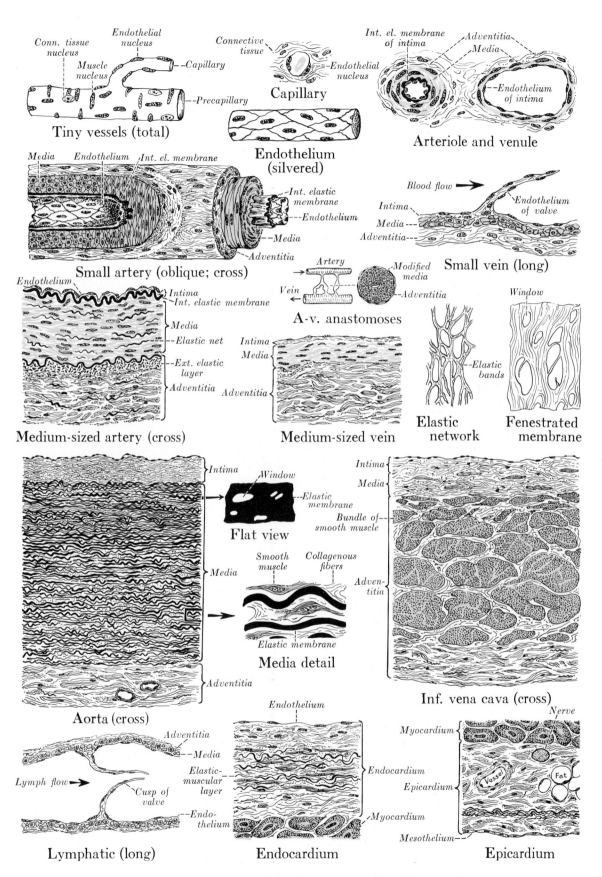

Tiny vessels (total)

Conn. tissue nucleus · *Muscle nucleus* · *Endothelial nucleus* · *Capillary* · *Precapillary*

Capillary

Connective tissue · *Endothelial nucleus*

Endothelium (silvered)

Arteriole and venule

Int. el. membrane of intima · *Adventitia* · *Media* · *Endothelium of intima*

Small artery (oblique; cross)

Media · *Endothelium* · *Int. el. membrane* · *Int. elastic membrane* · *Endothelium* · *Media* · *Adventitia*

Small vein (long)

Blood flow · *Endothelium of valve* · *Intima* · *Media* · *Adventitia*

A-v. anastomoses

Artery · *Vein* · *Modified media* · *Adventitia*

Medium-sized artery (cross)

Endothelium · *Intima* · *Int. elastic membrane* · *Media* · *Elastic net* · *Ext. elastic layer* · *Adventitia*

Medium-sized vein

Intima · *Media* · *Adventitia*

Elastic network

Elastic bands

Fenestrated membrane

Window

Aorta (cross)

Intima · *Media* · *Adventitia*

Flat view

Window · *Elastic membrane*

Media detail

Smooth muscle · *Collagenous fibers* · *Elastic membrane*

Inf. vena cava (cross)

Intima · *Media* · *Bundle of smooth muscle* · *Adventitia*

Lymphatic (long)

Adventitia · *Media* · *Lymph flow* · *Cusp of valve*

Endocardium

Endothelium · *Elastic-muscular layer* · *Endocardium* · *Endo-thelium* · *Myocardium*

Epicardium

Nerve · *Myocardium* · *Vessel* · *Fat* · *Epicardium* · *Mesothelium*

THE CIRCULATORY ORGANS

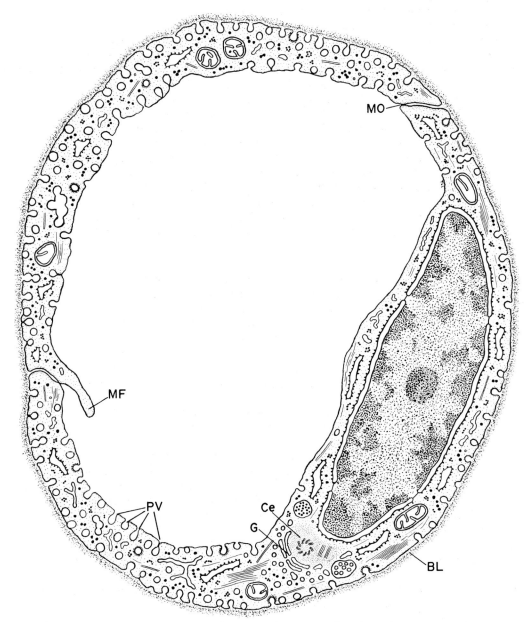

CAPILLARY.   This ordinary, unfenestrated capillary shows two endothelial cells meeting evenly on the right, with an overlapping marginal fold (MF) on the left. The abutting membranes fuse locally as tight junctions (MO). The nuclear membrane is interrupted by 'pores' and bears ribosomes. Nearby are a pair of centrioles (Ce), a Golgi membranous stack (G) and two multivesicular bodies. The cytoplasm also contains some smooth and rough endoplasmic reticulum, free ribosomes, small mitochondria, microtubules and filaments. The plasma membrane at both surfaces bears many invaginations, either open or detaching (PV), and similar free vesicles in the cytoplasm; they illustrate the mechanism of pinocytosis, transport and discharge. A basal lamina (BL) borders the external surface of each cell.

In general, arteries subjected to bending are reinforced by longitudinal and oblique muscle in the media; sometimes also by longitudinal muscle in the intima.

Example: common carotid; axillary; common iliac; popliteal.

The adventitia may contain longitudinal muscle.

Example: lingual; renal; splenic.

The wall may be relatively thin, with a reduction of some components.

In the pulmonary arteries this is correlated with lower blood pressure.

Arteries protected within the skull have the adventitia reduced, whereas elastic tissue is almost restricted to a thick internal elastic membrane.

Elastic tissue is highly developed in the renal and popliteal arteries.

By contrast, it is practically lacking in the umbilical arteries.

Cardiac muscle extends into the roots of the aorta and pulmonary artery.

Some small arteries contain longitudinal thickenings of the tunica intima.

Example: penile; prostatic; renal; thyroid; umbilical; nipple; nasal mucosa.

These are produced by prominent local concentrations of smooth muscle.

Such intimal cushions control blood flow by occluding the lumen.

Some specializations are associated with arrival at sexual maturity.

The deep penile arteries have longitudinal muscle in the intima.

Uterine arteries vary with the menstrual cycle and alter irreversibly in pregnancy.

5. Age changes.

Each artery has its characteristic pattern and schedule of change.

An early manifestation is an increase of connective tissue elements in the intima.

As the intima becomes thick, the internal elastic membrane fragments.

In elastic arteries the chief change is irregular thickenings in the intima.

In muscular arteries the chief change is calcification of the media.

6. Diagnostic features.

The following entries summarize the general characteristics of the arterial wall.

A. TUNICA INTIMA.

This ranges from very thin (arterioles) to fairly thick (elastic arteries).

An internal elastic membrane is always present, even in the smallest arterioles.

B. TUNICA MEDIA.

This middle coat equals, or exceeds, the adventitia in thickness.

In arterioles and small to medium-sized arteries it is dominantly muscular.

In the larger arteries of this category the media becomes increasingly elastic.

Elastic membranes and muscle layers then tend to alternate.

The largest arteries are dominantly elastic, having many elastic membranes.

C. TUNICA ADVENTITIA.

The external tunic is thinner than the media in arterioles and small arteries.

It equals, or nearly equals, the media-thickness in medium-sized arteries.

It is much thinner than the media in the largest arteries.

An elastic layer or external elastic membrane is present in many examples.

Exceptions are arterioles, some muscular arteries and aorta types.

D. OTHER FEATURES.

The wall is a robust tube, but its relative thickness varies.

The smaller an artery, the thicker is its wall (compared to the lumen).

Rigor mortis contractions tend to empty blood from the arterial lumen.

Hence sections of the arteries usually do not show much blood.

Thick elastic membranes are easily seen, even when unstained.

Fine networks are demonstrable only with special stains.

Most of the characteristics of arteries reflect a pressure-of-blood influence.

7. Functional correlations.

The heart delivers blood to the aorta in spurts and under considerable pressure.

The aorta and its elastic branches have two functions.

One is to expand as it receives more blood than it can otherwise contain.

This intermittent response to overfilling stores latent energy.

The second is to relax the stretched walls while the heart is filling again.

This passive return to unstretched elastic tissue releases kinetic energy.

It produces a more constant pressure and smoother flow of blood.

The elastic arteries are often termed *conducting arteries*.

This term emphasizes their conducting or 'piping' function.

The muscular arteries are able to regulate the amount of blood delivered to any part of the body, according to its changing needs.

This is done through nervous control of the muscle in the tunica media.

Hence these arteries are also called *distributing arteries*.

The arterioles have relatively thick walls and narrow lumina.

They are the prime controllers of systemic blood pressure and of local flow.

Hence only a gentle stream escapes into the delicate capillary beds.

Most of the fall in pressure occurs within the arterioles.

8. Carotid body.

Each is a small mass located at the bifurcation of a common carotid artery.

It contains epithelioid cells, dilated capillaries and many nerve fibers.

It is a sensory chemo-receptor in relation to the adjoining carotid sinus.

Similar masses, the *aortic bodies,* lie in relation to the arch of the aorta.

These organs are responsive to a reduction in the oxygen tension of the blood.

They play the important role of initiating respiratory reflexes.

F. VEINS:

Venous blood vessels are usually grouped into three classes:

1. Venules.

2. Small to medium-sized veins.

3. Large veins.

These divisions are often unsatisfactory as rigid categories.

Size and structure are not always well correlated.

There is more individual variation within a size-group than occurs in arteries.

Also the same vein may change structurally along its course.

Hence detailed generalizations are not so practical as with arteries.

1. Venules.

The diameter of these vessels lies between 0.2 and 1.0 mm.

A. TUNICA INTIMA.

The internal tunic is nothing more than an endothelium and its basement membrane.

(A subendothelial layer and internal elastic membrane are lacking.)

B. TUNICA MEDIA.

This is a very thin tunic, composed almost exclusively of smooth muscle.

Muscle cells are only 1 to 3 layers deep; elastic fibers are scanty or lacking.

C. TUNICA ADVENTITIA.

It is relatively thick in comparison to the very thin total wall.

This layer consists almost wholly of collagenous fibers, largely longitudinal.

2. Small and medium-sized veins.

The diameter ranges from 1 to 9 mm.

Included are: cutaneous branches; deeper veins of the forearm and leg; veins of the head, trunk and viscera (except main vessels and their tributaries).

A. TUNICA INTIMA.

Endothelial cells of veins of this size (and larger) have a short, polygonal shape.

The subendothelial layer is delicate and often lacking.

Bundles of longitudinal smooth muscle fibers occur in some vessels.

Elastic fibers vary from absence to a dense, net-like internal membrane.
Frequently this tunic is not clearly demarcated from the media.
B. TUNICA MEDIA.
Usually this is a weak layer; smooth muscle often occurs in plate-like bundles.
These muscle-masses are separated by collagenous fibers and elastic nets.
The media is best developed in the veins of the limbs (especially lower).
C. TUNICA ADVENTITIA.
This well developed, fibro-elastic coat forms the greater part of the wall.
Its inner region often contains some longitudinal smooth muscle.
There is no tendency to develop an external elastic layer or membrane.

3. *Large veins.*

This type includes: superior and inferior vena cava; portal vein.
Also the main tributaries to these trunks (including the upper arm and thigh).
A. TUNICA INTIMA.
The subendothelial layer is thicker than in smaller vessels.
It may contain scattered bundles of longitudinal muscle.
An internal elastic membrane is sometimes present, but is relatively delicate.
B. TUNICA MEDIA.
The smooth muscle is much reduced and may even be lacking (venae cavae).
At best this tunic is a relatively thin and feeble coat.
C. TUNICA ADVENTITIA.
This is by far the thickest of the three coats.
In it occur usually prominent bundles of smooth muscle, longitudinally arranged.
This muscle may occupy almost all of an extremely broad tunic.
There is no external elastic layer or membrane.

4. *Valves.*

Many small and medium-sized veins are provided with pocket-like valves.
They are especially well represented in the limbs.
They are absent in the cranium, and sparse in the thorax and abdomen.
Valves usually occur in pairs, facing each other on opposite sides of the lumen.
The free edges point in the direction of blood flow (*i.e.,* toward the heart).
They are usually located just distal to the entry of a tributary vein.
This position is favorable to prevent backflow (away from the heart).
Also they aid in moving blood toward the heart when veins become squeezed.
This occurs in many locations where veins lie between contracting muscles.
Structurally a valve is produced by a local folding of the intimal tunic.
Internally it contains a network of elastic fibers on the side facing the lumen.
It is covered with endothelium on both surfaces.

5. *Specialized veins.*

Some veins lack smooth muscle, and so are without a media.
Example: cerebral; meningeal; dural sinuses; veins of the retina, bones, splenic trabeculae and maternal placenta.
Some veins are rich in muscle.
Example: suprarenal; umbilical; uterine (of pregnancy); limbs (especially lower).
Some veins have muscle in all three coats.
Example: uterine (of pregnancy).
Longitudinal muscle bundles occur in the intima of some veins.
Example: limbs (some); mesenteric; uterine (of pregnancy); internal jugular.
Longitudinal muscle may occur in the internal layers of the media.
Example: limbs (some); umbilical.
Longitudinal muscle may constitute the bulk of the adventitia.
Example: veins of the belly cavity.
Longitudinal muscle may constitute all the muscle content.
Example: superior vena cava; inferior vena cava (in part).

Cardiac muscle extends for a distance into the adventitia.
Example: venae cavae; pulmonary.

6. Arterio-venous anastomoses.

In certain regions, arterioles and venules connect directly by cross-connections.
In such a bridge, endothelium lies directly on a specialized tunica media.
Modified smooth-muscle cells have become short and thick, forming a sphincter.
In section they resemble a stratified cuboidal epithelium.
The thick wall resembles an arteriole more than it does a venule.
One type of location for these anastomoses is the skin of exposed parts of the body.
Example: palm; sole; terminal phalanges; lips; nose; eyelids.
A second site is in tissues where metabolic activity is intermittent.
Example: mucous membrane of the gastro-intestinal tract; thyroid gland.
When the shunt is closed, arterial blood passes through the regular capillary bed.
When open, much of the blood by-passes directly across to the venule.
They can regulate venous pressure and serve organs having an intermittent function.
In exposed parts they can serve as protective devices.
They can increase the heat-loss and also prevent excessive local chilling.
COCCYGEAL BODY
This is a small mass, 2.5 mm. wide, located at the tip of the coccyx.
It consists of a group of arterio-venous anastomoses, with epithelioid muscle.
They are embedded in connective tissue representing an adventitial coat.
No special function is attributable to the coccygeal body.

7. Diagnostic features.

The following entries summarize the general characteristics of the venous wall.
A. TUNICA INTIMA.
In general, this tunic is thin.
Bundles of longitudinal muscle are present in some vessels.
This is especially true in large vessels.
An internal elastic membrane is an inconstant feature, never present in venules.
B. TUNICA MEDIA.
Smooth muscle and elastic tissue are relatively deficient.
The smooth muscle occurs mostly in flat bundles, circularly disposed.
C. TUNICA ADVENTITIA.
This is typically the thickest layer of a vein.
It commonly contains longitudinal bundles of smooth muscle.
An external elastic layer or membrane is lacking in all examples.
D. OTHER FEATURES.
The three tunics are frequently without clear boundaries.
The media, in particular, may not be distinguishable as such.
Collagenous tissue occurs in excess of all others.
The wall tends to be thin as compared with the size of the lumen.
It is loosely organized and flabby; hence an empty vein tends to collapse.
However, veins are often held open by accumulated blood.
(Venules packed with blood somewhat mimic nerve fascicles.)
The characteristics of veins are correlated with low pressure of their blood.

8. Functional correlations.

Blood in the venous system is under a pressure only one-tenth that in the aorta.
Hence it travels slowly, yet must replace the blood pumped out of the heart.
This is accomplished by using more vessels with relatively large lumens.
Since the venous pressure is low, thin walls are adequate.
Since the flow is constant, elastic tissue (for pulse absorption) is little needed.
Since veins do not control blood distribution, circular muscle is relatively sparse.
Longitudinal muscle is featured undoubtedly as a useful functional adaptation.

The proper interpretation of its specific local role is not wholly clear.

Raising blood against gravity is aided by the presence of valves.

Valves are more commonly present in vessels subject to external pressure or influenced by muscular movements.

Thin, weak walls correlate with the compression of veins by neighboring muscles.

This compressibility is a factor in promoting the venous circulation.

Also veins are easily distended; sometimes they act as reservoirs for blood.

G. REGENERATIVE ABILITY:

Blood vessels repair their local injuries and also participate in wound healing.

Vessels send solid endothelial sprouts into regenerating areas.

The sprouts hollow out; fibroblasts are at hand and myoblasts soon differentiate.

Accessory coats are laid down about the new endothelial tubes, as needed.

Transplanted segments of vessels, not from the same individual, are replaced slowly.

Endothelium grows into both ends and, meeting, serves as a first bridge.

Collagen then replaces all but the elastic tissue in the three coats.

Transplanted segments from the same individual remain as permanent replacements.

H. COMPARISON OF AN ARTERY AND VEIN OF THE SAME SIZE:

Paired vessels, encountered in sections, are usually identified easily as artery or vein.

Direct comparisons are then facilitated, especially in transverse sections.

But when a vessel is cut lengthwise, its mate often is not included.

Moreover, some structural features show to poor advantage in this plane.

The lumen of an artery is always smaller than that of its companion vein.

(Or the combined lumen of the companion veins, if there are two of these.)

The arterial wall is thicker and more rigid.

It holds its shape better and is less likely to collapse.

An artery is better supplied with elastic and muscular tissues.

Hence the media of an artery is usually the thickest coat.

Stronger postmortem contraction tends to force blood from the lumen.

Even the smallest arteries (arterioles) have a distinct internal elastic membrane.

Only some veins, larger than venules, are so supplied.

A vein is more loosely constructed than an artery and varies more from type.

The three tunics often lack clear boundaries.

Especially is the media inconspicuous or even absent.

The wall of a vein is relatively thin and its lumen relatively large.

A vein has collagenous tissue in excess of muscle and elastic tissue.

Hence the adventitia is usually the thickest coat.

Weaker postmortem contraction leaves blood in the lumen of a vein.

If blood has been drained away, veins collapse and the lumen becomes slit-like.

Veins are sometimes supplied with valves; arteries never have them.

However, valves are infrequently encountered in random sections of veins.

II. THE HEART

The heart is a highly specialized blood vessel that pumps 4000 gallons of blood daily.

There are the usual three coats of a blood vessel, but a distinctive name is given to each.

1. Endocardium.

The internal coat is homologous to a tunica intima.

Endothelium lies next to the central cavity of the heart.

The subendothelial layer is a thin sheet of fine white fibers.

With endothelium, it continues into the intima of vessels connecting with the heart.

Still deeper is a thick layer of fibro-elastic tissue and some smooth muscle fibers.

Farthest from the lumen is a loose connective-tissue layer.

This *subendocardial layer* binds the endocardium proper to the myocardium.
In the ventricles it contains the modified muscle of the impulse-conducting system.

2. Myocardium.

This is a middle coat that corresponds to the tunica media.
It is composed of cardiac muscle, much thicker in the ventricles than in the atria.
The *trabeculae carneae* are the only remnants of an embryonic spongy condition.
Cardiac muscle is arranged in dissectible sheets, separated by some fibrous tissue.
These wind around the atria and ventricles in complex, spiraling courses.
The spaces between muscle fibers contain reticular, collagenous and elastic fibers.
This endomysial tissue also carries vessels and nerves.

3. Epicardium.

The external coat is a serous membrane that substitutes for the tunica adventitia.
It is surfaced with mesothelium and supported by a thin fibro-elastic layer.
It affords a smooth, wet, slippery surface that minimizes friction.
Elastic fibers pass into the adventitia of vessels entering and leaving the heart.
A *subepicardial layer,* composed of areolar tissue, contains vessels, nerves and fat.
It attaches the epicardium to the myocardium.

4. Cardiac skeleton.

The central support of the heart is dense fibrous tissue, the *cardiac skeleton.*
It is a continuous 'fibrous base' on which cardiac muscle and valves insert.
The system consists mostly of two sets of *fibrous rings* related to two *fibrous triangles.*
One pair of rings surrounds the origin of the aorta and pulmonary artery.
Another pair surrounds the atrio-ventricular canals and joins the ventricular septum.
Both prevent these outlets from dilating when blood is forced through.
In old age the cardiac skeleton may calcify locally; it may even ossify.

5. Valves.

There are reduplications of endocardium about the cardiac orifices.
Each valve-fold is supported by an internal plate of dense fibro-elastic tissue.
At the base of a fold this fibrous tissue is continuous with a fibrous ring.
The ring is a component of the cardiac skeleton, already described.
The *bicuspid* and *tricuspid valves* connect with papillary muscles by fibrous cords.
These *chordae tendinae* attach to the free borders of the cusps.
Such guys restrain the cusps from everting when the ventricles contract.
The *semilunar valves* of the aorta and pulmonary artery have three cusps each.
The central, fibrous plate forms a thickening (*nodule*) at the free border of a cusp.

6. Impulse-conducting system.

Mammals possess a system of cardiac muscle fibers, specialized for impulse conduction.
This system has the function of co-ordinating the heart beat.
There are two parts to this functionally integrated, neuroid system.
The *sino-atrial node* is at the junction of the superior vena cava and right atrium.
Its specialized muscle fibers are the seat of impulse formation for the atrial beat.
From it the impulse spreads through ordinary cardiac muscle fibers.
It serves as a 'pacemaker', since this wave stimulates ventricular contraction.
The *atrio-ventricular node* is located in the median wall of the right atrium.
Its position is just below the orifice of the coronary sinus.
A common stem from this node begins the so-called *atrio-ventricular bundle.*
This stem gives off a branching trunk to each ventricle.
Its terminal twigs become continuous with ordinary cardiac muscle fibers.
The modified muscle fibers of the nodes and bundle-system are alike.
They are large, rich in sarcoplasm and poor in myofibrils (*Purkinje fibers*).
The bundles of fibers are more or less ensheathed by connective tissue.
They lie in the subendocardium, close to the myocardium.

7. Vessels and nerves.

The *coronary arteries* supply the heart, and *cardiac veins* drain it.
>The myocardium is profusely furnished with capillaries.
>This supply is about twice as rich as in skeletal muscle.

Lymphatics are abundant and intimately associated with muscle fibers.
The *nerve supply* is from the vagus and the autonomic system.
>Their functions are antagonistic: vagus, inhibiting; sympathetic, accelerating.
>Both sensory and motor fibers are contributed by the vagus.
>Small autonomic ganglia occur in the heart substance.

8. Regenerative ability.

The heart repairs injuries that are incurred by wounding or disease.
>This is done by filling-in the defect with fibrous tissue.

The regenerative capacity of cardiac muscle itself is negligible.

9. Diagnostic features.

The heart does not lend itself easily to generalized, diagnostic characterization.
>This is partly because of its wide regional differences in organization.
>Also the large size of the organ does not permit inclusive sections to be made.

The myocardium is unmistakable because of its massive content of cardiac muscle.
>Any trace of it makes the diagnosis of epicardium or endocardium much easier.

Endocardium or epicardium alone is not especially distinctive, respectively, over the tunica intima of large vessels or some serosal membranes elsewhere.
>Fat, sometimes abundant in the epicardium, helps to identify it.
>Smooth muscle and absence of fat indicate endocardium rather than epicardium.

III. THE LYMPHATIC VESSELS

These are closed tubes that collect excess tissue fluid and conduct it as *lymph*.
>Lymph drainage is a one-way flow, not a circulation.

Distally, lymphatics form networks, whose capillaries end blindly or in loops in connective tissue.
Centrally, the converging lymphatic vessels empty into the great veins, near the heart.
Only a few organs lack lymphatic capillaries and larger vessels.
>Example: brain; spinal cord; eyeball; internal ear; bone marrow.

1. Capillaries.

Lymph capillaries are somewhat broader than blood capillaries.
>They are not uniform in caliber but bear dilatations and constrictions.
>They branch profusely and anastomose freely with one another.

The capillaries form dense networks, roughly co-extensive with blood capillaries.
>They often run in company with blood capillaries.

Near surfaces they frequently begin as loops or as blind, swollen tubules.
>Such surfaces are the skin and internal membranes.
>Here the lymphatic capillaries lie at a deeper level than do blood capillaries.

The wall is composed of endothelium alone, even lacking investing pericytes.
>The endothelial cells are large, thin and delicate; their junctions may bear gaps.
>Pinocytotic pits and vesicles occur; a basal lamina is discontinuous or absent.

2. Collecting vessels.

Lymphatics larger than capillaries have the endothelium reinforced by auxiliary tissue.
>These are connective tissue and scanty smooth muscle.

Vessels of about 0.3 mm. begin to have three tunics, and then resemble a vein.
>However, these coats are indistinct and poorly demarcated.
>Also, their walls tend to be thinner than a vein of equal size.

The largest of these collecting vessels are usually less than 1 mm. in diameter.

A. TUNICA INTIMA.

An endothelium lies upon a delicate network of longitudinal elastic fibers.

B. TUNICA MEDIA.

Smooth muscle occurs in thin layers: inner, circular; outer, longitudinal.

A few elastic fibers lie between muscle bundles.

C. TUNICA ADVENTITIA.

This thickest coat consists of interlacing, longitudinal collagenous and elastic fibers.

Peripheral fibers are continuous with those of adjacent connective tissue.

Longitudinal bundles of smooth muscle occur in the adventitia.

D. VALVES.

Lymphatic valves are much more closely spaced (up to 2 mm. apart) than in veins.

Between the valves the vessels are swollen, giving a beaded appearance.

They occur in opposed pairs, their free edges directed with the current flow.

A valve is a pocket, formed by a local fold of the tunica intima.

3. *Main lymphatic trunks.*

These are the thoracic and the right lymphatic ducts, and their tributaries.

The structure is much like that of a vein of equal size.

But the three coats are even less distinctly demarcated.

Also, they vary more, at different levels, in thickness and internal organization.

The structure of the *thoracic duct* (4 to 6 mm. wide) is best known for details.

The *intima* has some longitudinal muscle and a thin, inconstant, elastic membrane.

It is well provided with valves; fibrous tissue supports the intimal fold.

The *media* is the thickest coat; it has more muscle than a vein of equal size.

The muscle occurs in well spaced bundles that have a circular arrangement.

The best organized vessels have inner and outer longitudinal layers also.

The *adventitia* is not well defined and blends into the adjacent connective tissue.

It contains a few bundles of longitudinal muscle.

4. *Blood vessels and nerves.*

Blood vessels supply the wall of the thoracic duct, much as they do in veins.

Nerve fibers, both motor and sensory, are found in the wall of larger vessels.

5. *Regenerative ability.*

Injuries to lymphatics can be replaced by outgrowths from existing capillary vessels.

The process is similar to that in blood vessels (p. 137), but slower.

6. *Diagnostic features.*

Capillaries are large and irregularly swollen, in contrast to blood capillaries.

Collecting vessels are thinner-walled than blood vessels of the same size.

Their tunics are less well defined; they are more subject to collapse.

Valves are encountered more frequently than in veins.

The vessel is commonly bulbous in the intervals between two sets of valves.

This feature is apparent in longitudinal sections only.

Collecting vessels often accompany an artery and vein.

There are often several in close association with a vein.

This makes comparison and diagnosis easier.

The main trunks (*i.e.*, thoracic duct) resemble a vein of equal size.

But they have more muscle in the media than do comparable veins.

It is mostly circular, but is broken into well spaced bundles.

The typical content in the lumen of lymphatics is a granular or fibrinous coagulum.

Lymphocytes occur sparingly; other leucocytes rarely; red corpuscles, almost never.

In clotted lymph the leucocytes tend to lie at the periphery of the clot.

7. *Functional correlations.*

Material, escaped from blood capillaries, must be returned to the blood stream.

Among these transudates in the tissue spaces there is some protein.

If left, such colloid would bind increasing amounts of water and produce edema.
Only lymphatic capillaries are able to recapture this colloid material.
Lymphatic capillaries also provide the chief route for uptake of particulate matter.
Moreover, they convey a larger part of the fat absorbed from the intestine.
In general, these vessels specialize in taking up substances of large molecular size.
Lack of a basement membrane and pinocytosis (p. 16) may assist this transport.
Flow is promoted by compression from adjoining muscles and pulsating blood vessels.
Among other possible factors, muscular propulsion by the vessel wall is uncertain.
The valves seem to be the dominant feature in controlling the direction of flow.
Valves also occur at the junction of the main trunks with systemic veins.
These act to prevent a backflow of blood into lymphatic trunks.
Injected dyes appear in the thoracic duct promptly (in 10 sec. from the foot of a dog).
Discharge from the human thoracic duct averages 1 ml. per min., but is variable.
The pressure is quite low in comparison to the blood pressure in veins.
Lymph, in its onward passage beyond capillaries, encounters interposed lymph nodes.
It percolates through these organs, thereby being filtered but gaining lymphocytes.
Lymphatic endothelium is not normally phagocytic.

Chapter XIV

The Lymphoid Organs

Certain regions or organs contain accumulations of a material called *lymphoid tissue.*
    Alternative names for this substance are *lymphatic tissue* and *adenoid tissue.*
Simpler types of organization are in close relation to epithelial membranes.
    Example: diffuse lymphoid tissue; solitary nodules; aggregate nodules; tonsils.
There are more highly organized structures that comprise separate organs.
    Example: lymph node; spleen; thymus.
All these can be arranged in a series based on increasing complexity of organization.

I. LYMPHOID TISSUE

Lymphoid tissue consists of two primary tissue-elements, intermingled in intimate association:
    (1) *Reticular tissue;* (2) *cells,* chiefly lymphocytes, in the reticular interstices.
The crowded lymphocytes tend to conceal the reticular-tissue component.
This common association of cells and reticulum makes a sort of elementary building material.
    Since it occurs in various organs, it is for convenience spoken of as a tissue.
    When it is dominant in an organ, such is called a *lymphoid organ.*
    Lymphoid tissue, as a whole, constitutes one of the largest tissue-masses of the body.
        Some believe it exceeds the liver in bulk, or is at least 1 per cent of body weight.
The reticular-tissue component has the structural features already described (p. 51).
    The *reticular cells* may seem to constitute a syncytium, but actually they only touch.
        Some have little cytoplasm and are relatively undifferentiated, like mesenchymal cells.
            These are the *primitive reticular cells.*
        Others have acquired more cytoplasm and have gained phagocytic abilities.
            These are *fixed macrophages* which, on detachment, become *free macrophages.*
            Both the fixed and free macrophages can increase by cell division.
    The *argyrophil fibers* are wrapped about, at least in part, by reticular cells.
The *free cells* are of several types.
    Commonest are the small lymphocytes.
        Medium-sized lymphocytes and large lymphocytes are much less abundant.
            Those of medium size are commonly called large when seen in circulating blood.
        Also all intergrades in size can be found in-between these three types.
    Large lymphocytes divide into medium-sized, and medium-sized into small lymphocytes.
        Small lymphocytes can then grow into larger forms, but this is uncommon.
    Free macrophages occur, especially in the sinuses of lymph nodes and in splenic pulp.
    Plasma cells and granulocytes are also found at times.

A. Diffuse Lymphoid Tissue:

    This is the simplest manifestation of lymphoid tissue.
    It occurs as an infiltration into the lamina propria of a mucous membrane.
        The chief locations of these lymphoid drifts are the alimentary and respiratory tracts.
        In the intestine the composite is not a pure lymphoid tissue.
            Collagenous and elastic fibers may be present also.
            Other cells, less typically associated (plasma cells; eosinophils), may occur.
    There is no special organization since the cell-fiber distribution is fairly uniform.
        Proliferation occurs, essentially in the manner to be described for the nodule.

B. LYMPH NODULES:

Other names in use are *lymphatic follicle* and *primary nodule*.
Nodules are dense aggregations of lymphoid tissue arranged in rounded masses.
  Such a mass (up to 2 mm. in diameter) is visible to the unaided eye.
Many occur as *solitary nodules*, most commonly embedded in diffuse lymphoid tissue.
  Example: in the intestinal lining there are some 30,000 of these nodules.
Others occur as components of specific lymphoid organs (tonsil; lymph node; spleen).
  Here they constitute a kind of structural building unit.

1. General features.

A nodule may be homogeneous throughout, the small lymphocyte predominating.
But often there is a darker-staining *cortex* and a lighter *germinal center*.
  The cortex consists of small lymphocytes, at times in concentric zones.
  The center consists mostly of cells that are larger and paler-staining.
The reticulum is denser in the cortex and is concentrically arranged there.
  This is caused by cells being crowded away from the center by growth.
  At the periphery the reticulum continues into that of adjacent diffuse tissue.
Lymph nodules are not constant features, either in structure or in position.
  They (and their centers) appear, remain for a time, and then disappear.
  New nodules may arise at any time or place in diffuse lymphatic tissue.

2. Germinal centers.

The lighter-staining *centers* (also called *secondary nodules*) are inconstant features.
  They arise after birth, decline in advancing years and lack in old age.
  They also appear and disappear periodically.
A typical center is rather sharply demarcated from the more peripheral cortex.
  It measures up to 1 mm. in diameter.
  Most of the cells are larger, with more cytoplasm and paler-staining nuclei.
    Hence, the whole central area appears lighter in stained sections.
Most of the free cells are medium-sized lymphocytes.
  These are the most actively dividing elements.
  Some large lymphocytes, macrophages and plasma cells are also seen.
Reticular-tissue cells are found here (and elsewhere) in the nodule.
  Their nuclei are pale, oval and wrinkled; the cytoplasm is not well defined.
  Occasionally these cells divide also.

3. Proliferative cycle.

Lymph nodules, in a state of relative rest, do not posses germinal centers.
  Such a nodule consists mainly of small lymphocytes.
But periodically the central cells may begin a phase of mitotic activity.
  The dominant central cells are proliferative, medium-sized lymphocytes.
    By growth some of them transform into large lymphocytes.
  Primitive reticular cells give rise to some medium-sized lymphocytes.
    This activity is in addition to their production of macrophages.
  Thus the *center* organizes and acquires its characteristics.
During an active phase, small lymphocytes are the most abundant product.
  They are mostly the daughter cells of the medium-sized lymphocytes.
  To a lesser degree they are derived from large lymphocytes.
  Also some trace origin indirectly to primitive reticular cells.
    This is through the latter elements giving rise to medium-sized lymphocytes.
These activities at the expanding center create pressure in a peripheral direction.
  The small lymphocytes, adjoining the center, are crowded into a peripheral zone.
  This compact region comes to be the *cortex*, well demarcated from the center.
After a time the center approaches a new period of inactivity.

Mitotic divisions diminish in frequency and finally come to a virtual halt.
Such an inactive center contains mostly reticular cells and macrophages.
As the center becomes inactive, the former growth pressure subsides.
This removes the sharp boundary between germinal center and cortex.
New small lymphocytes then mingle with older ones.
Thus the nodule may even return to a homogeneous state, without a center.
The formation of lymphocytes is not wholly confined to the center.
It occurs in the cortex and in diffuse lymphoid tissue as well.

4. Reaction centers.

In certain inflammatory states, nodules have central areas of a different kind.
The cells are free macrophages and reticular cells.
In such pale areas new lymphocytes are not being produced.
These areas are called *reaction centers*, created by toxic and other stimuli.
Reaction centers are frequently observed in the tonsil and appendix.

5. Vessels and nerves.

An *arteriole* and a *venule* supply the nodule, forming a peripheral plexus.
Another plexus supplies the germinal center, when this region is present.
Lymph capillaries envelop the exterior of the nodule, but do not invade it.
Nerve fibers are apparently all vasomotor.

6. Diagnostic features.

The darkly stained, basophilic mounds are prominent even to the naked eye.
Sections, outside the midplane, may fail to include the pale germinal center.
Such a section is unreliable evidence for or against the presence of a center.
Any rounded, sizable mass of lymphocytes is, however, recognizable as a nodule.
Reticular cells have pale, wrinkled nuclei; the cytoplasm is indistinct.
Indistinct cytoplasm is explained by its ensheathing relation to reticular fibers.
Medium-sized and large lymphocytes have nuclei with somewhat more chromatin.
Cytoplasm and its limits are plainer because these cells are free.
Small lymphocytes have checkered, dark nuclei and show little or no cytoplasm.

7. Functional correlations.

An obvious function of lymphoid tissue is the production of new lymphocytes.
Some of these cells migrate into blood capillaries.
Others enter the sinuses of lymph nodes and spleen in large quantities.
(Under abnormal conditions, lymphoid tissue can also produce granulocytes.)
Also plain are the phagocytic potentialities of free and fixed macrophages.
This activity is directed against bacteria, spent blood cells and foreign matter.
The macrophage system of lymphoid tissue filters tissue fluid, lymph or blood.
The particular fluid, so treated, depends on where the filtering is done.
Lymphocytes are believed to be associated with the production of immunity.
More specifically, plasma cells are the chief producer of antibodies.
It is the germinal center that seems to specialize in antibody production.

II. THE AGGREGATE NODULES

1. Structural plan.

These aggregations in the intestinal lining attain a small degree of organization.
Each is a closely grouped mass of lymph nodules that has fairly sharp limits.
Its appreciable size and its response to growth pressure produce a slight, visible bulge
(toward the lumen) in the intestinal lining.
These masses, also called *Peyer's patches*, are located primarily in the lamina propria.

They occur mainly in the ileum, but some may lie at higher levels.
A Peyer's patch is an oval group of closely associated, pear-shaped nodules.
   It is always located in a position opposite to the attachment of the mesentery.
   The long axis of a patch runs lengthwise of the intestine.
The total number of patches, larger than 25 sq. mm., is 25 to 50.
   They vary in size; a large patch can measure several centimeters in length.
   The lymph nodules of a fairly large patch will total into the hundreds.
      They lie close together and commonly show germinal centers.
The broad bases of the expanded nodules burst through the muscularis mucosae.
   They thus encroach on the submucosa and compress it.
      There is, however, no definite encapsulation of the massed nodules.
   The nodules commonly merge, except at their apices, thus becoming confluent.
The top of the nodule, facing the lumen, is covered with intestinal epithelium.
   This surface is smooth, because here the villi have been largely effaced.
   Emigrating lymphocytes infiltrate the epithelium profusely.
Intestinal glands are distorted or obliterated locally where nodules occur.
The patches are seemingly rather permanent until senile involution overtakes them.

2. *Diagnostic features.*

An aggregate of lymph nodules lies largely in the mucosa of the intestine.
   The superficial surface is covered by a simple columnar epithelium.
   The deep surface encroaches on the submucosa of the intestine.
Where nodules occur, the villi and glands tend to be suppressed through pressure.
   But remnants of these, or adjoining intact tissue, identify an intestinal site.

3. *Functional correlations.*

Aggregate nodules are supplied solely by efferent lymphatics.
   (The same is true of diffuse tissue, solitary nodules and tonsils.)
   All such serve as filterers of local tissue fluids.
No distinctive function can be ascribed to aggregate nodules.
   It is commonly said that they act in some way protectively against bacteria.
   Yet they are the chief seats of ulceration in typhoid fever and local tuberculosis.
Neither can their choice of the ileum as a preferred location be explained adequately.

III. THE TONSILS

Three tonsillar groups form a lymphoid ring about the entrance of the throat.
   There is structural similarity in all these types located in the mucous membrane.
Some advances in organization contrast with the simpler aggregate nodules.
   These are: epithelial inpocketings; encapsulation; and a coarse internal framework.

A. Palatine Tonsil:

The location of these organs is at the entrance to the throat, one on each side.
   Each tonsil lies between two arching folds of the pharynx.
   This relation gave the fanciful name of tonsilla, 'a mooring stake.'
A tonsil is ovoid, with its long axis paralleling the long axis of the body.
   Each measures about 1×0.5 in.
The medial surface is freely exposed, and sometimes bulging.
   This surface is studded with pits, which are mouths of distinctive pockets (*crypts*).

1. *Structural plan.*

A tonsil is a dense mass of diffuse and nodular lymphoid tissue.
   It is a specialized region of the pharyngeal mucous membrane.
It is loosely *encapsulated* and is subdivided by *septa*.

The free surface is covered with *epithelium,* continuous with that of the pharynx. Invaginated, epithelial pockets (called *crypts*) invade the tonsillar substance.

2. *Detailed structure.*

A. FRAMEWORK.

Fibrous tissue, adjacent to the deepest portions of the tonsil, is compacted.
This results from pressure from the expanding organ on the submucosa.
Such compressed tissue produces a poorly organized, thin *capsule.*
The capsule covers the base and most of the sides of the tonsil.
Continuations of the capsule extend, as *septa,* into the interior of the tonsil.
These plates separate incompletely some 10 to 20 regions.
Such regions, or *lobules,* have an individual crypt as an axis.
The fibrous septa bind the tonsil firmly to its capsule.
As a result, the tonsil can be removed surgically as a unit.
Various cell types are found in the septa: lymphocytes; mast cells; plasma cells.
Neutrophils, present in excess numbers, are indicative of inflammation.
Reticular fibers are continuous with the capsule and septa.
They permeate the parenchyma everywhere as a delicate, intimate support.

B. EPITHELIUM AND CRYPTS.

The free surface is covered with a *stratified squamous epithelium.*
This is continuous with the lining of the mouth and pharynx.
The epithelium rests upon a *basement membrane,* under which, in some places, there may be a little ordinary connective tissue.
About 40 epithelial *crypts* penetrate into the interior of the tonsil.
Some are simple tubules, but many branch complexly and extend far inward.
All open on the surface; only the larger ones are easily noticeable pits.
The lumen of a crypt contains material that may even form cheesy plugs.
Included are: emigrated lymphocytes and plasma cells (living and dead); desquamated epithelial cells; micro-organisms; cellular debris.
The surface area of the crypt systems of both tonsils totals some 90 sq. in.
This is twelve times the exposed surface-area of the entire pharynx.

C. LYMPHOID TISSUE.

The general *lymphoid tissue* is a fairly dense cellular mass.
It borders the surface epithelium in a layer 1 to 2 mm. thick.
This layer also follows the epithelium wherever it dips inward as crypts.
Hence a fold of lymphoid tissue is bordered by epithelium on the crypt side and by a connective-tissue septum on its deeper side.
(Slanting sections exaggerate the real thickness of the lymphoid layer.)
Lymph nodules occur abundantly in the general sheet of lymphoid tissue.
They usually lie in a single layer, paralleling the epithelium.
Germinal centers are unusually large; see *reaction centers* (p. 144).

D. LEUCOCYTIC INFILTRATION.

Emigrating lymphocytes are seen in the surface epithelium and especially within the epithelial lining of the crypts.
In addition, plasma cells and polymorphonuclear leucocytes may emigrate.
The invasion of the epithelium may involve only a scattering of lymphocytes.
By contrast, the infiltration is frequently so intense that many pockets form.
In this instance the epithelium is largely destroyed locally.
Usually, however, a few layers of cells remain at the original surface.
Also, the basement membrane is usually still recognizable.
Highly eroded and nearly intact areas of epithelium often exist side by side.
Many migrant-lymphocytes escape and appear in the saliva.
Added to other cells occurring there, they are known as *salivary corpuscles.*

E. ASSOCIATED STRUCTURES.

Mucous glands lie in the submucosa, beneath the tonsil and its capsule.
Their ducts empty into the cavity of the pharynx.

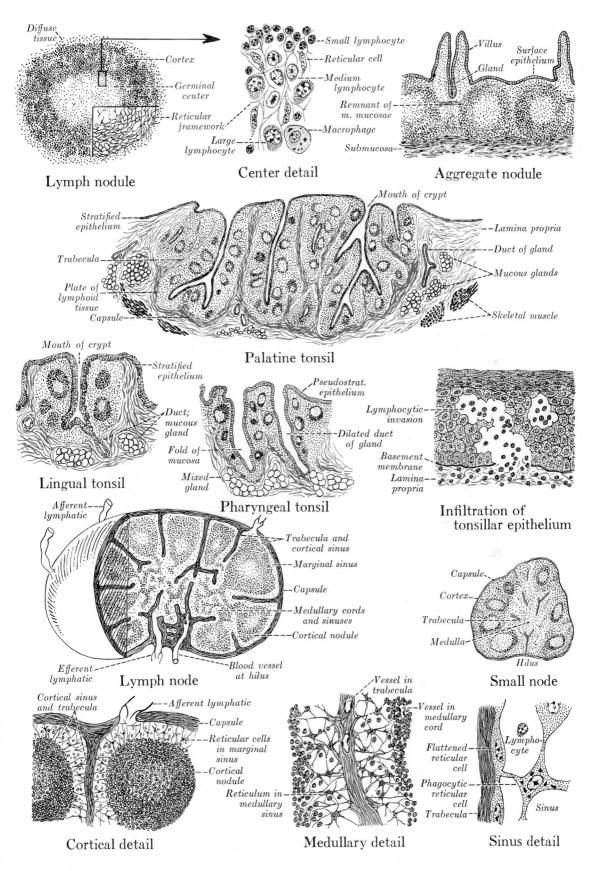

Diffuse tissue

Cortex

Germinal center

Reticular framework

Lymph nodule

Small lymphocyte

Reticular cell

Medium lymphocyte

Macrophage

Large lymphocyte

Center detail

Villus

Gland

Surface epithelium

Remnant of m. mucosae

Submucosa

Aggregate nodule

Stratified epithelium

Trabecula

Plate of lymphoid tissue

Capsule

Mouth of crypt

Lamina propria

Duct of gland

Mucous glands

Skeletal muscle

Palatine tonsil

Mouth of crypt

Stratified epithelium

Duct; mucous gland

Lingual tonsil

Pseudostrat. epithelium

Fold of mucosa

Dilated duct of gland

Mixed gland

Pharyngeal tonsil

Lymphocytic invasion

Basement membrane

Lamina propria

Infiltration of tonsillar epithelium

Afferent lymphatic

Trabecula and cortical sinus

Marginal sinus

Capsule

Medullary cords and sinuses

Cortical nodule

Efferent lymphatic

Blood vessel at hilus

Lymph node

Capsule

Cortex

Trabecula

Medulla

Hilus

Small node

Cortical sinus and trabecula

Afferent lymphatic

Capsule

Reticular cells in marginal sinus

Cortical nodule

Cortical detail

Vessel in trabecula

Vessel in medullary cord

Flattened reticular cell

Phagocytic reticular cell

Trabecula

Reticulum in medullary sinus

Medullary detail

Lympho cyte

Sinus

Sinus detail

SMALL LYMPHOID ORGANS

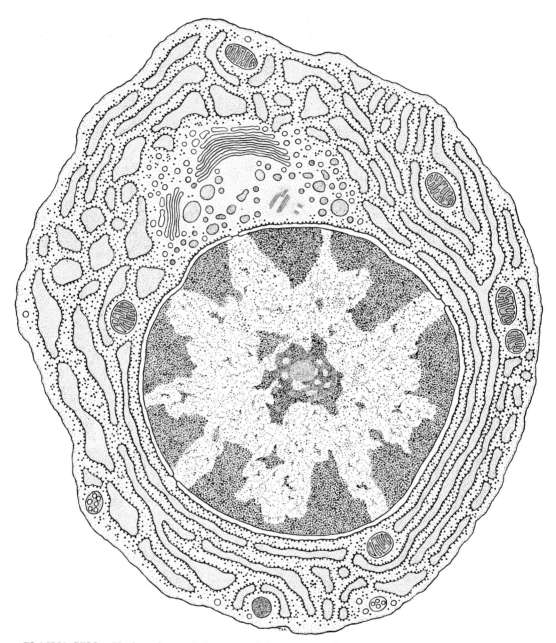

PLASMA CELL.   Nuclear chromatin is arranged characteristically in a central mass and in numerous radial masses at the double-layered, fenestrated nuclear membrane. The adjacent cytoplasm contains a pair of centrioles and, nearby, Golgi membranous stacks and vesicles. Rough endoplasmic reticulum is extensive and dilated with amorphous antibody-material. Between these cisternae are free ribosomes, mitochondria and an occasional lysosome or multivesicular body.

These openings are on the surface of a tonsil, or near its periphery.

Only rarely does a duct open into a crypt, and then near its mouth.

Skeletal muscle underlies the capsule and mucous glands.

A little of it may be encountered in sections of an excised tonsil.

Sometimes small islands of cartilage (or even bone) lie near the tonsils.

These are probably inconstant derivatives of the embryonic branchial arches.

B. LINGUAL TONSIL:

This organ is located on the root of the tongue, behind the vallate papillae.

It is an aggregation of epithelial pits, each surrounded by lymphoid tissue.

In all, there are between 35 and 100 of these tonsillar units.

In surface view, each unit is a low mound with a central crater — like a dimple.

The pit is a simple *crypt* which, however, sometimes bifurcates.

It is lined with a continuation of the surface *epithelium* (stratified squamous).

Leucocytic infiltration is usually less severe than in the palatine tonsils.

The mound-like elevation is due to a mass of *lymphoid tissue* 1 to 5 mm. in diameter.

This surrounds the crypt and is ovoid to inverted-conical in shape.

It contains usually a single layer of *lymph nodules* with germinal centers.

Bordering each unit is a thin connective-tissue *capsule*.

Ducts of underlying *mucous glands* open either into the crypts or onto the surface.

C. PHARYNGEAL TONSIL:

The clinical name is *adenoids*, especially when overgrowth occurs.

This organ comprises an accumulation of lymphoid tissue, about 3 cm. long.

It is located in the median dorsal wall of the nasopharynx.

At the tonsillar site, the pharyngeal lining makes a series of longitudinal *folds*.

Sections cut across them look like longitudinal sections of a series of crypts.

However, this is a deception, and true, pocket-like crypts are lacking.

The *epithelium* is pseudostratified, with cilia and goblet cells.

There are some islands of stratified epithelium, especially in the adult.

Infiltration of epithelium by migratory leucocytes occurs and can be extensive.

The *lymphoid tissue* occupies a layer about 2 mm. thick.

It contains *lymph nodules*, usually with germinal centers.

A thin *capsule* underlies the tonsil and sends *septa* outward into the folds.

Mixed *sero-mucous glands* are plentiful beneath the capsule.

Their *ducts* open into the trough-like downfoldings and onto the alternating crests.

Most of these ducts widen surfaceward into prominent, long funnels.

They resemble unbranched crypts and seem, additionally, to serve the same purpose.

D. VESSELS AND NERVES:

Blood vessels course in the capsule and septa, and supply the lymphoid tissue.

Lymphatic vessels form plexuses about the lymphoid mass, but do not invade it.

Nerves follow the blood vessels into the septa and parenchyma.

E. INVOLUTION:

Tonsils, in general, reach their maximal development in childhood.

The *pharyngeal tonsil* begins to decline at about the time of puberty.

In the adult it is usually atrophic to a marked degree.

The pseudostratified epithelium has been replaced largely by stratified squamous.

The time when *palatine tonsils* begin to involute is not generally agreed upon.

Different observers favor middle childhood, puberty or adulthood.

This divergence of opinion probably reflects an inherent variability in the onset.

In advanced age tonsils become replaced to a large degree by fibrous tissue.

The *lingual tonsils* mature slowly, and involution begins later than in other tonsils.

F. Regenerative Ability:

Both the palatine and pharyngeal tonsils have marked regenerative capacity.
Incomplete removal may be followed by extensive regrowth.

G. Diagnostic Features:

Dense lymphoid tissue, with nodules, is bordered on one surface with epithelium.
Lingual and *palatine tonsil* epithelium is stratified; *pharyngeal tonsil*, pseudostratified.
Lymphocytic infiltration is characteristic, but variable in extent and intensity.
The surface epithelium dips into pockets; these are surrounded with lymphoid tissue.
In the *lingual tonsil* the crypt is single, and each tonsil unit is small.
In the *palatine tonsil* many of the crypts are long and branched.
Numérous branches are cut so as to appear isolated in the lymphoid tissue.
In the *pharyngeal tonsil* a series of folds, when cut across, resembles crypts.
These do not feature branching, as do true crypts of the palatine tonsil.
Still more crypt-like are dilated ducts from glands located beneath the tonsil.
Glands and skeletal muscle underlie all three types.
Only the pharyngeal tonsil has mixed muco-serous (rather than pure mucous) glands.
Only the lingual tonsil has its associated muscle interlaced in three planes.

H. Functional Correlations:

The several tonsils constitute a discontinuous lymphoid ring about the pharynx.
They are situated favorably so as to guard the entrance to the pharynx.
Lymphocyte production, however, is the only obvious function known.
Such activity is generally held to be a defense maneuver against bacteria.
Yet epithelial erosion by lymphocytes enhances an invasion by micro-organisms.
At least, the tonsils are frequent portals of infection.
The tonsils are involved in the production of antibodies.
Possibly bacteria, gaining entrance, are made less virulent and vaccines are produced.
It might follow that bacteria in the crypts become detoxified.
Glands opening into the crypts of the lingual tonsil presumably flush them clean.
Perhaps this is why this organ is rarely diseased.

IV. THE LYMPH NODES

These lymphoid organs show four distinct advances over those previously considered.
There is a supporting framework consisting of a complete *capsule* and beam-like *trabeculae*.
The lymphoid tissue exhibits two different regions, a *cortex* and a *medulla*.
Lymphatic vessels open freely into the organ; other lymphatics drain it.
There is a system of internal *lymph sinuses*, adapted for filtering lymph.
Lymph nodes are so named because they resemble knots at intervals on lymphatic vessels.
They were also called *lymph glands* because they generate cells, as do some other glands.
Lymph nodes, interposed in the lymph stream, are restricted to mammals.
They usually occur in chains or groups, and are numerous in definite regions of the body.
Example: prevertebral region; mesentery; vicinity of large joints; along large arteries.
The stated total of some 500 lymph nodes in the body is believed to be too low.

A. Structural Plan:

A *lymph node* is an ovoid or bean-shaped body, ranging from 1 to 25 mm. in diameter.
It has a convex contour except at an indented region named the *hilus* (or hilum).
A fibrous *capsule* encloses the entire gland and gives it shape.
It is continuous with an internal trestlework of *trabeculae*.
These, in turn, connect with a much finer spongework of *reticular-tissue*.
The *parenchyma* (lymphoid tissue) is specialized into two regions.
Beneath the capsule there is a solider *cortex*, characterized by *lymph nodules*.
At the hilus the cortex is lacking.
The interior of the gland is the *medulla*, characterized by *medullary cords*.

Cortex and medulla are not sharply demarcated, but blend irregularly.
Extensive *lymph sinuses* bound the parenchyma and also penetrate it.
They constitute a communicating system of cortical and medullary channels.
Afferent lymphatic vessels open into the sinus system at multiple points.
They are located on the convex surface of the node, opposite the hilus.
Efferent lymphatics drain the sinuses in a restricted area at the hilus of the node.
Blood vessels and *nerves* enter and leave at the hilus.
Neither arteries nor veins communicate directly with the sinus system.

B. DETAILED STRUCTURE.

1. Framework.

A. CAPSULE.

There is a firm external envelope, convex except at the indented hilus.
At the hilus this *capsule* is thick and, in a sense, intrudes into the organ.
It is composed mostly of densely packed collagenous fibers.
Scattering elastic fibers and some smooth-muscle fibers are present also.
Muscle fibers are located noticeably around the orifices of lymphatic vessels.
On its external surface, the capsule is uneven or rough.
This is because fibers pass from it to the surrounding connective tissue.

B. TRABECULAE.

At intervals, fibrous *trabeculae* project vertically inward from the capsule.
They stake off the cortex into incomplete compartments, 1 mm., or more, wide.
Each space is bluntly pyramidal in shape and contains a lymphoid mass.
Such trabeculae are broad interrupted bands, rather than complete partitions.
In the medulla, trabeculae lose even these membranous tendencies.
Here they become truly beam-like, and are irregular and branching.
They converge toward the hilus and connect with the thickened capsule there.
Each trabecula is completely surrounded by a space belonging to the sinus-system.
All trabeculae resemble the capsule structurally.

C. RETICULUM.

This tissue extends as a delicate, spidery meshwork throughout the node.
Its fibers blend with the collagenous fibers of the capsule and trabeculae.
Many of the reticular-tissue cells are fixed phagocytes (macrophages).
These cells belong to the category called the reticulo-endothelial system.
Some are primitive reticular cells, relatively undifferentiated (p. 46).

2. Cortical parenchyma.

In nodes rich in trabeculae, each *cortical nodule* (and the diffuse lymphoid tissue about it)
is marked off by a set of cortical trabeculae.
These nodules underlie the capsule, and often cause it to bulge locally.
Each nodular mass is attached to the nearby capsule and trabeculae by reticulum.
It is, in a sense, largely suspended in the sinuses that border it intimately.
In man there are fewer trabeculae; the nodular masses are more irregular in shape.
Several then unite by their lateral surfaces and occupy a larger compartment.
Each cortical nodule is about 0.5 mm. in diameter.
Nodules usually show *germinal centers,* but these features are impermanent (p. 143).
In nodes of the inguinal region, centers are never well developed.
It is also said that the whole nodule may disappear as such, and reform.
Associated with lymphocytes are plasma cells, macrophages and monocytes.

3. Medullary parenchyma.

In the medulla the lymphoid tissue takes the form of dense strands or plates.
These *medullary cords* branch and anastomose, thereby making a loose spongework.
Some are continuous with the deep surface of the cortical lymphoid masses.
Other cords end blindly near the hilus.
Still others form loops by joining with neighboring (otherwise loose) ends.
Medullary cords are entirely surrounded by medullary sinuses.

Reticulum, bridging the sinuses, attaches each cord to adjacent trabeculae.
The cellular components of cords are like those in a cortical nodule.
However, these cords are the chief site of plasma cells and their production.
Also, germinal centers never occur in medullary cords.

4. Lymphatic vessels and sinuses.
A. LYMPHATIC VESSELS.
No other organ is similarly inserted into the course of lymphatic vessels.
That is, none other is supplied with afferent and efferent lymphatics.
Afferent vessels pierce the half of the convex capsule, opposite the hilus.
They enter slantingly at various points, encircled by a little smooth muscle.
Efferent vessels are fewer, but larger, and are restricted to the hilus-region.
They penetrate the thickened muscle-containing capsule, and then emerge.
Valves restrict the flow of lymph to an onward direction, as in all lymphatics.
B. LYMPH SINUSES.
Every node contains a tortuous system of irregular channels, named *sinuses*.
They are a looser or more open sort of lymphoid tissue.
Such labyrinthine channels both widen and slow the lymphatic stream.
Lymph sinuses differ from lymphatic vessels in structure.
They are not lined with endothelium; on the contrary, they are *sinusoids*.
These particular ones are merely washed-out spaces in lymphoid tissue.
Some are probably impermanent channels.
Their 'lining' is furnished by flattened reticular cells.
These cells make an incomplete layer.
Hence lymph seeps into the parenchyma and lymphocytes escape.
The sinus is criss-crossed by a meshwork of typical reticular tissue.
Some of the cells stretched along the fibers are *primitive reticular cells*.
Others are *fixed macrophages* (reticulo-endothelium).
A varying number of transient cells occur in the spaces of this spongework.
These cells are mostly lymphocytes, but there are some free macrophages.
In addition, a few granulocytes and red corpuscles may be seen at times.
One border of the sinus-system underlies the capsule and follows all trabeculae.
The other border bounds all cortical nodules and medullary cords.
Hence all trabeculae and lymphoid masses are anchored in a lymph stream.
Thus three parts of the sinus system are distinguished.
The *marginal sinus* (or subcapsular sinus) underlies the capsule.
It separates the capsule from the cortical parenchyma.
Cortical sinuses lie between cortical trabeculae and cortical nodules.
Medullary sinuses lie between medullary trabeculae and medullary cords.

5. Blood vessels and nerves.
Arteries enter the lymph node at the hilus and tunnel within trabeculae.
Some branches continue to run in trabeculae, and ultimately reach the capsule.
Other branches leave the trabeculae, enter the medullary cords, course axially in
them, and finally reach and supply each cortical nodule.
Dense capillary plexuses supply the medullary cords and cortical nodules.
Small lymphocytes pass through the endothelium and enter the parenchyma.
Many lymphocytes emigrate from postcapillaries, which continue into venules.
Veins return blood to the hilus over the same general route taken by arteries.
Nerves, which are at least mostly vasomotor, follow the blood vessels.

6. Structural variations.
Lymph nodes are highly variable, depending on their locations within the body.
A node may be much simpler than the ordinary type.
This is especially true of the very small ones.
On the other hand, any of the structural constituents may be reduced or exaggerated.

Example: hilus; trabeculae; sinus extent; cortical parenchyma; medullary cords.
The relative amount of cortex and medulla, and their inter-relations vary widely.
   The cortical nodules may be several layers deep.
   The cortex may surround the medulla completely or only partially.
   The cortical and medullary components may even lie at opposite poles of the node.
   Either the cortex or medulla may be lacking, or unrecognizable as such.
   Nodes of the peritoneal cavity are rich in medullary cords and sinuses.
(In some animals nodules occur in both cortex and medulla.)

C. INVOLUTION:

After puberty the cortex of lymph nodes tends to decrease progressively.
   With this decline goes a regression of the germinal centers.
   Eventually the medulla may reach to the marginal sinus in some places.
In some nodes these changes are relatively slight.

D. REGENERATIVE ABILITY:

Young animals may replace excised glands from local tissue.
   This capacity is lost rapidly as age advances.
Local injuries to nodes are usually healed by the differentiation of scar tissue.

E. DIAGNOSTIC FEATURES:

The encapsulated organ possesses a cortex and medulla, not sharply demarcated.
   The cortex consists of lymph nodules, usually with germinal centers.
      (A single section naturally misses some of the centers.)
   The medulla consists of lymphoid strands, appearing like a network.
Lymph sinuses border the cortical nodules and medullary cords.
   They are variable in abundance, but usually are more numerous in the medulla.
The lymph node is the only organ in the body that contains lymph sinuses.
   The free cells are mostly small lymphocytes.
   The sinuses do not contain other leucocytes or erythrocytes in significant numbers.

F. FUNCTIONAL CORRELATIONS:

Relative to size, a lymph node is the most active lymphopoietic organ in the body.
   Lymphocytes enter the sinuses partly by amebism and partly by crowding pressure.
      Some lymphocytes enter directly into blood capillaries of the lymphoid tissue.
         In doing this they bypass the ordinary lymphatic route of exit.
      Part of the lymphocytes in sinuses entered the node as recycling lymphocytes (p. 63).
   Lymph is not cellular to any extent until it passes through lymph nodes.
      Many more lymphocytes leave a node than enter it.
   In some abnormal conditions, lymph nodes may produce myeloid elements.
A lymph node is the only organ in the body acting as a filterer of lymph.
   Favoring this is the reticular tissue, crossing and lining the system of sinus-channels.
   Also favorable is the slow trickle of lymph percolating through these passages.
   It is believed that all the returning lymph of the body passes through at least one node
      before entering the blood stream.
Filtration depends on the phagocytic ability of fixed and detached reticular cells.
   Fixed cells are fixed macrophages; detached cells are ordinary free macrophages.
   Cells located in sinuses are especially active because of their favorable position.
   Dust, carbon, bacteria and degenerating cells are ingested by the phagocytes.
   Bronchial lymph nodes are even blackened by carbon storage.
Lymphatic vessels provide paths for the spread of cancerous cells from a primary focus.
   Within lymph nodes their proliferation leads to the setting up of secondary centers.
   This is abetted by the slowness of passage through the sinus-labyrinth.
Antibodies are elaborated, and the node is important in producing immunity.

V. THE HEMAL NODES

The term *hemolymph node* is also used, but this is not generally appropriate.
Hemal nodes are poorly understood, and there are many conflicting opinions concerning them.
They are characterized by a rich content of red blood corpuscles within sinuses.
   Accordingly, the organ is red, or dark, in color.
True hemal nodes occur along the ventral side of the vertebrae in various mammals.
   They are distinct entities in ruminants, such as the sheep and ox.
   On the other hand, their presence in the prevertebral tissue of man is doubtful.
      Alleged nodes may have been abnormal lymph nodes or accessory spleens.

1. Structure.

   The size ranges up to that of a pea.
   The general organization is much like a lymph node.
      However, the *sinuses* are purely blood sinuses; there is no lymphatic supply.
      Trabeculae are greatly reduced, and sinuses may be diminished also.
      Typical *lymph nodules*, with or without germinal centers, do not occur.
   The blood vessels are not known definitely to communicate directly with sinuses.
      Some claim that perforations exist in the vessel wall, but others deny this.
      Yet red corpuscles must emerge in some way and gain entrance into the sinuses.
         The problem, not fully solved, is much like that in the spleen (p. 156).
   In structure a hemal node approaches the relations existing in the spleen.
      The hog has a type midway between a lymph node and an ordinary hemal node.
         The contents both of blood vessels and of lymphatics mingle in the sinuses.
         In this instance, the term 'hemolymph node' is appropriate.
      A structural series would then run: ordinary lymph node; hemolymph node (of hog);
         hemal node; spleen.

2. Diagnostic features.

   Trabeculae are rudimentary; cortical nodules and germinal centers are lacking.
   The presence of red blood corpuscles in the sinuses is positively diagnostic.
      Inflamed, hemorrhagic lymph nodes, showing sinus blood, must be excluded.
      (Moreover, the sinuses of normal lymph nodes contain a few red corpuscles.)

3. Functional correlations.

   Activities resemble those of the spleen, on a small scale.
   A hemal node is lymphopoietic and a filterer of the blood.
   It destroys many red blood corpuscles; these are probably nearing death.

VI. THE SPLEEN

This largest of all lymphoid organs is ovoid in shape and about the size of the fist.
   After death it expels blood and loses up to three-fourths of its live weight.
The spleen is much like a huge, congested hemal node, interposed in a blood stream.
   But it has developed a peculiar kind of storage-sinus for blood.
   It is the only human organ that is unquestionably specialized for filtering blood.
   The spleen is located between the stomach, left kidney and diaphragm.

A. STRUCTURAL PLAN:

   The soft spleen is surrounded by a fibrous *capsule*, surfaced with peritoneum.
   Many *trabeculae* pass from the capsule to the interior.
   There is a long, deep *hilus* where blood vessels enter and leave the large trabeculae.
   The parenchyma *(splenic pulp)* is of two distinct types.
      These masses are distributed throughout the spleen as fairly discrete entities.

White pulp surrounds and follows the arteries, like a sheath.
At intervals it thickens into ovoid masses, the *splenic nodules*.
Red pulp is more abundant; it occurs in irregular masses, known as *pulp cords*.
Splenic sinuses are sausage-shaped channels that intervene between arteries and veins.
Sinuses and terminal blood vessels are embedded in a common mass of red pulp.

B. Lobulation:

Primary trabeculae mark out the spleen into many pyramidal compartments.
Each of these *lobules* is about 1 mm. in diameter and is bounded by several trabeculae.
It receives a terminal arterial branch, with a splenic nodule about it.
It is drained by veins that leave the lobule within the trabeculae that bound it.
Such lobulation is indicated on the surface by a faint mottling.
This *primary lobule* is subdivided (actually imperfectly demarcated) by smaller trabeculae.
About ten *secondary lobules* are created in this manner.
Terminal arterial twigs vascularize each of these ultimate 'compartments.'
Splenic lobulation is imperfect and is demonstrable locally only in favorably cut sections.
It is of academic, rather than practical, value.
Yet it is interesting that an approach to orderly, unit organization does exist.

C. Detailed Structure:

1. Framework.

A. Capsule.

This is tough, but elastic, and is firmly anchored by trabeculae.
In man the *capsule* is relatively thin (0.1 to 0.15 mm.), except at the hilus.
It is heaviest at the hilus, where it supports the large splenic vessels.
The capsule contains dense fibro-elastic tissue and scanty smooth-muscle fibers.
Some mammals possess a rich content of smooth muscle, even in layers.
Superficially the capsule is covered with reflected peritoneum.
Hence there is a layer of mesothelium at the actual free surface.

B. Trabeculae.

Massive *trabeculae* radiate inward from the hilus and subdivide repeatedly.
Other trabeculae extend perpendicularly inward from the capsule.
Branching and anastomosis produce a complex trestlework throughout the interior.
On the whole, the splenic trabeculae are notably robust.
The largest are easily visible to the naked eye.
Trabeculae are similar to the capsule in composition.
Elastic fibers are even more numerous than in the capsule.

C. Reticulum.

Splenic pulp is supported throughout by a fine spongework of *reticular fibers*.
Both the red and white pulp are permeated with them.
The reticulum blends insensibly into the trabeculae, vessels and capsule.
Ensheathing *reticular cells* accompany the reticular fibers.
Some of them, as elsewhere, are like primitive, multipotent mesenchyme.
Others are fixed macrophages that can detach and become free macrophages.

2. White pulp.

One component of the *white pulp* is represented by elongate, branching, strands.
Such a lymphoid cord ensheathes a *central arteriole* coursing in solitary manner.
The adventitia of these vessels is largely replaced by reticular tissue.
This modified meshwork is infiltrated with lymphocytes, most of which are small.
These lymphocytes constitute the great majority of free cells in white pulp.
Less frequent types include plasma cells and macrophages.
A second component is the *splenic nodule*, also called 'Malpighian corpuscle.'
These occur at intervals along the cords as thicker accumulations of white pulp.
They are interconnected by the more slender cylinders of ordinary white pulp.
Splenic nodules are spindle-shaped, but become spheroidal where arterioles branch.

Their diameter averages about 0.5 mm.; hence they are visible to the naked eye.
They are typical lymph nodules that enclose an unusually prominent arteriole.
From this vessel nutrient twigs pass to the tissue of the nodule; some, beyond.
The supporting *reticulum* makes a denser basketwork peripherally in the nodule.
The number of splenic nodules before adulthood ranges from 100,000 to 200,000.
They are said to disappear and organize anew from time to time.
The *germinal center* of a nodule is a similarly inconstant feature.
The *central arteriole* is really eccentric; it avoids the germinal center.
Frequently a splenic nodule is located in the crotch of a branching vessel.
In such instances two (or more) arterioles pierce the nodule.

3. *Marginal zone.*

At the periphery of white pulp there is a shell of tissue called the *marginal zone*.
It is looser in texture than white pulp and is transitional into red pulp cords.
It receives blood directly from some central arteriolar branches opening there.
Venous sinuses of the red-pulp type are lacking.

4. *Red pulp.*

This is a pasty, dark-red mass that can be scraped from a freshly cut surface.
Its density and firmness vary with the amount of blood contained.
After death it looks compact because of the collapse of sinusoids.
Structurally, red pulp is a modification of white pulp and blends into it at marginal zones.
It is looser in texture, owing to an abundant tissue-fluid.
It is infiltrated with all elements of the circulating blood.
The support of pulp is a typical *reticulum* and its associated reticular cells.
Red pulp occupies all space not utilized by sinuses, white pulp and trabeculae.
Its tissue is tunneled by innumerable venous sinuses.
On section, the intervening pulp gives the appearance of cellular cords.
These *pulp cords* are actually a continuous system of joined plates and masses.
Red pulp shows variations in composition among different mammalian groups.
Its density and erythrocyte content vary widely.
Many mammals have some marrow cells in their red pulp, as did the human fetus.
Among the free cells of red pulp the nongranular leucocytes are commonest.
A. LYMPHOCYTES.
All sizes intermingle; they are relatively less numerous than in white pulp.
Many came from white pulp by amebism; others were brought by the blood stream.
Once in the red pulp the larger ones continue to multiply there.
Modified cells of the lymphocyte-line occur as *plasma cells*.
B. MONOCYTES.
These fairly numerous elements were once called *splenic cells*.
Some are brought by the blood stream; others arise locally from hemocytoblasts.
All are capable of self-proliferation.
Monocytes have phagocytic potentialities, and may become vigorous scavengers.
Such enlarged phagocytes become indistinguishable from other macrophages.
C. FREE MACROPHAGES.
The spleen is the greatest producer of macrophages.
These ameboid elements are descended from primitive reticular cells.
They are similar to the fixed macrophages still attached to the reticulum.
Evidences of phagocytosis are often seen within their cytoplasm.
Red corpuscles are digested; their iron pigment is stored for a time.
D. GRANULOCYTES.
Neutrophils, eosinophils and, rarely, basophils are all represented.
They are blood cells that have taken temporary residence in the red pulp.
E. ERYTHROCYTES.
These are abundant in red pulp and give it a characteristic red color.
Normally neither red cells nor granulocytes arise in the pulp.

5. *Blood vessels.*

The vascular arrangement is of great importance in the spleen.

It determines the distribution and inter-relation of both red and white pulp.

It also determines the structural plan of the spleen as a whole.

The terminal vessels are peculiar in structure and in their inter-relations.

A. ARTERIES.

These vessels are especially associated with white pulp.

They enter at the hilus and follow the larger trabeculae for a short distance.

As the trabeculae branch, the arteries subdivide also.

They are distinguished from veins by their muscular coat and small lumen.

When reduced to a diameter of 0.2 mm., they leave the trabeculae as arterioles.

Passing into the splenic parenchyma, the adventitia changes in character.

It loosens and becomes a mesh, composed largely of reticular tissue.

Infiltration by lymphocytes produces the ensheathing white pulp.

These *central arterioles* supply capillaries chiefly to the white pulp.

Arterioles about 50 μ in diameter lose their investment of white pulp.

In so doing, they necessarily enter the red pulp.

Here each subdivides into several branches that diverge like a fan.

This cluster is named a *penicillus* (*i.e.*, brush).

Each branch of a penicillus shows three successive segments:

First is the pulp arteriole, which branches and rapidly narrows to 15 μ.

It still retains a thin layer of smooth muscle.

Next are *sheathed arterioles* (30 μ), with a markedly thickened wall.

These spindle-shaped *ellipsoids* are composed of reticular cells and fibers.

Finally are *terminal capillaries*, whose manner of ending is disputed.

Each set of arterioles within the splenic pulp is a functional 'end artery.'

That is, if such a vessel is blocked, the tissues served by it suffer.

The impairment results from lack of an adequate collateral supply of blood.

B. VENOUS SINUSES.

The so-called *sinuses* constitute a system of tunnels within the red pulp.

They occupy more space than do the 'pulp cords' between them.

Actually the 'sinuses' are specialized sinusoids of the pulp.

The branching and anastomosing sinuses are highly distensible (2 to 100 μ).

Their appearance after death is one of relative collapse.

The sinus wall is not endothelium, but specialized reticular cells.

They are fixed macrophages (reticulo-endothelium), greatly elongated.

Normally they are much less actively phagocytic than those of the red pulp.

The rod-like reticular cells course lengthwise of the sinus.

In the region of the nucleus the cell bulges farther into the lumen.

The cells rest upon a *basement membrane* that is highly fenestrated.

Branching reticular fibers encircle the sinus externally and support it.

The light microscope shows the cells in transverse section as cuboidal blocks.

These are arranged loosely in a circle, with gaps intervening.

Longitudinal sections show them as the loosely fitting staves of a barrel.

Electron micrographs show the cells touching, but without desmosomes or cement.

The cells separate easily since blood cells slip through readily.

(Hence the slits commonly seen are presumably technique-artifacts.)

C. VEINS.

The venous sinuses connect by a gradual transition with the so-called *pulp veins.*

These are true endothelial tubes that begin much like postcapillaries.

They are supported by reticulum and then by white and elastic fibers.

Leaving the parenchyma, the veins continue within trabeculae.

Here they consist of bare endothelium, buried in trabecular tissue.

Veins run longer distances in trabeculae than do most arteries.

Hence they are the only vessels present within the smaller trabeculae.

The *trabecular veins*, on reaching the hilus, drain into the splenic vein.

D. THE ARTERIO-VENOUS JUNCTION.

The manner of junction or union has long been a subject of dispute.

Some claim that arterial capillaries open freely into the splenic pulp.

Blood then enters the sinuses indirectly; it is an *open circulation.*

Others hold for a primarily continuous system, or *closed circulation.*

That is, arterial capillaries communicate directly with venous sinuses.

Still others think that both types of circulation (open and closed) exist.

A final decision still awaits crucial evidence, generally acceptable.

In any event, cellular interchange between red pulp and sinuses occurs.

6. Lymphatics.

Efferent vessels, but not afferents, are present in the capsule and larger trabeculae.
They also occur to some extent in white pulp, coursing toward trabeculae.

7. Nerves.

Unmyelinated nerve fibers follow the arteries and end in their smooth muscle.
Sparse myelinated fibers occur; they are probably sensory in function.
Some fibers enter both the red and white pulp, but their endings are unknown.

D. AGE CHANGES:

The amount of white pulp decreases in old age, as does lymphoid tissue generally.
The number and size of splenic nodules also diminish with advancing age.
Germinal centers are numerous in the young, fewer in the adult and absent in old age.

E. REGENERATIVE ABILITY:

The spleen is able to heal local injuries.
This it does through the formation of scar tissue at the site of the wound.

F. DIAGNOSTIC FEATURES:

The spleen has lymph nodules scattered widely in a pulp that contains red corpuscles.
It is characterized negatively by the lack of a cortex and medulla.
The smooth capsule is surfaced with peritoneum (and hence mesothelium).
The trabeculae are conspicuously robust—more so than in any other lymphoid organ.
Splenic nodules, with prominent eccentric arterioles, are specifically diagnostic.
The venous sinuses, interspersed with red pulp, are exclusively characteristic.
Blood sinuses do not exist surely in any other human lymphoid organ.

G. FUNCTIONAL CORRELATIONS:

Splenic activities are incompletely understood.
The spleen is not essential to life; the body withstands its extirpation successfully.
Readjustment is made through the compensatory growth of lymphoid tissue elsewhere.
Phagocytic functions are then carried out by the macrophages of other organs.
The spleen is an elastic, controllable reservoir that is important in adjusting the volume of the circulating blood to changing needs.
In life the spleen undergoes both rhythmic and passive contractions.
In part this activity is attributed to the smooth muscle in its framework.
But the major control of size is regulated through changes in its blood-volume.
The spleen is expansible because of its abundant elastic tissue.
Especially does it store, temporarily, red corpuscles in the sinuses and red pulp.
The spleen is an important hemopoietic organ, generating both lymphocytes and monocytes.
Lymphocytes are formed in both types of pulp, but chiefly in the white pulp.
Thence they pass to the red pulp, and so into the sinuses and splenic vein.
Monocytes differentiate from hemocytoblasts in the red pulp and splenic sinuses.
Pathologically the spleen may come to resemble bone marrow and imitate its functions.
It can then generate all types of blood cells (as in early fetal life).

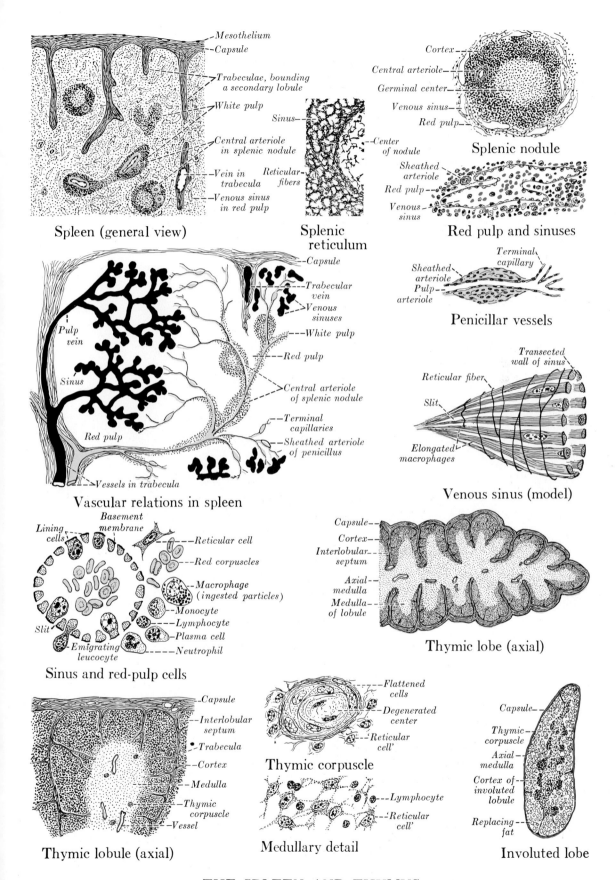

Mesothelium
Capsule
Trabeculae, bounding a secondary lobule
White pulp
Central arteriole in splenic nodule
Vein in trabecula
Venous sinus in red pulp

Spleen (general view)

Sinus
Center of nodule
Reticular fibers

Splenic reticulum

Cortex
Central arteriole
Germinal center
Venous sinus
Red pulp

Splenic nodule

Sheathed arteriole
Red pulp
Venous sinus

Red pulp and sinuses

Capsule
Trabecular vein
Venous sinuses
White pulp
Red pulp
Central arteriole of splenic nodule
Terminal capillaries
Sheathed arteriole of penicillus
Vessels in trabecula

Pulp vein
Sinus
Red pulp

Vascular relations in spleen

Terminal capillary
Sheathed arteriole
Pulp arteriole

Penicillar vessels

Transected wall of sinus
Reticular fiber
Slit
Elongated macrophages

Venous sinus (model)

Basement membrane
Lining cells
Reticular cell
Red corpuscles
Macrophage (ingested particles)
Monocyte
Lymphocyte
Plasma cell
Neutrophil
Slit
Emigrating leucocyte

Sinus and red-pulp cells

Capsule
Cortex
Interlobular septum
Axial medulla
Medulla of lobule

Thymic lobe (axial)

Capsule
Interlobular septum
Trabecula
Cortex
Medulla
Thymic corpuscle
Vessel

Thymic lobule (axial)

Flattened cells
Degenerated center
Reticular cell'

Thymic corpuscle

Lymphocyte
Reticular cell'

Medullary detail

Capsule
Thymic corpuscle
Axial medulla
Cortex of involuted lobule
Replacing fat

Involuted lobe

THE SPLEEN AND THYMUS

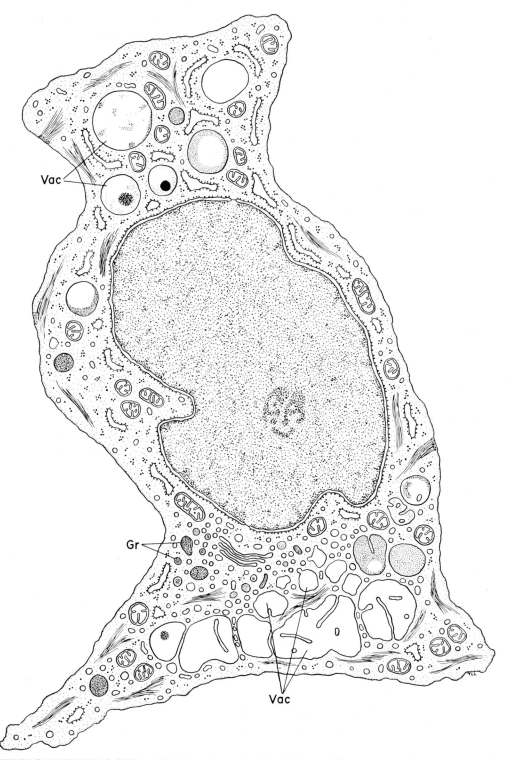

THYMIC EPITHELIAL CELL. This type, characteristic of the medulla, occurs in clusters or strands, and varies in shape. Its nuclear chromatin is highly dispersed. The cytoplasm contains dense granules (Gr), the small and less dense ones lying near the Golgi complex. Additionally there are rough endoplasmic reticulum, clusters of free ribosomes and bundles of tonofilaments; some of the latter insert on desmosomes which form connections with other cells. Vesicles coalesce and form vacuoles (Vac); some of these contain varying amounts of dense material, while others have a content of low density and show microvilli protruding inward. These cells are believed to produce a material that induces lymphocyte proliferation in other organs.

It is a filterer of the blood; phagocytosis is actively engaged in by the free and fixed macrophages of the red pulp and, to a lesser degree, by the lining cells of the sinuses.

Red corpuscles, leucocytes, bacteria, and other particles are ingested.

They are then digested, destroyed or stored.

Iron, extracted from disintegrating red corpuscles, is stored for a time in macrophages.

It is then given up as needed and re-utilized in forming hemoglobin.

The hemoglobin, also made available, is converted into bile pigments.

For a time the spleen is the most important organ in the production of antibodies.

Evidence indicates that plasma cells, as specialized lymphocytes, are the main source.

The spleen is also active in defense against air-borne infections.

It produces the most macrophages, and the most active ones in any filtering organ.

Its macrophage system is surpassed in size by that of the liver alone.

Endocrine functions, such as depressing marrow activity, remain unaccepted.

The spleen has no cellular element that is not shared by other lymphoid organs.

Hence the cellular basis for the elaboration of a distinctive hormone is lacking.

VII. THE THYMUS

The *thymus* is a broad, flat, bilobed mass of lymphoid tissue.

Its location is beneath the upper sternum, in the anterior mediastinum.

A. STRUCTURAL PLAN:

The thymus consists of two halves, or *lobes*, thus retaining its original double origin.

The two parts, however, are closely applied and united by connective tissue.

A lobe is subdivided into thousands of *lobules*, each with a cortex and medulla.

All lobules, however, are incomplete on their deep (or central) side.

The *medulla* is a central core that sends a lateral projection into each lobule.

Thymic corpuscles (of Hassall) are a characteristic constituent of the medulla.

The *cortex* surrounds the lateral extensions of the medulla as so many local caps.

There is a rather sharp demarcation between cortex and medulla.

A *capsule* encloses each lobe, and extensions of it (*septa*) stake off the lobules.

Trabeculae come off at right angles from the capsule and septa.

They traverse the cortex, but do not continue into the medulla.

B. LOBULATION:

Each *lobe* is subdivided into thousands of *lobules*, each 0.5 to 2 mm. in greatest dimension.

A *lobule* is a representative sample of both the cortex and medulla.

It is encapsulated by connective tissue except on its central side.

Here the medulla of the lobule becomes continuous with the main medullary axis.

This axial strand, or medulla proper, is not a part of the system of lobules.

The main medulla forms a continuous central axis, or core, within each lobe.

It sends a bud-like, lateral offshoot into each lobule.

Hence the lobules radiate about the central medullary axis.

Each lateral bud of medullary tissue is surrounded by a cap of cortical tissue.

This thimble-shaped cap abuts against the capsule and septa of a lobule.

In sections, many lobules are cut across their axes and appear like closed compartments.

That is, the encapsulated cortex surrounds completely the medullary bud.

(Only sections cut through the axis of a lobule show its true relations.)

C. DETAILED STRUCTURE:

1. Framework.

The thin *capsule* is composed of collagenous and some elastic fibers.

It surrounds the lobe, and extensions from it *(septa)* continue as far as the medulla.

In doing so, these *interlobular septa* largely separate the lobules from each other.

Intralobular trabeculae extend perpendicularly from the capsule through the cortex.

They end abruptly at the junction of cortex and medulla.
The entire parenchyma is supported by a 'reticulum' of peculiar, stellate cells.
They resemble reticular cells in shape, but not in origin or function.
They take form by a loosening-up of the cells constituting the embryonic thymus.
(The original, paired primordia were solid masses of entodermal epithelium.)
These branching *epithelio-reticular cells* form a meshwork called a *cytoreticulum.*
Branches of different cells make contact but do not merge as a syncytium.
They produce differentiations that are characteristic of epithelial cells.
Such are tonofibrils, desmosomes and cytoplasmic vesicles.
On the contrary, they are completely lacking in fibrils of the reticular type.
Also they do not store dyes, like true reticular cells (of mesenchymal origin).
The only typical reticular tissue that occurs came in with invading blood vessels.

2. Cortex.

The parenchyma consists of lymphocytes of all sizes, densely and uniformly packed.
They occupy the spaces in the open cytoreticular meshwork and largely obscure it.
Lymphopoiesis is active, and the small lymphocyte is the commonest type seen.
These are said to migrate into the medulla and leave by the medullary veins.
The origin of the thymic lymphocyte in late fetal and postnatal life is in dispute.
Usually these cells are now viewed as invading, special lymphocytes.
Such lymphocytes, of bone-marrow origin, are the short-lived type (p. 62).
Some have believed them to be derivatives of the entodermal cytoreticulum.
Yet young thymic transplants, if screened, never give rise to 'thymocytes.'

3. Medulla.

This region is much lighter staining and less compact than the cortex.
In children it is sharply demarcated from the cortex; in adults, less so.
Lymphocytes are not so numerous as in the cortex.
Consequently, the epithelio-reticular cells are prominent and predominant.
These constitute an apparent syncytium, with large pale nuclei.
Some macrophages and plasma cells are additional constituents.
Thymic corpuscles (of Hassall) are characteristic and diagnostic features.
During childhood these total about 1,500,000.
Each is a nest of epithelioid cells, arranged like a layered ball.
Their size is large (mostly 20 to 150 μ), and it increases with age.
A thymic corpuscle is in direct continuity with the nearby cytoreticulum.
The component cells are acidophilic, and often strongly so.
The central cells are larger and form a core to the total mass.
They are surrounded by flattened cells, arranged concentrically.
There is much hyalinization and degeneration, especially at the center.
The origin of corpuscles is from enlarged, compacted epithelio-reticular cells.
They increase in size with aging, as more cells are added peripherally.

4. Vessels and nerves.

Arteries enter along the medullary core and distribute largely to the cortex.
Capillaries have a thick basement membrane and a unique cellular envelope.
The latter sheath consists of epithelio-reticular cells.
This produces a sort of *blood-thymus barrier*, but not a wholly complete one.
It acts to protect lymphocytes from antigens carried in the blood.
Interlobular *veins* drain the cortex; medullary veins drain the medulla.
Lymphatics lie mainly in the interlobular connective tissue.
Afferent vessels and lymph sinuses are wholly absent.
Nerves are furnished by the vagus and sympathetics.
They are, at least mainly, vasomotor.

D. INVOLUTION:

The thymus reaches its maximum size at puberty, and then begins to wane.

Wasting, or involution, continues even into old age, but the organ still functions.
Involution is more severe than that occurring in other lymphoid organs.
The cortex loses density; the cortico-medullary boundary thereby becomes less sharp.
The medulla also declines progressively in the postpuberal years.
Fat replaces the degenerated lymphocytes and epithelio-reticular cells.
The thymic corpuscles are spared longest; their remains are identifiable in the aged.

E. REGENERATIVE ABILITY:

The regenerative capacity of the thymus has not been studied adequately.
The normal decline of the organ reflects an early inability to maintain itself.

F. DIAGNOSTIC FEATURES:

The thymus is a highly lobulated organ; it is the only plainly lobulated lymphoid organ.
The medulla is continuous from lobule to lobule by way of a common axial strand.
There is a fairly sharp and even demarcation of cortex from medulla in each lobule.
After childhood this clear-cut boundary is progressively lost.
A fibrous-tissue framework is associated with the cortex alone.
There are neither lymph nodules nor sinuses; it is the only lymphoid organ lacking both.
The thymic corpuscle is specifically diagnostic; it stains well with acid dyes.
(Small blood vessels, full of blood, may resemble them somewhat at low magnifications.)

G. FUNCTIONAL CORRELATIONS:

Lymphopoiesis is more vigorous in the fetus and infant than in all other lymphoid organs.
Plasma cells are also produced, but in small numbers.
The involution curve suggests that the thymus functions chiefly in the prepuberal years.
The onset of involution correlates with the rise of gonadal hormone in puberty.
This timing may be significant; at least steroid hormones induce involution.
The thymus is not essential to life in experimental adult animals.
Thymus removal at birth results in severe lymphocyte deficiency and antibody lack.
Such animals do not repel invading micro-organisms or reject foreign grafts.
Some attribute these deficiencies to a failure of 'thymocytes' to emigrate and colonize the
spleen and lymph nodes, which then fail to develop significantly.
Yet there is evidence that the thymus secretes an effective humoral factor into the blood.
This stimulates the production of lymphocytes and plasma cells in other organs.
These cells are the source of immunologic competence in the body.
The epithelio-reticulum is the presumptive source of this humoral substance.
It is suggested that even the thymic corpuscles participate in secretory activity.
In any event, the thymus does exert a control over the immunity mechanisms.
This is done despite its not producing a significant amount of antibody.
Perhaps this deficiency correlates with the absence of thymic germinal centers.

Chapter XV

Moist Membranes and Glands

Certain structural and functional units enter into the composition of many organs.

    Important among these are the moist, *internal membranes* and various kinds of *glands*.

It is advantageous to introduce these topics before describing the remaining organs.

    After this is done, in subsequent chapters only the special features of the membranes and glands in any particular region will need to be brought to attention.

    That is, by presenting the fundamental information now, later repetitions can be avoided.

I. THE MOIST MEMBRANES

These membranes are the joint product of an epithelium and its underlying connective tissue.

    They are kept moist either by a watery exudate or by a slimy secretion.

    On this basis they are named *serous membranes* and *mucous membranes*, respectively.

A. SEROUS MEMBRANES:

1. Occurrence.

    Each of the closed body cavities is bounded by a membranous sheet, or *tunica serosa*.

        These membranes are specifically named the *pericardium, pleurae* and *peritoneum*.

    A *parietal portion* lines the external wall of each of the body cavities.

    A *visceral portion* envelopes various organs of the body.

        It also provides mesenterial supports for some of these organs.

2. Structure.

    A *serous membrane* consists of mesothelium lying upon a connective-tissue layer.

    The *mesothelium* consists of simple, squamous, cellular plates.

        Their serrated edges interlock and their surface bears short, scattered microvilli.

        Minute apertures (*stomata*) can be found between some cells of the omentum.

            They are apparently temporary openings caused by outwandering cells.

        A *basement membrane* is present, but it is not an obvious feature.

    A layer of delicate connective tissue underlies mesothelium and gives it support.

        The thickness and density of this *lamina propria* vary regionally.

        In some regions (visceral pleura; mesenteries) it is quite elastic.

        It contains abundant blood vessels and lymphatics, but no glands.

        The cellular population includes a considerable range of cell types.

            The *milky spots* of the omentum and lungs feature massed macrophages.

    Beneath freely movable regions of serous membranes there is lax areolar tissue.

        This constitutes a *subserous layer* (tela subserosa).

    The serous cavities contain a small amount of watery fluid.

        This *serous transudate* suspends various kinds of free cells.

            Included are detached mesothelial cells, macrophages and lymphocytes.

    A *mesentery* (including omenta) is a double membrane whose laminae propriae fuse.

        Hence there is mesothelium on each free surface, and connective tissue between.

        Such double structures contain fat, and some of them enclose lymph nodes.

3. Regenerative ability.

Denuded areas are resurfaced by spreading and proliferation of mesothelial cells.
The omentum, when excised, does not regenerate to any significant degree.

4. Diagnostic features.

A serous membrane is a thin layer in vertical section.
Its surface epithelium appears as scarcely more than a bordering line.
Occasionally flattened nuclei make bead-like bulges along it.
The lamina propria is not distinctive, except negatively for the lack of glands.
A lax subserosa is a feature that is present only in some locations.
Identifying the exact location of a serous membrane, by itself, is impossible.
It can be done only when clues are furnished by associated organs or parts.

5. Functional correlations.

Serous membranes cover all surfaces that face upon the coelom in any way.
They constitute a protective and barrier layer.
Mesenterial and 'ligamentous' extensions of the layer pass to some organs.
These provide obvious support and permit some freedom of movement.
They also provide thoroughfares for the passages of vessels and nerves.
Mobility of a membrane is correlated with its composition in any local region.
Conducive to mobility is an increased elastic content.
Additionally important is the presence of a stretchable subserosa.
The lymph-like transudate moistens and lubricates the free surfaces of serosae.
This facilitates free play between the individual visceral organs.
It also permits the viscera to glide against the body wall; both are slippery.
The serous transudate, though normally small in amount, undergoes rapid turn-over.
Pathologically the amount may become very large.
In conditions of inflammation it then contains many neutrophils.
The omentum, in particular, is an efficient absorptive organ.
It is the direct avenue from the peritoneal cavity to the blood stream.
The macrophages, especially in 'milky spots,' are important in defense activities.
They take care of inert particles and of bacteria in infections.

B. Mucous Membranes:

These membranes (*tunicae mucosae*) are mucus-secreting sheets in the interior of the body.
All are in communication, mostly indirectly, with the exterior of the body.
Mucous membranes constitute the lining of various hollow organs, including small tubes.
Subject to distention in most locations, they tend to fold when relaxed.
A few membranes in this category do not secrete mucus, but are otherwise typical.
Example: bladder; vagina; ductus deferens.
Membranes, in general, use several methods of increasing their effective free surface:
Folds. Rather extensive wrinkling of the sheet (stomach rugae; intestinal plicae).
Evaginations. Local elevations above the general surface (various villi).
In this outpocketed fold the bases of opposed epithelial cells face each other.
Invaginations. Local inpocketings into the subjacent connective tissue (glands, varying from simple tubes to complex, tree-like branchings).
In this type of local fold the tops of opposed epithelial cells face each other.

1. Occurrence.

Alimentary tract (and large glandular ducts opening into it).
Respiratory tract (and associated accessory sinuses).
Auditory tube; tympanic cavity.
Urinary and genital tracts.
Conjunctiva.

2. Structure.

The *mucous membrane*, or tunica mucosa, consists typically of four layers.
A. EPITHELIUM.
This layer may be simple, pseudostratified or stratified.
In man, the stratified type is never fully cornified.
The epithelium is moistened and lubricated by a mucous secretion.
This may be produced by ordinary surface cells or specialized *goblet cells*.
Or it may be produced by multicellular glands opening onto the epithelium.
B. BASEMENT MEMBRANE (MEMBRANA PROPRIA).
The thickness of this supporting membrane varies within wide limits.
Example: trachea, thick; intestine, thin; urinary passages, extremely thin.
C. LAMINA PROPRIA MUCOSAE.
Attached to the basement membrane is a bed of connective tissue.
Areolar tissue is commonest, but reticular tissue is utilized also.
The name of this sheet is commonly shortened to *lamina propria*.
Glands, frequently located in this layer, open onto the surface epithelium.
The lamina propria may become variably infiltrated with lymphocytes.
D. LAMINA MUSCULARIS MUCOSAE.
Sometimes smooth muscle marks exactly the deep boundary of the lamina propria.
The name of this sheet of muscle is commonly shortened to *muscularis mucosae*.
It may be arranged longitudinally, or circularly and longitudinally.
When both layers are present, the one nearer the epithelium is circular.
E. TELA SUBMUCOSA.
The mucous membrane commonly rests upon a deeper, fibrous layer.
This *submucosa* consists of loose areolar tissue, and is rich in vessels.
It may contain glands (that drain to the free surface) and fat cells.
A demarcation from the lamina propria is distinct only when a muscularis mucosae is
present to delimit the latter.
In some regions a submucosa is unrecognizable as a definite entity.
The submucosa commonly is more lax than the mucosa, and affords it mobility.
It also serves to bind the mucosa to deeper, firmer structures.
This connection may be to a muscular wall, cartilage or bone.

3. Regenerative ability.

The epithelium restores the continuous, normal loss of covering and gland cells.
Local destruction of the membrane can be followed by complete regeneration.
Even glands differentiate from the still unspecialized, replacing epithelium.

4. Diagnostic features.

A mucous membrane lines all internal, hollow organs that connect with the exterior.
Its surface epithelium may be simple, pseudostratified or stratified.
The epithelium is soft and moist; it is almost always slimy.
Typically the epithelium has either gland cells in it or glands beneath it.
Both conditions may exist in the same membrane.
A basement membrane may or may not be recognizable as such.
A lamina propria is always present and usually has considerable thickness.
But its composition and special features are subject to local adaptations.
Glands and lymphoid infiltration are commonly present.
The deep surface of the muscularis mucosae establishes the limit of the membrane.
In its absence, the junction of the mucosa and submucosa is usually ill defined.
In some instances the submucosa is considered to be lacking.
This, however, can be a matter of individual opinion, since the presence of a looser
texture and a richer content of vessels are quantitative features.

5. Functional correlations.

A mucous membrane serves as a boundary and barrier between the body and the exterior.

It is also secretory and self-lubricating; it may be highly absorptive.
Slimy mucus protects surfaces against mechanical irritation and drying.
It entangles foreign particles, and is possibly bactericidal.
Increased mucus-flow, following irritations, tends to clean surfaces.
Ordinary mucus is inert chemically; it is a good lubricant for chafing-surfaces.
The mucus discharged on the epithelial surface varies in amount.
There is more mucus where mechanical irritation is greatest.
Example: gastro-intestinal tract; respiratory tract.
Mucus may even be lacking in some locations.
Example: urinary tract (moistened by passing urine).
A mucous membrane may also elaborate a secretion of a more watery nature.
These serous secretions typically contain chemically active enzymes.
Example: enzymic juices of gastric and intestinal glands; tears.
Absorption is a primary function of the gastro-intestinal mucosa.
Its epithelium notably elaborates microvilli for this purpose.
The muscularis mucosae accomplishes local movements of the mucous membrane.

II. THE GLANDS

Certain cells create and expel materials not related to their ordinary metabolic needs.
Such cells are specialized in the direction of glandular activity.
It is customary to distinguish glandular products as secretions or excretions.
Secretion involves constructive metabolism, synthesis and the release of formed products.
Raw materials obtained from the blood are elaborated into nonliving substances.
This requires work on the part of cells, and the use of DNA and RNA.
These manufactured products of a new sort are of use to the organism (or to its young).
Example: digestive enzymes; hormones; mucus; milk (useful to young).
Certain glands produce whole cells as their product.
Example: lymphocytes; sex cells (useful, not to the organism, but to the race).
Excretion sifts waste products from the circulating blood, without significant expenditure of energy.
Example: bile pigments; urea; carbon dioxide.
Excess useful materials in the blood are also eliminated as excretions.
Example: water; salts; glucose; hormones (synthesized secretions).
Secretory activity is a function displayed most commonly by epithelium.
Cells of nervous- and connective-tissue origin are more rarely concerned.
Example: oxytocin (nerve tissue); testosterone, muco-polysaccharide (connective tissue).
Some epithelial sheets not only are protective but they also secrete and absorb.
The body, however, requires more secretory products than simple sheets can supply.
Aslo, specialization for complex secretion tends to omit other types of differentiation.
Hence some surface epithelia develop downgrowths that become specialized as glands.
These lodge in the underlying connective tissue which then give them support.
A *gland* is an aggregation of cells, specialized as an organ of secretion or excretion.
Some single cells act as independent glandular units, but they are not organs.

I. BASES OF CLASSIFICATION

Glands can be classified in several different ways:

1. By cell numbers.
A. UNICELLULAR. Single cells within epithelial sheets act as complete glandular units.
Example: goblet mucous cell; mucoid cells of uterine tube.
B. MULTICELLULAR. Many cells co-operate in producing a gland-complex.
This type commonly organizes as tubes or sacs, opening onto the parent surface.
Example: uterine glands; sweat glands; salivary glands; mammary glands.
(Endocrine glands, however, do not maintain this relation to a parent surface.)

2. By kind of secretion.

A. MUCOUS. Slimy, chemically inert mucus (palate; colon; uterine cervix).

B. SEROUS. Watery, albuminous discharge; usually containing enzymes (parotid; pancreas), but not necessarily so (mammary glands; olfactory glands).

C. SERO-MUCOUS. Mixed discharge, owing to the presence of both cell types in the same or different alveoli (labial gland; submandibular gland).

D. CELLULAR. Blood cells (hemopoietic organs) and sex cells (gonads).

E. MISCELLANEOUS. The secretion differs from the common types already listed.

The product may be watery (sweat; urine; most hormones); viscid (seminal vesicle); greasy (sebum); waxy (cerumen); etc.

3. By manner of release.

A. WITH RESPECT TO THE PLACE OF DISCHARGE.

1. *Exocrine.* Onto the epithelial surface from which the gland developed.

In general, the secretion reaches the outside of the body directly (skin glands) or indirectly (digestive, respiratory, and urogenital glands).

2. *Endocrine.* Into the blood or lymph streams (hormones).

3. *Acrine.* No discharge of the elaborated product from the cells that synthesize it.

Example: granular leucocytes, whose granules are enzyme-containing lysosomes.

B. WITH RESPECT TO THE METHOD OF INITIAL TRANSPORT.

1. *Through a duct.* 'Duct-glands' (all ordinary multicellular glands).

2. *By diffusive transfer.* 'Ductless glands' (hormone-secreting glands).

C. WITH RESPECT TO GLAND-CELL PARTICIPATION.

1. *Merocrine.* The cell remains essentially intact.

Release is accomplished by the synthesized, secretory materials passing through the cell membrane without rupturing it (p. 166).

Example: most of the common glands, such as serous and mucous types.

2. *Apocrine.* Some of the apical cytoplasm of the gland cell detaches, along with each secretory droplet that collects there.

Example: mammary gland; some specialized sweat glands.

3. *Holocrine.* The entire cell is discharged during secretion.

Proliferated cells may be discharged intact; such glands are called *cytogenic.*

Example: hemopoietic organs; sex glands.

The cell may die, disintegrate and thereby liberate the secretion.

Example: sebaceous glands, whose cells undergo fatty degeneration.

II. THE EXOCRINE GLANDS

I. UNICELLULAR GLANDS

Single specific secretory cells may be scattered throughout an epithelial sheet.

Example: intestine; uterine tube.

The commonest type is the *goblet mucous cell* of the respiratory and intestinal tracts.

In the resting condition it is an ordinary-looking columnar cell.

At the beginning of activity, droplets of *mucigen* (*i.e.*, premucin) appear in the cytoplasm.

They collect in the upper part of the cell and distend it progressively.

(For the characteristics of mucigen and its end-product, *mucin,* see p. 167.)

Experiments show that the turn-over of secretion can be rapid.

Radioactive sulfate is taken up and discharged as labeled mucus in 24 hours.

By contrast, the basal end often remains slender; the whole cell takes on a goblet shape.

In the base is found the main mass of unaltered cytoplasm.

Here also is the nucleus, sometimes pressed downward and flattened against the base.

The events leading to the release of mucin are similar to those occurring in serous cells (p. 166).

Goblet cells usually have a single, relatively long cycle and discharge continuously.

Yet in the intestine they are cast off and replaced every few days.

Replacements come from other cells which move in from some distance away.

When a goblet cell discharges explosively, it collapses and is compressed by its neighbors.

Presently synthesis resumes and the cell refills.

The goblet-cell shape occurs only when mucous cells are interspersed in an epithelium.

The goblet shape is gained by crowding and distorting neighboring, ordinary cells.

When every cell in an epithelium is mucus-secreting, then no goblet shape occurs.

This is the case in the surface lining of the stomach and of the uterine cervix.

DIAGNOSTIC FEATURES.

The goblet cell occurs in either a simple columnar or pseudostratified epithelium.

The goblet- to barrel-shape of this bloated cell is distinctive.

If mucigen is preserved, it stains fairly well with basic dyes in general.

If mucigen fails to stain, then three possibilities exist.

The cell may have discharged recently, and is now temporarily empty.

The mucigen may have been dissolved by an improper fixing agent.

The stain may be inappropriate to demonstrate mucigen.

In ordinary preparations, inactive and early-regenerating stages are not conspicuous.

II. MULTICELLULAR GLANDS

All the cells of an epithelium may become secretory units.

This arrangement can be called a secretory epithelial sheet.

Example: surface layer of the stomach, uterus and choroid plexus.

Intermediate between unicellular and multicellular glands are the pit-like, intra-epithelial glands that lie wholly within a generalized epithelial layer.

Example: nasal mucosa; urethra; efferent ductules.

In general, multicellular glands arise as invaginations into vascularized connective tissue.

Most of them have an *excretory duct*, which is a nonsecretory drainage tube.

The functionally active portion of the gland consists of secretory *end-pieces*.

The simplest glandular invaginations have a secretory portion, but lack a separate duct.

Example: intestinal 'crypt.'

More complex glands have a single, unbranched excretory duct.

Example: duodenal gland.

The most complex glands have a branched, tree-like system of ducts.

The branching may be slight (labial gland) or extensive (kidney; parotid).

The secretory end-pieces of a gland are named according to their shapes.

Tubular refers to a blindly ending, hollow cylinder.

Alveolar (or *acinar*) refers to a globular to pear-shaped ending, with a small lumen.

Tubulo-alveolar refers to a tubule with *alveoli* inset at the end, sides or both.

It also may refer to the presence of separate tubules and alveoli.

Saccular refers to a pouch-like ending, with a relatively large lumen.

A. ANATOMICAL CLASSIFICATION:

1. Simple glands.

The excretory duct, when present, is single and unbranched.

A. TUBULAR.

1. Straight tubular (*e.g.,* intestinal crypts).
2. Coiled tubular (*e.g.,* ordinary sweat glands).
3. Branched tubular.
   a. Without an excretory duct (*e.g.,* stomach; uterus).
   b. With an excretory duct (*e.g.,* small glands of mouth and esophagus; deep glands of the duodenum; axillary sweat glands).

B. ALVEOLAR.

Unbranched alveolar (*e.g.,* tarsal glands).

C. SACCULAR.

1. Unbranched saccular (*e.g.,* seminal vesicle).
2. Branched saccular (*e.g.,* sebaceous glands).

2. Compound glands.

Such a gland consists of several to many component *lobules*.

Each lobule is a unit that is the equivalent of a simple, branched gland.

The several lobular ducts join and finally unite into one main excretory duct.

Four subtypes are based on the shape of the secretory end-pieces.
>   A. TUBULAR.
>>   Example: kidney (blind tubules); testis (anastomosing tubules).
>   B. ALVEOLAR.
>>   Example: some of the simpler glands of the respiratory tract.
>   C. TUBULO-ALVEOLAR.
>>   Example: large salivary glands; pancreas; large glands of the esophagus and respiratory tract; lacrimal gland.
>   D. SACCULAR.
>>   Example: mammary gland.

B. CHARACTERISTICS OF SECRETORY CELL-TYPES:

Most of the exocrine glands are composed of serous cells, mucous cells, or both types.

1. Serous cells.

This type discharges a clear, watery, albuminous secretion, elaborated from granules.
The secretory end-pieces are tubules or rounded to pear-shaped alveoli.
>   The single layer of wedge-shaped cells surrounds a notably narrow *lumen.*
>>   Such a lumen is adequate to conduct a watery, free-flowing secretion.
>>   The lateral boundaries between adjacent cells are indistinct.
>   *Secretory canaliculi* course between the gland cells and reach the alveolar lumen.
>>   They are merely grooves between the plasma membranes of abutting cells.
>>   In some instances the groove is continuous with the intracellular tubules.
>>>   These are invaginations of the plasma membrane into the cell-cytoplasm.
>>   The Golgi silver-technique demonstrates these tiny canaliculi well.
All serous cells exhibit a characteristic internal organization.
>   The nucleus is rounded and located nearer the base of the cell.
>   Cytoplasm above the nucleus contains the Golgi complex and *secretion granules.*
>>   In many glands such granules are enzyme precursors (*zymogen granules*).
>>   Formol fixation and some basic dyes (*e.g.,* neutral gentian) stain them well.
>>   So-called secretion granules are actually droplets coagulated by fixatives.
>   Cytoplasm of the cell-base contains endoplasmic reticulum, studded with *ribosomes.*
>>   Their presence relates to the synthesis of proteinaceous secretion droplets.
>>   This synthesizing complex, staining with basic dyes, is called *ergastoplasm.*
>>>   It sometimes bears vertically oriented *basal striations.*
>>>   These are produced by mitochondria and infoldings of the plasma membrane.
>   Synthesis is carried out according to instructions supplied by nuclear genes (p. 26).
>>   The protein-product moves within the endoplasmic channels to the Golgi complex.
>>   Transported as droplets (*intermediate vesicles*), it is concentrated there, packaged into membrane-bounded vesicles and then discharged.
>   Release is achieved by a droplet's membrane first touching the cell's plasma membrane.
>>   The two membranes then merge and the droplet escapes without membrane rupture.
>>   The secretion contains salts, protein and, often, an enzyme.
>   The speed of synthesis has been determined by administering radioactive amino acids.
>>   In five minutes it has been detected over the ergastoplasm; in 20 minutes over the Golgi region, and in 60 minutes at the cell apex (or discharged).
>   At the end of a synthetic phase, the serous cells are distended and ready to discharge.
>>   Cell boundaries are indistinct and the lumen of the alveolus is of minimal size.
>>   As the discharge continues, the cells shrink and the lumen enlarges somewhat.
>>   At the close of normal emptying, only a few secretory droplets remain in the cell.
>   A cell, depleted of its secretory content, is small and has dark-staining cytoplasm.
>>   The cytoplasm straightway enters upon a new constructive period.
>>   The synthesized product appears as droplets in the cytoplasm above the nucleus.
>>>   As they accumulate, the cytoplasm between them reduces to a spongework.
>>   The nucleus may be forced to the base of the cell, but it does not flatten.
>   During a cycle there is a waxing and waning of certain cell-components.
>>   These include the ergastoplasm, Golgi apparatus and nucleolus.

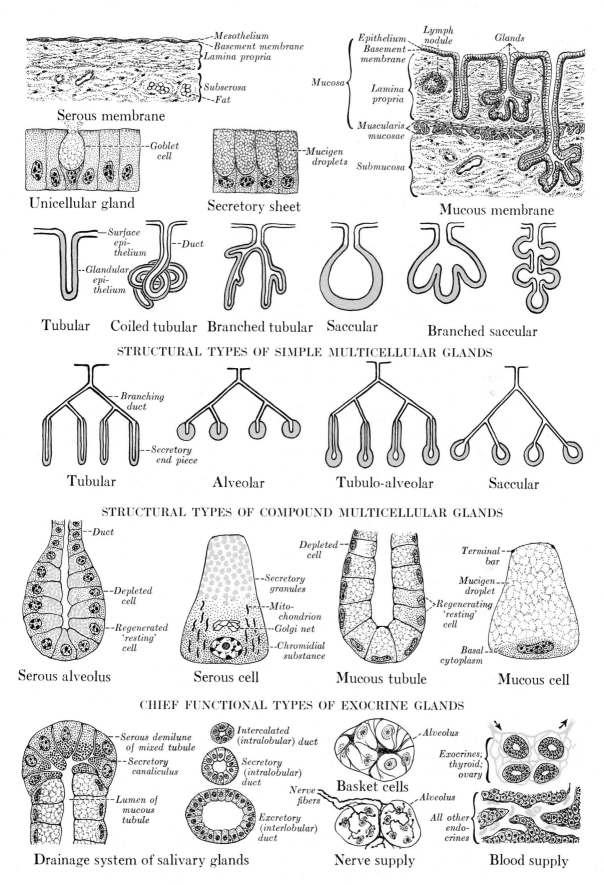

Serous membrane

Unicellular gland

Secretory sheet

Mucous membrane

Tubular   Coiled tubular   Branched tubular   Saccular   Branched saccular

STRUCTURAL TYPES OF SIMPLE MULTICELLULAR GLANDS

Tubular   Alveolar   Tubulo-alveolar   Saccular

STRUCTURAL TYPES OF COMPOUND MULTICELLULAR GLANDS

Serous alveolus   Serous cell   Mucous tubule   Mucous cell

CHIEF FUNCTIONAL TYPES OF EXOCRINE GLANDS

Drainage system of salivary glands   Basket cells   Nerve supply   Blood supply

MOIST MEMBRANES AND EXOCRINE GLANDS

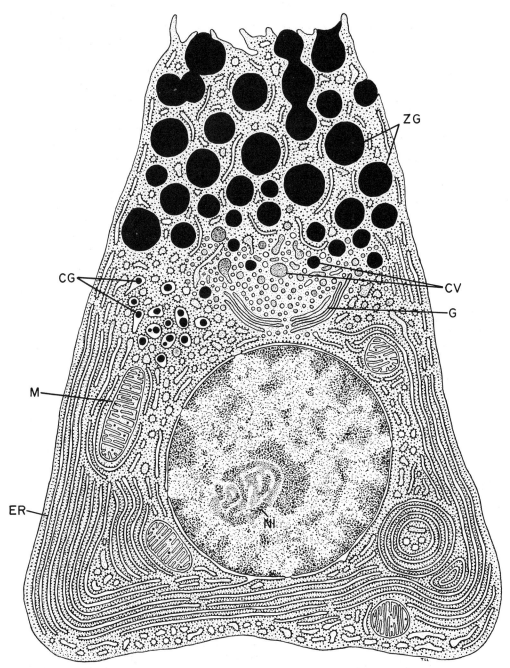

PANCREATIC EXOCRINE CELL. The basal half of this cell contains an extensive system of rough endo-plasmic reticulum (ER), concerned with protein synthesis. Free ribosomes and mitochondria (M) occupy regions between the membrane-pairs. The Golgi complex (G) is prominent, its concavity facing stages ranging from small vesicles to condensing vacuoles (CV) in the formation of dense zymogen granules (ZG). Granule release occurs when part of the granule membrane fuses with the plasma membrane and this region opens. Some dense granules, similar to zymogen granules, occur in the higher endoplasmic channels; these are called cisternal granules (CG). The outer, ribosome-studded layer of the nuclear membrane is continuous (basally) with a cisterna of the endoplasmic reticulum. The nucleolus (Nl) is channeled and prominent.

2. Mucous cells.

This type discharges a viscid, mucous secretion, formed as droplets in the cytoplasm.
The secretory end-pieces are tubules, made of a single layer of wedge-shaped cells.
   The lateral membranes, between cells, show as well defined boundaries.
      The cell-tops are usually encircled by sets of terminal bars.
   The lumen of the tubule is wide, thus facilitating the flow of thick mucus.
      Secretory capillaries, such as occur in serous alveoli, are lacking.
A mucous cell has a characteristic internal structure.
The cytoplasm above the nucleus contains *mucigen*, a proteinaceous elaboration.
   The exact chemical nature of mucigen varies considerably in different glands.
      This may also be true of different tubules in the same gland.
      It may even occur in different regions of the same tubule.
   Mucigens are glycoproteins that vary in composition, but commonly are acidic.
      Such acidic products stain well with some basic dyes, such as thionin.
      They stain specifically with mucicarmine (pink) or muchematin (purple).
      With ordinary stains they respond poorly; cells may appear to be empty.
   The mucigen droplets are hard to preserve satisfactorily in fixed tissues.
      The droplets are destroyed and dissolved by aqueous fixatives.
         The cytoplasm then appears as a honeycomb that stains like mucin.
         This is because a cytoplasmic spongework has mucigen precipitated on it.
      Alcoholic fixatives preserve mucigen somewhat better.
The cytoplasm below the nucleus contains *ergastoplasm*, as in serous cells.
   This material (endo. reticulum and ribosomes) engages in the synthesis of mucigen.
   The events are essentially like those already described for serous cells (p. 166).
      But the polysaccharide component of mucigen is added by the Golgi complex.
The membrane-bounded mucigen droplets collect first near the free end of the cell.
   They then progressively invade deeper parts of the cytoplasm.
   Accumulating droplets push the nucleus steadily downward.
      Finally it more or less flattens against the cell base.
   When the cell contains much mucigen, only a little basal cytoplasm remains.
When the synthetic phase ends and the cell is 'ripe,' the mucigen droplets escape.
   Discharge through the cell apex is like that used by serous cells (p. 166).
   When liberated, mucigen imbibes water and is then known as *mucin*.
      This is a thick, viscid, glairy secretion.
   Having acquired inorganic salts and other additions, it is often called *mucus*.
   Mucus is chemically inactive, but is important for protection and as a lubricant.
If all the mucigen is emptied, the cell collapses and reverts to a slender shape.
   The nucleus rises higher in the cell and becomes rounded again.
   The cytoplasm then regenerates and fills out the cell.
   Until the synthesis of mucigen resumes, the cell somewhat resembles a serous cell.
If discharge of mucigen is but partial, the events of recovery are not so plain.

3. Mixed sero-mucous tubules.

Some serous cells also stain slightly with mucicarmine.
   They are sometimes designated as sero-mucous cells.
Quite different are glands that have both cell types in at least some of the tubules.
   If the mucous cells dominate a tubule, the serous cells occur in groups.
   They either occupy the distal end of a mucous tubule, or overlap it there.
      More rarely the serous group outpockets from the side of a tubule.
   These oval-shaped, serous patches are called *demilunes* or *crescents*.
The serous cells of a demilune are smaller than the mucous cells of the tubule.
   Intercellular *secretory canaliculi* connect such serous cells with the lumen.

4. Diagnostic features.

Secretory *end-pieces* appear as circular to elongate groups of epithelial cells.
   When the lumen is cut across, the cells are wedge-shaped and radially arranged.
   When the lumen is cut axially, the cells are cuboidal to columnar in shape.
   (Most of the end-pieces become cut across somewhat obliquely.)

Serous cells usually stain fairly well with ordinary dyes, especially at their base.

The cytoplasm is distinctly granular; cell boundaries are not clear.

Specific zymogen granules may show distinctly in some ordinary preparations.

As a whole, they stain with some acid dyes and some basic dyes.

Nuclei may lie at the cell base, but they are not flattened.

The alveolar lumen is small, or not even noticeable.

Mucous cells commonly remain pale after ordinary fixation and staining.

If the mucigen is partially preserved, a reticulum can be seen.

It stains moderately well with basic dyes.

Nuclei are basal in position and tend to be definitely flattened.

The alveolar lumen is conspicuous; cell boundaries are sharply defined.

Demilunes may appear to be separate, or a patch applied onto a mucous tubule.

These appearances are largely owing to the obliquity of the section.

C. STRUCTURAL PLAN:

1. Secretory end-pieces.

The secretory epithelium of a gland is arranged as specialized *end-pieces*.

These attach to the terminal ducts.

Their shape may be that of a tube, long-necked flask, berry or sac.

The lumen is variable in size, depending on the type of gland.

The component cells of an end-piece are almost always but one layer deep.

They are most commonly shaped like truncated pyramids.

A *basement membrane* separates epithelium from connective tissue.

Basket (or *basal*) *cells* frequently occur about secretory end-pieces or small ducts.

These are scattered, stellate, flat cells; ordinary stains show them poorly.

They lie between the gland cells and the basement membrane.

In section they appear thin, with dark, flat nuclei.

They are clasping elements, with internal fibrils of a contractile nature (actin).

For this reason they are also known as *myo-epithelial cells*.

2. Ducts.

The ducts are primarily drainage tubes of different sizes.

The duct systems of small and large glands compare as does a shrub to a tree.

In a large gland the ducts located outside of lobules may number 1500.

A duct is lined with a very regular epithelium, showing distinct cell boundaries.

The epithelium of small ducts is frequently clasped by basket cells.

The duct system reaches its highest specialization in the major salivary glands.

An *intercalated* (or *intermediate*) *duct* attaches to the alveolus.

Its cells are of a low, cuboidal type.

Secretory ducts, next in order, are peculiar to the salivary glands.

Their columnar cells bear vertical basal-striations; another name is *striated ducts*.

This appearance is produced in part by parallel rows of mitochondria.

Also many infoldings of the basal plasma membrane pass into the cytoplasm.

Such ducts are said to secrete water and salts.

Excretory ducts are the largest branches (and also the main trunk) of the duct-system.

In general, they are lined with a high columnar epithelium.

The main trunk of some of them has a pseudostratified epithelium.

In some locations the region of the outlet changes to a stratified epithelium.

The several ducts are sometimes designated as being *interlobular* and *intralobular*.

These terms refer merely to a location between or within lobules, respectively.

Excretory ducts are preponderantly interlobular in position.

Intercalated ducts are wholly intralobular, and secretory ducts almost always so.

3. Framework and lobulation.

A definite fibro-elastic *capsule* surrounds many of the larger glands.

Fibrous *septa* divide large, compact glands into *lobules* (and sometimes into *lobes*).

Each lobule is arranged about a branch of the duct-system and its twigs.
It represents a somewhat independent unit of glandular organization.
The septa contain the larger ducts; also blood vessels, lymphatics and nerves.
Fat cells may occur in the septa, and even within the lobule.
Delicate connective tissue within a lobule forms a *stroma* that embeds the alveoli.

4. Vessels and nerves.

Blood vessels follow the connective-tissue septa and ducts.
Rich capillary networks form about secretory end-pieces and terminal ducts.
Lymphatics are said to be scarce in many glands.
Secretory *nerve fibers* form plexuses of bare filaments beneath the epithelium.
Extensions penetrate between the cells and make simple or branched endings.

D. REGENERATIVE ABILITY:

Mucous cells show mitoses rarely, and there are few signs of degeneration.
Serous cells, under normal conditions, undergo mitoses occasionally.
In general, replacements come from cells recruited from the adjoining ducts.
Some glands regenerate rather well after incurring considerable gross loss.

E. DIAGNOSTIC FEATURES:

All but the simplest glands appear as multiple, closely packed, epithelial islands.
These are set in a small amount of delicate, connective-tissue stroma.
The continuity and unity of the system is not apparent in a random, single section.
The larger glands are subdivided into lobules by coarse connective tissue.
This interlobular tissue often is subject to marked shrinkage.
The epithelial *end-pieces* are circular, ovoid or tubular in section.
A lumen may or may not be seen; it varies greatly in size.
The variation is correlated with the type of gland and its functional state.
For the characteristic features of mucous and serous alveoli, see pp. 166, 167.
Other types of glands will be considered under the several organ systems.
Intercalated ducts are much smaller than alveoli, and hence are rather inconspicuous.
They are easiest seen when traceable to alveoli as small tubules.
Their epithelium is scarcely thicker than the contained nuclei.
Secretory ducts, when present, are the most conspicuous structures within a lobule.
This is because of their fair size, bright acidophilic coloration, precisely regular proportions and prominent lumen.
The lumen is somewhat the same diameter as the thickness of the duct wall.
The component columnar cells show vertical basal-striations.
The epithelium frequently shrinks away from its basement membrane.
Excretory ducts course in the connective tissue between lobules.
This location and their large size readily identify them.
The epithelium is usually tall columnar or pseudostratified; it is not striated.
The lumen tends to be definitely wider than the wall.

III. THE ENDOCRINE GLANDS

This group has no ducts of any kind; secretion is released directly into the blood stream.
Hence these glands are designated as *ductless* or *endocrine* (internally secreting).
It follows that the vascular supply to these organs must be both rich and intimate.
Each cell abuts upon either a sinusoid or capillary.
Most of the endocrine glands are separate entities, recognizable as distinct organs.
Example: thyroid; suprarenals; hypophysis; parathyroids.
These have a connective-tissue capsule and a delicate internal stroma.
Some endocrine tissue, however, occurs as scattered masses within an exocrine gland.
Example: pancreatic islands; interstitial cells of testis; corpus luteum of ovary.
These combined exocrine-endocrine organs are sometimes spoken of as *mixed organs.*

The endocrine tissue may be distributed so diffusely that it is not regarded as an 'organ.'
    Example: cells in the lining of the duodenum produce three different hormones.
In general, endocrine tissue has undergone detachment from its parent epithelium.
    Some representatives become secondarily an epithelium with a free surface.
        Example: thyroid follicles; ovarian follicles.
    Others are composed of atypical epithelium that lacks a free surface.
        Example: parathyroids; adenohypophysis; pancreatic islands.
    Still others are not even epithelial in origin.
        Example: nervous (neurohypophysis); connective tissue (interstitial cells of testis); neural crest (suprarenal medulla).
Endocrine glands, as a group, have a simpler organization than exocrine glands.
    This is largely because they lack the organization imposed by a duct-system.
        As a result, the gland cells must abut directly against vascular channels.
    Most of this group of glands are arranged in cords or plates of atypical epithelium.
        These cords are separated by sinusoids or broad capillaries.
            Example: suprarenal; parathyroid; pancreatic islands; hypophysis; corpus luteum.
    A few glands consist of typical epithelial sacs, surrounded by a vascular plexus.
        Example: thyroid; ovarian follicles.
The secretion-products of endocrine glands are named *hormones*.
    A hormone is capable of eliciting a specific response from a target organ at some distance.
        The response is usually an activation (including the maintenance of function).
        On the contrary, the effect is sometimes to inhibit activity or arousal.
        The responsive target may be a tissue, an organ or the body as a whole.
    Only a minute quantity of a hormone is required to produce an optimum effect.
        Its action is essentially like that of a chemical catalyst.
    Some glands produce only one hormone; others elaborate several.
Secretion granules (hormone precursors) are synthesized by all endocrine glands.
    The method of synthesis and packaging of the products is essentially as in exocrine glands.
    Little is known, however, of the methods of release and entry into capillaries.
    The granules, for the most part, are plainly demonstrable only by special techniques.
    Yet steroid products (forming in agranular reticulum) do not have demonstrable precursors.
All endocrine organs store their secretory products to some extent.
    Storage is usually within the cells of origin; notably so in the pancreatic islands.
        Yet in the suprarenal cortex, secretion is released almost as fast as it is formed.
    By contrast, storage may be in a pool enclosed by the glandular cells.
        In this instance the epithelium takes the form of sacs (*e.g.*, thyroid).
The group of endocrine glands constitutes an organ system.
    Their mode of secretion and target effectiveness are characteristics shared in common.
    These organs not only integrate other parts but interact to regulate themselves.
The individual endocrine glands will be described in the following chapter.

Chapter XVI

The Endocrine Glands

An introduction to the endocrine organs has been presented in the preceding chapter.
The present accounts will discuss in detail those glands that are separate organs.
Several other endocrines are contained within organs of a wholly different type.
   Such include pancreatic islands, gonadal tissue and gastro-intestinal epithelium.
   These will be described with the major organs of which they are a part.

I. THE THYROID GLAND

The *thyroid* arose as an epithelial bud detaching from the floor of the pharynx.
   The meaning is 'shield-shaped,' in reference to its relation to the upper trachea.
The main bulk of the organ consists of a *lateral lobe*, on each side of the trachea.
   These two lobes are connected by a narrow *isthmus* in front of the trachea.
Each main lobe is roughly the size of half a golf ball.

A. STRUCTURAL PLAN:

An enveloping *capsule* is continuous externally with the tissue of the deep cervical fascia.
   This outer, looser fascia separates easily from the thinner capsule proper.
Capsular tissue continues inward as *septa* which subdivide the thyroid mass.
   The *lobules*, thus formed, are incompletely surrounded with connective tissue.
   The uncovered regions of parenchyma interconnect at intervals.
The gland consists of enormous numbers of closed epithelial sacs, or *follicles*.
   Each lies separately in a common, connective-tissue *stroma*.
   Each contains little to much stored secretion, known as *colloid*.

B. DETAILED STRUCTURE:

1. Framework.

A fibro-elastic *capsule* sends delicate *septa* inward, delimiting *lobules* incompletely.
Areolar and reticular-tissue provide a thin, highly vascular *stroma*.
   In this bed lie myriads of individual *thyroid follicles*.

2. Follicles.

The structural and functional unit is a closed, single-layered epithelial sac, the *follicle*.
The size of a normal follicle in the adult varies from 50 to 500 μ in diameter.
   This range depends on the degree of distention by secretion.
Normally the smaller follicles are more numerous than the larger ones.
   The total number of follicles is, perhaps, 20 millions.
The shape of a follicle is spheroidal, or sometimes elongate.
   Occasionally there are constricted, twisted or bizarre shapes.
A. EPITHELIUM.
   The shape of the component cells varies about a mean, which is cuboidal.
      The cells are low when the gland is underactive (much stored colloid).
      The cells are high when the gland is overactive (little stored colloid).
      However, cell height also varies with age, sex, diet, season, etc.

The epithelium lies upon a thin, wholly inconspicuous *basement membrane.*
Cell height in any follicle is quite uniform; the arrangement of cells is regular.
    The cells show a definite polarization with respect to their components.
        The nuclei are relatively large and open-structured.
            They lie centrally to somewhat basally, in an even row.
                Above the nucleus are the *Golgi net, centrioles* and most *mitochondria.*
The cytoplasm of the follicular epithelium is finely granular and palely basophilic.
    At the cell-top the cytoplasmic border projects as submicroscopic *microvilli.*
    Droplets of colloid (recovered from the pool?) may occur in the cytoplasm.
    So-called 'colloid cells' are degenerating elements, with pyknotic nuclei.
        Their cytoplasm is strongly acidophilic and often contains colloid droplets.
Sparse *pale cells* lie between the epithelium proper and the basement membrane.
    These large *parafollicular cells* are migrants from embryonic pharyngeal pouches.
    They are unlike the thyroid cells in structure and function (p. 173).

B. Colloid.

The thyroid is a gland that is notable for its storage of reserve secretion.
    This reserve is the semifluid *colloid* that fills the follicular lumen.
    Fresh colloid is homogeneous, clear and viscous.
Colloid consists chiefly of *thyroglobulin,* a glycoprotein.
    Its amount and consistency vary normally between wide limits.
        A large amount indicates glandular inactivity; such colloid is a stiff jelly.
        An active gland contains a small amount of thin, more fluid colloid.
Colloid does not stain identically in all follicles.
    It may even stain differently in local regions of the same follicle.
    In active follicles (rapid turn-over) the colloid is definitely basophilic.
    Inactive follicles have acidophilic (or very weakly basophilic) colloid.
Sections often show vacuoles in the colloid and a detached, scalloped border.
    Both are artifacts, caused by shrinkage, but have some significance.
    The scallops (former vacuoles) are most striking in active follicles.
        Probably the colloid in these areas was more fluid.
        That is, it was ready for resorption, but was lost in section-making.

3. Secretion and storage.

The process of secretion is complicated by the temporary storage of its product.
Thyroid cells remove iodine rapidly from the blood stream and concentrate it.
    It is then combined into a protein-bound iodide, the storage substance.
    Both processes have been followed by using radioactive iodine and leucine.
The normal direction of secretion is first into the lumen of the follicle, exocrine style.
    Here the synthesized substance joins the colloid-pool and is stored.
    The storage-form is *thyroglobulin* (amino acids conjugated with a globulin).
For release into the blood, thyroblogulin is first recovered from the colloid pool.
    This is accomplished by pinocytosis, whereupon *colloid droplets* are demonstrable in
        the cytoplasm of follicle cells.
    Hydrolyzing enzymes from lysosomes split thyroglobulin into other products.
        Most abundant (90 per cent) is *thyroxin*; another is the more potent *tri-iodothyroxin.*
        These hormonal substances leave the cells and enter adjoining capillaries.
        Both products have been isolated in pure crystalline form.
Thus secretion is reversible, and it can proceed in both directions simultaneously.
    Under excess stimulation, secretion is chiefly direct—into the blood.

4. Vessels and nerves.

Blood vessels and *lymphatics* form intimate plexuses about follicles.
Arterio-venous anastomoses are common.
Capillaries about the follicles are of the thinned, rapid-transport type (p. 128).

The thyroid is about the best vascularized organ of the body.
Thyroxin is demonstrable in both veins and lymphatics, but chiefly in veins.
Most of the *nerve fibers* are vasomotor in function.
A few fibers end about follicles, but their secretory function is not proved.

C. REGENERATIVE ABILITY:

There is normal loss and replacement of thyroid cells, but the details are disputed.
Tissue lost by excision is not replaced significantly by cellular proliferation.
Former total size, however, can be regained by the hypertrophy of remaining tissue.

D. DIAGNOSTIC FEATURES:

Sections show crowded epithelial rings, set in a scanty stroma.
These rings (follicles) are of assorted sizes, the largest being macroscopic.
What seem to be small follicles may be only border slices off larger ones.
Solid epithelial disks represent tangential shavings from follicles.
There is a superficial resemblance to the active mammary gland and prostate.
The lining epithelium of a follicle is a simple layer, usually of cuboidal cells.
Homogeneous, eosinophilic colloid fills the follicles.
With some compound stains, colloid colors variously in different follicles.
Colloid commonly is shrunken in sections, and has a spiny border.
Fractured colloid in sections is the thicker, inactive type.

E. FUNCTIONAL CORRELATIONS:

The thyroid is an important gland, but not essential to life.
One-fifth of the gland suffices to maintain its normal functioning.
The thyroid regulates the metabolic rate; thyroxin increases cell metabolism.
It also is concerned with development, differentiation and growth.
A congenital thyroid deficiency leads to a condition known as *cretinism.*
This is a complex that includes dwarfism and impaired mentality.
The thyroid is a notably labile gland that varies greatly in size and structure.
Undersecretion, after childhood, leads to simple *colloid goiter* and *myxedema.*
In this type of goiter colloid collects in excess, but it lacks iodated protein.
Hence available hormone is deficient and functions are slowed.
Myxedema is characterized by muco-polysaccharides accumulating in connective tissues.
Oversecretion is associated with overgrowth of the follicular epithelium.
Follicles are large and folded, and the cells are tall and active.
The secretion is in excess, yet it may or may not be rich in thyroxin.
Typically the metabolic processes increase; body weight diminishes.
The parafollicular cells, outside the follicle proper, secrete the hormone *calcitonin.*
This reduces blood-calcium level and offsets the influence of the parathyroids (p. 175).
Thyroid secretion affects variously certain other endocrine glands.
Interaction with the hypophysis maintains balanced functional responses in both.
An hypophyseal hormone (*thyrotropin*) stimulates the release of thyroxin.
But thyroxin in the blood exerts a restraint on thyrotropic production.

II. THE PARATHYROID GLAND

There are typically four brownish, *parathyroid glands.*
Two are attached to the back of the capsule of each lateral thyroid lobe.
Other, accessory, glands occur frequently (30 per cent of individuals).
The glands are ovoid in shape; each is about the size of an apple seed.

A. STRUCTURAL PLAN:

Each gland has a thin *capsule*, from which delicate *septa* extend inward.

The *parenchyma* takes the form of solid cell plates that interconnect.
> The appearance is one of compact epithelial tissue, but without a free surface.
> Between the cell plates there are broad capillaries.
> Some clumps of *acidophilic cells* usually occur among the preponderant, *pale cells.*

B. Detailed Structure:

1. Framework.

The fibro-elastic *capsule* is a delicate layer.
Thin *septa* penetrate into the gland and divide it incompletely into *lobules.*
> This invasion begins some time after birth and continues as age advances.
> In this way the parenchyma increasingly is reduced to plate-like strands.
A basketwork of reticular tissue supports the cell plates as a delicate *stroma.*
Fat cells collect in the connective tissue increasingly, beginning at puberty.

2. Parenchyma.

The *epithelium* is a type that has secondarily lost its free surface.
> It was originally a part of the pharyngeal lining, but became detached and buried.
The epithelium takes the form of irregular, connecting masses of cells.
> This total epithelial mass is channeled by capillaries.
> It is claimed that each cell abuts against a capillary.
> > (When uninjected, capillaries are inconspicuous and tend to escape notice.)
The plates and cords are surrounded by an inconspicuous basement membrane.
Two main cell types, each well segregated, are recognized.

A. Chief Cell.

This is the fundamental and most abundant kind of cell component.
> They are the only cells seen until middle childhood.
> These small cells are arranged in plates and cords.
> With ordinary staining the cytoplasm is pale and 'empty'; nuclei are vesicular.
> > The slightly acidophilic cytoplasm tends to shrink during fixation.
> > The cytoplasm contains *secretion granules*, demonstrable by silver stains.
> Two subtypes of chief cells are recognized, but intermediates exist.
The *light chief cells* are slightly larger and are the most numerous type by far.
> The nucleus is relatively large; the cytoplasm is clear, but rich in glycogen.
> Secretory granules are rare or lacking; the cell is inactive or resting.
The *dark chief cells* differ from the pale chief cells quantitatively.
> They are somewhat smaller and have slightly smaller and darker nuclei.
> The cytoplasm is very finely granular; it contains many secretory granules.
> These cells are held to be in the active, secreting state.
Small, colloid-containing follicles are seen occasionally.
> These are especially noticeable after thyroid removal and in old age.
> The 'colloid' has no functional relation to the colloid of the thyroid.
Parathyroid cells resist postmortem autolysis better than other moist epithelia.

B. Oxyphil Cell.

This type first appears in childhood and becomes abundant in old age.
> The *oxyphil cell* is characteristic of man, but is absent in almost all mammals.
> The common arrangement of these cells is in small and large groups.
Oxyphil cells are much larger than chief cells because of their abundant cytoplasm.
> The cytoplasm is plainly granular and definitely acidophilic.
The ordinary oxyphil is deeply acidophilic, with a small dark-staining nucleus.
> Mitochondria pack the cytoplasm; other organelles and secretory granules lack.
> These cells appear to be senile; there is no evidence of functioning.
There are also pale oxyphil cells with lighter staining nuclei and cytoplasm.
> These are intermediate between the chief and oxyphil types.

3. Vessels and nerves.

The *blood supply* is fairly rich, the larger vessels following the septa.

The parenchyma is channeled by broad, irregular capillaries.
The presence of *lymphatics* is asserted, but details are few.
Nerve fibers, probably vasomotor, are scanty.

C. REGENERATIVE ABILITY:

The chief cells are seemingly the only ones that proliferate, and they do so rarely.
The parathyroid transplants readily, but fails to regenerate significantly.

D. DIAGNOSTIC FEATURES:

The general picture is of a densely cellular organ, arranged in masses and cords.
    Both capsule and septa are subordinated, and are often a minor feature.
The parenchyma consists of closely packed epithelial cells.
    These fit together in a mosaic of polyhedrons.
    Interspersed are capillaries (most of which are collapsed and inconspicuous).
Most numerous are pale cells, with a small amount of clear cytoplasm.
    Their closely spaced nuclei give an appearance somewhat like lymphoid tissue.
        But the cells are much larger and have more cytoplasm.
Conspicuous are irregularly distributed groups of larger cells (especially in adults).
    Their cytoplasm is abundant, granular and acidophilic.
    The cell nucleus is relatively small, shrunken and dark.

E. FUNCTIONAL CORRELATIONS:

The parathyroid hormone has been isolated in pure chemical form.
    Its normal effect is to cause the withdrawal of calcium from bones.
        The liberated calcium then accumulates in the blood plasma.
    An increasing calcium level in the plasma depresses parathyroid activity.
    These balanced effects maintain blood calcium at a nearly constant level.
    It is claimed that the hormone does not act by dissolving bone directly.
        Rather, the influence is exerted primarily upon cells (osteoclasts?).
Experiments have established the existence of a counterbalancing hormone, *calcitonin*.
    Its secretion is induced when the calcium level becomes high.
    The effect is to depress the level of blood-calcium by suppressing bone resorption.
    Calcitonin, first ascribed to parathyroids, is now known to reside in the thyroid (p. 173).
Atrophy or removal of the parathyroids is followed by a fall in blood calcium.
    This is accompanied by nervous hyperexcitability and muscular spasms.
    This condition, known as *tetany*, will lead to death unless intervention occurs.
    The administration of calcium or parathyroid extract affords relief.
Underactivity of the parathyroids has a marked effect on the developing skeleton.
    Calcification of the teeth and bones may be seriously impaired.
Overactivity of the glands occurs when there is calcium deficiency, as in rickets.
    The glands enlarge and their cells proliferate in attempting to compensate.
Overactivity can also result from hyperplastic or tumorous growth of parathyroid tissue.
    This may lead to extensive resorption of bone, and hence to elevated blood-calcium.

III. THE HYPOPHYSIS

The meaning is 'a sprout beneath' (the brain); an alternative name is the *pituitary body*.
It is a compound gland, made up of two wholly unlike parts.
    An *epithelial portion* originates from a sac pinched off from the primitive mouth.
    A *neural portion* is a downgrowth from the floor of the brain.
The hypophysis is largely buried in a fossa of the sphenoid bone.

A. STRUCTURAL PLAN:

The *hypophysis* is about the size of a small, somewhat flattened grape.
A pinkish portion is designated as the *adenohypophysis*, or epithelial hypophysis.
    It consists of glandular tissue, derived as a sac from the oral epithelium.

This portion is subdivided by the *residual lumen* into very unequal parts.
>   The lumen represents remnants of the cavity of the embryonic sacculation.
The larger part is in front of these clefts; it is the *pars distalis.*
>   An extension that surrounds the neural stalk is the *pars tuberalis.*
>   Both are composed of epithelial cords and sinusoids.
The smaller part, behind the clefts, is very thin; it is the *pars intermedia.*
A second, whitish, fibrous portion is designated as the *neurohypophysis.*
>   It consists of three component parts:
>>   One is the *pars nervosa*, fused to the epithelial portion of the total gland.
>>   The second and third parts are, respectively, the *infundibular stalk* (which extends
>>>   upward from the pars nervosa) and the *median eminence* of the brain.
Often the terms 'anterior lobe' and 'posterior lobe' are employed, for convenience.
>   Exact usage differs, but reference is especially to the two most important regions.
>>   *Anterior lobe* refers particularly to the pars distalis.
>>   *Posterior lobe* refers particularly to the pars nervosa.

B. DETAILED STRUCTURE:

1. Framework.

>   The fibro-elastic *capsule* is merely an innermost part of the neighboring dura mater.
>>   It is thickest where it encloses the anterior lobe.
>   *Trabeculae*, bearing blood vessels, radiate from one point into the pars distalis.
>   A meshwork of *reticular tissue* supports the cords and sinusoids of that lobe.

2. Pars distalis.

>   This portion constitutes about three-fourths of the organ (exclusive of its stalk).
>   Its epithelium is arranged in anastomosing cords and plates; it is the *parenchyma.*
>>   Epithelial vesicles, filled with a colloid substance, occur occasionally.
>   The epithelial parenchyma is supported by a *basement membrane.*
>>   Between the cords are dilated, sinusoidal capillaries.
>   The component epithelial cells are of two main types, unequal in numbers.
>>   The cell shape is ovoid to polyhedral; nuclei vary somewhat in the cell types.
>>   But the cytoplasm is the differential feature that distinguishes the two types.
>>>   One group responds feebly to stains, and is named *chromophobes.*
>>>   The other group has strong staining affinities, and is called *chromophils.*
>   A. CHROMOPHOBE CELLS.
>>   These faintly staining elements are degranulated, exhausted cells.
>>>   They are inactive phases of the other main group (chromophils).
>>>   It is possible that some represent unspecialized stem-cells.
>>   They tend to be located in clusters, more axially within the cell cords.
>>>   That is, they do not border on sinusoids, as active cells do.
>>   The chromophobe cell is smaller than the chromophils and is the commonest (50%).
>>>   Its cytoplasm is scanty, stains lightly and at best has but few granules.
>>>   Cell boundaries are not seen in ordinary preparations.
>>>   The nuclei are closely spaced because there is little cytoplasm.
>   B. CHROMOPHIL CELLS.
>>   These cells are larger than chromophobes, and their cell boundaries are distinct.
>>>   The cytoplasm is definitely granular and readily stainable.
>>   This quality makes chromophils far more conspicuous than chromophobes.
>>   Chromophils tend to lie at the surface of cell cords, next to the sinusoids.
>>>   There is evidence that the granules are actual precursors of secretions.
>>>   The degree of granularity varies with the functional state of a cell.
>>>   There are two cell types: *acidophils* and *basophils.*
>>>>   Their distribution differs regionally, and varies locally.
>>>>   Also cell ratios are modified by pregnancy, castration, etc.

The *acidophil cells* comprise 35 per cent of all cells in the pars distalis.
> They are more numerous in the center of each half-lobe, and posteriorly.
> Acidophils take on acid dyes, but also stain with safranin, a basic dye.
>> (Hence some prefer to call them *alpha cells,* but this is confusing since a subtype is also so named.)
> Their specific granules are abundant; they differ in size in each subtype.
> Two cell-types are distinguishable on the basis of granularity and staining.
>> They are *alpha cells* (orangeophils) and *epsilon cells* (carminophils).

The *basophil cells* total 15 per cent of all cells in the pars distalis.
> They are more numerous in the midplane and the antero-lateral margins.
> In general, basophils stain with basic dyes, but not greedily with most.
>> In addition, the granules stain with aniline blue, an acid dye.
>> (For this reason some prefer to call this category *beta cells,* but confusion exists with a subtype also so named.)
> Basophils tend to be appreciably larger than acidophils.
>> Their granules are smaller and fairly uniform in size in the subtypes.
>> At comparable stages the granules are fewer than those of acidophils.
> Three cell types are recognized with the electron microscope and staining.
>> These are named *beta-, gamma-* and *delta cells.*

c. SECRETORY CYCLE.
> Mitoses are rare; therefore, the cells must pass through repeated cycles.
> The relations between the cell-types have seemingly been solved (in the rat).
>> The chromophobes are inactive resting cells, of two distinguishable types.
>> As they approach a new phase of activity, granules appear in them.
>>> The granules are of two different kinds, and two cell-types differentiate.
>>> One type becomes acidophils; the other type becomes basophils.
>> Engorged cells then secrete and return to their chromophobic, inactive state.

3. Pars tuberalis.
> There are cell groups and short cords, set in a well vascularized reticulum.
> Some of the cells are finely granular and faintly basophilic.
> There is a tendency toward the formation of cysts with 'colloid' in them.

4. Residual lumen.
> The *lumen* is typically an epithelial-lined cleft.
>> It is well represented in most mammals, including young children.
>> In adult man it may be entirely obliterated or may persist as remnants.
>>> Such cystic cavities frequently possess a ciliated lining.

5. Pars intermedia.
> In most mammals this portion is a narrow, but definite, layer.
>> It is located behind the residual lumen and is several cells deep.
>> Its polyhedral cells stain with basic dyes.
>>> Secretory granules have been described in them.
>> Cysts are common, filled with a colloid or hyaline material.
> In man and apes, the pars intermedia is usually an ill-defined region.
>> This is because the residual lumen is virtually obliterated as a cleft.
>> The pars intermedia is probably the most variable organ of the body.
>> A thin layer of *cells* and *colloid cysts* occurs next to the neural lobe.
>>> Portions of this tissue project backward into the neural lobe.
>>> Some cells are pale-staining; others are granular and basophilic.
>>>> The basophils are prone to invade the neural lobe by migration.

6. Neurohypophysis.
> It is now recognized that the solid *pars nervosa* belongs to a larger entity.

This is a complex that can be named the *neurohypophysis*.

Besides the pars nervosa it also includes the *infundibular stalk* and *median eminence* of the diencephalon.

All three portions have the same neuroglial cell-types, a common blood and nerve supply, and contain the same active hormonal principles.

In the median eminence are specialized nerve cells, neurosecretory in function.

Their unmyelinated axons, some 100,000 in number, descend into the pars nervosa.

These fibers constitute the *hypothalamo-hypophyseal tract.*

Intermingled with the nerve fibers are distinctive cells, the *pituicytes*.

There are four subtypes, but all are regarded as specialized neuroglia.

The main nerve tract descends from the brain and branches in the pars nervosa.

Each bundle of nerve fibers forms the core of a 'lobule.'

The nerve fibers terminate in swollen endings at the periphery of a lobule.

Their parallel arrangement produces a regular palisade pattern.

Capillaries lie in close association with the enlarged nerve terminations.

A selectively stainable substance occurs in nerve cells, fibers and swollen endings.

It is secreted by the nerve cells in the brain, is passed down within the nerve fibers and accumulates in the fiber terminations.

The endings of some axons become enormously expanded with stored secretion.

Such microscopically visible pools have long been known as *Herring bodies*.

Precursor granules of the secretion are demonstrable in nerve cells and fibers.

There is indication of the presence of two different kinds of granules.

The secretion of these neurons contains two specific hormone-principles.

7. *Vessels and nerves.*

The plan and richness of *vascularization* is not constant throughout the organ.

One arterial source supplies the pars tuberalis with capillaries.

Extensions pass to the median eminence and infundibular stalk.

This plexus is drained by veins that supply the sinusoids of the pars distalis.

These vessels constitute a true portal system between two capillary beds.

The pars nervosa has an independent arterial supply (and drainage).

Its vascularity is good, but much inferior to that of the pars distalis.

Some of its branches extend through the pars intermedia and open into the capillaries of the pars distalis.

Hence the pars distalis is fed both by arterial and by venous vessels.

The capillaries of both lobes have thin, fenestrated regions (p. 128).

Lymphatics have never been demonstrated in relation to the gland.

There is a thick *nerve bundle* that descends into the pars nervosa (see above).

Some of its fibers enter the anterior lobe and terminate close to gland cells.

Stimulation of the tract in the rabbit is effective (inducing ovulation, etc.).

This is not true of mammals in general, which ovulate spontaneously.

Yet various functions of this lobe do depend on hypothalamic connections.

Other fibers end in the pars intermedia, but the great majority terminate within the neurohypophysis, and especially in the pars nervosa.

Autonomic fibers supply the vessels of the anterior and posterior lobes.

Secretion in the pars distalis is not related to the few nerve fibers found there.

Neurons in the median eminence emit releasing factors that stimulate the gland cells.

These factors reach the pars distalis through the portal system of vessels.

C. REGENERATIVE ABILITY:

The pars distalis can compensate in size for fairly extensive losses.

The pars nervosa heals injuries by scar-like tissue, as do other parts of the brain.

D. DIAGNOSTIC FEATURES:

A section through a total gland displays two quite different regions.

There is a larger, highly cellular part, that represents the anterior lobe.

A smaller, fibrous-looking part is the pars nervosa of the posterior lobe.

The pars distalis stains well (largely acidophilic); the pars nervosa is relatively pale.

Epithelial-lined clefts tend to separate the two regions.
The *pars distalis* consists of short cords, interspersed with capillaries.
  The frequency-ratio of acidophils and basophils varies regionally.
  Acidophilic cells are prominent, and are the most abundant elements seen.
    They stain well with eosin.
  Basophils tend to stain weakly with hematoxylin.
  Chromophobes are easily identified as groups of closely spaced, nearly naked nuclei.
    They lie within cords, and their cytoplasm is not well seen.
The region of the residual lumen and *pars intermedia* is distinctive.
  It is dominated by cyst-like spaces and cells with basophilic coloration.
The *pars nervosa,* with ordinary stains, has a pale, fibrous appearance.
  It resembles the texture of unmyelinated-nerve tissue.

E. FUNCTIONAL CORRELATIONS:

The hypophysis is the master endocrine organ, also controlling other endocrines.
  Six hormones have already been obtained from it in rather pure form.
The physiological effects of an endocrine organ can be ascertained by experiment.
  A gland can be removed and the resulting functional loss noted.
    Administering an extract of the gland should then promote functional recovery.
The cell-type responsible for a particular effect may also become known.
  — Removal of a target organ may lead to an increase in the number of those cells responsible
      for elaborating the associated hormone.
  — Pathology of a cell-type may accompany abnormal functioning of an organ.
  Regional abundance or lack of a cell-type may correlate with hormone assays there.

1. Anterior lobe.

A. PARS DISTALIS.

The growth hormone is known technically as *somatotropin (STH).*
  It stimulates general body growth, and especially at epiphyses.
  Undersecretion leads to *dwarfism* of the midget type.
  Oversecretion prolongs growth and produces *gigantism*; in adults, *acromegaly.*
  Evidence implicates a particular type of acidophil (orangeophil) as the source.
Three hormones influence the gonads, and are hence called *gonadotropes.*
  The *follicle-stimulating hormone* (FSH) promotes growth of ovarian follicles.
    In the male it activates the testis to produce spermatozoa.
      Hence *gametokinetic hormone* would be a better general name.
    The delta basophil seems to be the source of the hormone.
  The *luteinizing hormone* (LH) is the decisive factor in producing ovulation.
    It also converts the ruptured follicle into a corpus luteum.
    In the male it incites the interstitial cells of the testis into function.
      For this it is sometimes called, more appropriately, ICSH.
    The gamma basophil is associated with the elaboration of the hormone.
  The *luteotropic hormone* (LTH) makes the corpus luteum secrete progesterone.
    It has also been called the *lactogenic hormone* (or prolactin).
      It activates the secretion of milk by the properly developed breast.
    A particular acidophil (carminophil) is thought to produce the hormone.
The *thyrotropic hormone* (TSH) maintains and stimulates the thyroid epithelium.
  Evidence points toward the beta basophil as the cell of origin.
The *adreno-cortico-tropic hormone (ACTH)* maintains the suprarenal cortex and con-
    trols the secretion of its products.
  A relationship to a subtype of the beta basophil is suggested.
Chromophobes are believed not to be active hormone producers.
  Tumors occur that feature these cells, with a loss of the other cell types.
  Such excessive growths do not produce any specific symptoms.

B. PARS TUBERALIS.

No specific hormonal function has been assigned to its cells.

2. Pars intermedia.

A *melanocyte-stimulating hormone (MSH)* is produced by the pars intermedia.
> In lower vertebrates it expands the mobile pigment in pigment cells.
> In mammals its physiologic role is not clear.
> Injection into man causes hyperpigmentation, much as in Addison's disease.
Correlated with the irregular dispersion of the pars intermedia in man is the
> presence of MSH in neighboring pars distalis and pars nervosa.

3. Neurohypophysis.

Two active factors have been extracted from all three parts of this organ.
> Both of these hormonal substances have also been synthesized.
One, the *antidiuretic hormone*, exerts its effect on the kidney tubules.

ADH = vasopressin!

> They are influenced to reabsorb water from the provisional urine.
>> This salvage prevents the voiding of large quantities of dilute urine.
> High dosage raises blood pressure (by constricting arterioles).
>> Because of this influence the hormone is also called *vasopressin*.
The second hormone *(oxytocin)* contracts smooth muscle in certain locations.
> One is the smooth muscle of the uterine wall (induced by distention).
> Another is the muscular elements in the sacs and ducts of the mammary glands.
>> This response, and the resulting ejection of milk, is induced by sucking.

Total 9 hormones

IV. THE SUPRARENAL GLAND

An older name, the *adrenal gland*, is unofficial but often used.
Each gland has the shape of a flattened, triangular cocked-hat; its size is $5 \times 3 \times 1$ cm.
> Each perches upon the cranial pole of a kidney and adapts itself to that contour.
A sectioned, fresh gland presents two different regions (three, by color).
> The *cortex* is firm; it is yellow externally and reddish brown internally.
> The *medulla* is thinner, softer and dark gray.
> These two regions are wholly different in origin, structure and function.
Development proves that these regions are separate components, united secondarily.
> The cortex grows from peritoneal mesothelium.
> The medulla differentiates from primitive autonomic-ganglion tissue.
Comparative anatomy shows their presence as separate organs in fishes.
> In amphibians and reptiles the two components intermingle.
> In mammals alone is the medullary tissue concentrated into a separate central mass.
Accessory suprarenal tissue (usually cortex) may occur nearby or at a distance.

A. STRUCTURAL PLAN:

A robust *capsule* sends delicate, radial *trabeculae* inward toward the medulla.
The *cortex* consists of epithelial columns, arranged radially like a palisade.
> Three concentric *zones* (but not separate layers) can be recognized in it.
>> These are based on three different patterns of cell arrangement.
The thinner *medulla* is spongy and more irregularly arranged.
> Its epithelium takes the form of hollow cylinders, enclosing vascular channels.
There is a *hilus* where a large vein leaves the gland.

B. DETAILED STRUCTURE:

1. Framework.

The *capsule* is a rather thick, fibro-elastic covering.
> Its inner zone is looser and more vascular.
Slender *trabeculae* extend from this inner capsule radially through the cortex.
> They consist mainly of reticular fibers; sinusoidal vessels accompany them.

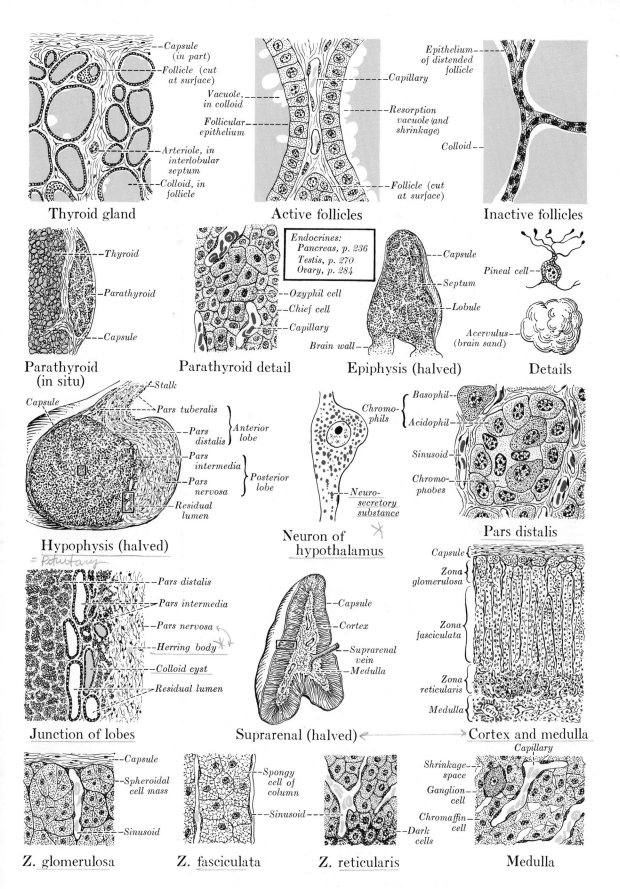

Thyroid gland

- Capsule (in part)
- Follicle (cut at surface)
- Vacuole, in colloid
- Follicular epithelium
- Arteriole, in interlobular septum
- Colloid, in follicle

Active follicles

- Capillary
- Resorption vacuole (and shrinkage)
- Follicle (cut at surface)

Inactive follicles

- Epithelium of distended follicle
- Colloid

Parathyroid (in situ)

- Thyroid
- Parathyroid
- Capsule

Parathyroid detail

Endocrines:
Pancreas, p. 236
Testis, p. 270
Ovary, p. 284

- Oxyphil cell
- Chief cell
- Capillary

Epiphysis (halved)

- Capsule
- Septum
- Lobule
- Brain wall

Details

- Pineal cell
- Acervulus (brain sand)

Hypophysis (halved)

- Capsule
- Stalk
- Pars tuberalis
- Pars distalis } Anterior lobe
- Pars intermedia
- Pars nervosa } Posterior lobe
- Residual lumen

Neuron of hypothalamus

- Chromophils
- Neurosecretory substance

Pars distalis

- Basophil
- Acidophil
- Sinusoid
- Chromophobes

Junction of lobes

- Pars distalis
- Pars intermedia
- Pars nervosa
- Herring body
- Colloid cyst
- Residual lumen

= Pituitary

Suprarenal (halved)

- Capsule
- Cortex
- Suprarenal vein
- Medulla

Cortex and medulla

- Capsule
- Zona glomerulosa
- Zona fasciculata
- Zona reticularis
- Medulla

Z. glomerulosa

- Capsule
- Spheroidal cell mass
- Sinusoid

Z. fasciculata

- Spongy cell of column
- Sinusoid

Z. reticularis

- Dark cells

Medulla

- Capillary
- Shrinkage space
- Ganglion cell
- Chromaffin cell

THE ENDOCRINE GLANDS

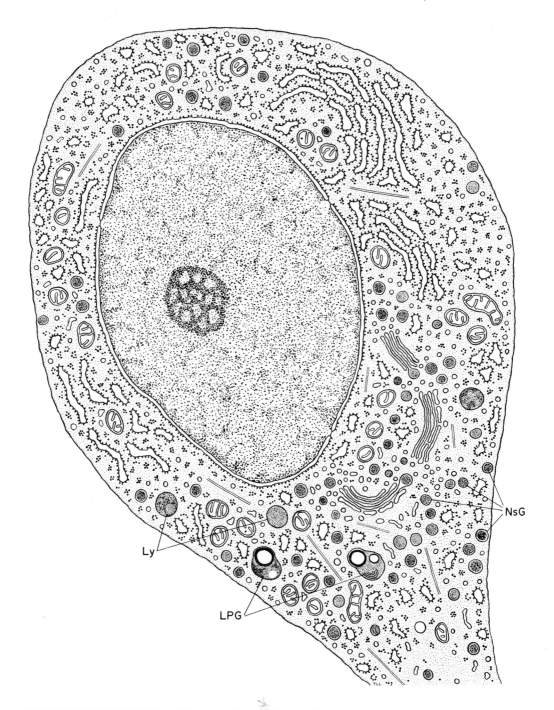

NsG

Ly

LPG

NEUROSECRETORY CELL. This hypothalamic cell resembles a neuron, but also synthesizes neurosecretory granules (NsG). The site of synthesis of the hormonal product is the rough endoplasmic reticulum, which aggregates as the Nissl bodies. Condensing and packaging into membrane-bounded secretory granules takes place in the immediate vicinity of an elaborate Golgi apparatus. The cytoplasm also contains free ribosomes, small mitochondria, lysosomes (Ly) and lipofuchsin pigment (LPG). Size distinguishes lysosomes and pigment bodies from the smaller neurosecretory granules. The nucleus has its chromatin dispersed, but the nucleolus is conspicuous.

vesicular [L *vesicula* a little bladder] Comprised of or relating to small, sac-like bodies

Through their influence the cortex is divided into cell cords or columns.
The *medullary reticulum* forms coarser baskets about the parenchymal masses there.

2. Cortex.

The radial, cellular *cords* are relatively long, slender and well demarcated.
    Thin trabeculae, with sinusoidal capillaries, separate them from each other.
    For the most part the cords are two cells thick.
        The cytoplasm is acidophilic and each cell abuts on a sinusoid.
There are three poorly demarcated layers in the cortical parenchyma.
    These strata are arranged concentrically and blend without sharp boundaries.
        They are more uniform and well demarcated in laboratory mammals.
    The cords of each zone continue as cords in the other zones.
A. ZONA GLOMERULOSA.
    This is a thin layer, located just beneath the capsule.
    Its cells are arranged mostly as arches, but without a significant lumen.
        Some arches, cut slantingly, appear as cellular balls.
    The component cells are columnar in shape, with deeply staining nuclei.
        The lightly staining cytoplasm contains some lipid droplets.
B. ZONA FASCICULATA.
    This middle layer is much the widest and is regularly arranged.
        It takes the form of long, parallel cords of roughly cuboidal cells.
        The cells are relatively large; the nuclei (frequently two) are vesicular.
    In the outer two-thirds of the zone the cytoplasm contains many lipid droplets.
        Cholesterol is most abundant, but fatty acids and neutral fat occur also.
        Lipid extraction leaves thin plates of cytoplasm, bordering cavities.
            Hence these vacuolated cells are sometimes called *spongiocytes*.
    The inner third of the zone is poor in lipids and stains darker.
C. ZONA RETICULARIS.
    This layer is intermediate in thickness between the other two.
        Its cords take irregular courses and anastomose into a meshwork.
    Near the zona fasciculata, the component cells are much like those of that zone.
        Yet, as a detail, they contain still fewer lipid droplets.
    Near the medulla there is an intermixture of '*dark cells*.'
        These have deeper staining, acidophilic cytoplasm and shrunken nuclei.
            The cytoplasm contains large lipid droplets.
            After puberty, it also acquires a yellow-brown pigment.
        Both the light and dark cells are perhaps senescent elements.
            They differ only in degree from dying cells, also seen here.
    The demarcation between cortex and medulla is irregular, but fairly sharp.
D. HISTOLOGICAL ZONES.
    The three zones just considered are based on different arrangements of cells.
    From the standpoint of similarity of cell structure there are four zones:
        1. Zona glomerulosa (and a transitional region of the z. fasciculata).
        2. Outer two-thirds of the z. fasciculata; a region of marked spongiocytes.
        3. Inner third of the z. fasciculata and outer half of the z. reticularis.
            A region poor in lipids and less basophilic.
        4. Inner half of the z. reticularis (juxtamedullary portion).
            A region characterized by pigment and senescent, dark cells.

3. Medulla.

In man this region is thin; it comprises only about 10 per cent of the whole organ.
    In the lateral wing-like expansions of the gland, medullary tissue often fails.
    Here connective tissue and vessels may occur alone.
The medullary cells are polyhedral in shape, but shrink irregularly in sections.
    They have basophilic cytoplasm and large, vesicular nuclei.
    The cytoplasm contains variable numbers of specific secretory granules.
        They are actual precursors of hormone substance (largely *epinephrine*).

Medullary cells are arranged in tubular formations around postcapillary venules.
    One end of each cell abuts on such a venule; the other end on a capillary.
The cell is definitely polarized with respect to this vascular relationship.
    The capillary end receives the terminations of sympathetic nerve fibers.
        The nucleus is also located toward this end of the cell.
    The venous end contains the Golgi apparatus and precursor granules.
        Here the secretion-granules collect and discharge into the venules.
There are two different kinds of medullary cells containing catecholamine granules.
    One secretes *epinephrine;* the other the closely related *norepinephrine.*
    These have different (and opposite) pharmacological effects on tissues.
    The respective granules also differ histochemically and in autofluorescence.
The granules of both cell types are browned readily by a bichromate solution.
    This results from the oxidation of the granules by the bichromate.
    Such an effect is known as the *chromaffin reaction.*
        Also cells responding in this way are called *chromaffin cells.*
        (Actually, any appropriate oxidizing agent will produce similar results.)
A few autonomic ganglion cells also occur in the medulla.

4. Vessels and nerves.

The *vascular supply* is perhaps the richest of any organ in the body.
The cortex receives blood from multiple arterioles in the capsule.
    On entering, these become sinusoids which pass downward between cell columns.
The medulla receives its blood from two different sources.
    The major source is venous blood from the cortical sinusoids, just mentioned.
        On reaching the medulla, these connect promptly with postcapillaries.
    A lesser supply is from arterioles that pass directly from capsule to medulla.
        In the medulla they open into a capillary plexus located there.
        This meshwork is in intimate relation with the medullary parenchyma.
        Its terminations also open into the postcapillary collecting venules.
All the blood of the medulla drains into small collecting veins.
    These, in turn, open into a main, central vein that leaves at the hilus.
    The main vein and its larger tributaries are atypical.
    They have much longitudinal muscle in the adventitia.
Lymphatics occur in the capsule and in association with medullary veins.
Unmyelinated *nerves*, from the solar plexus, enter the capsule in small bundles.
    Following trabeculae, some end in the cortex; most end about medullary cells.
        The latter are like preganglionic fibers, the medullary cells taking the place of autonomic ganglia in the ordinary autonomic-system arrangement.
    Stimulation of the splanchnic nerves produces a heavy discharge of hormone.

C. Postnatal Involution:

Within two weeks after birth the suprarenal glands lose one-third of their weight.
    This is due to the degeneration of the bulky *fetal cortex*, bordering the medulla.
Outside the fetal cortex, at birth, is the thin representative of the *permanent cortex.*
    This consists of the z. glomerulosa and part of the z. fasciculata.
    All layers of the final cortex are represented before the first year has elapsed.
The fetal cortex apparently is dependent on placental gonadotropic hormone.
    The tissue seems competent functionally and is believed to secrete androgens.
    Cessation of such hormonal influence at birth leads to involution.

D. Regenerative Ability:

Cells of the z. glomerulosa and of the outermost, transitional region of the z. fasciculata are commonly held to proliferate steadily, thereby compensating for cell losses.
    Daughter cells would then be progressively pushed downward toward the medulla.
    In the z. reticularis they decline, die and are removed mainly by macrophages.
On the other hand, some mitoses are discernible at all levels.

For this reason, the preceding migration hypothesis has been challenged.
Cortical cells are easily injured by infections, toxins, narcosis, etc.
  Repair follows unless the damage leads to scar-formation or eventual death.
  In experiments a cortical mass will regenerate from traces of the z. glomerulosa.
Medullary cells show little sign of either degeneration or regeneration. *(makes sense - is derived from nervous tissue)*

E. DIAGNOSTIC FEATURES:

It is a parenchymatous organ, without ducts, having an obvious cortex and medulla.
  The medulla is largely missing in the compressed 'wings' of the gland.
The *cortex* is arranged in a palisade of radial, epithelial cords.
  Three concentric zones, with different cell arrangements, are fairly well shown.
  Sometimes sections contain seeming islands of cortex within the medulla.
    These are junctional portions of the cortex that bulged into the plane of section.
The *medulla* consists of cell groups arranged irregularly as masses and cords.
  Such cell groups are highly vascularized, the larger vessels being conspicuous.
  In some regions, veins are about the only medullary component seen.

F. FUNCTIONAL CORRELATIONS:

The cortex and medulla are functionally distinct, like separate organs.
  This is consonant with different developmental origins and cytological structure.
The *cortex* is essential to life, although nine-tenths can be removed safely.
  Cortical destruction by tuberculosis (Addison's disease) has a fatal expectancy.
    Death can be averted by the administration of the cortical extract.
  The cortex is necessary in order to maintain a variety of vital functions.
    1) It maintains the electrolyte and water balance in the body.
        Otherwise there is a concentration of the plasma, a shift of water from tissue
          spaces into cells, and deranged kidney function.
    2) It maintains the proper carbohydrate balance in the body.
        With derangement of this control, the glycogen stores are depleted.
          Protein fails to convert into carbohydrate.
    3) It maintains resistance to stress (temperature extremes; fatigue; trauma).
      It maintains properly the intercellular substances of the body.
  4) Forty steroid compounds have been isolated from the cortex.
      Seven have marked cortex-like activity; others have sex-hormone activity.
      But no single one has all the properties of a crude, cortical extract.
    There is some evidence pointing to a functional specialization of the zones. *in class:*
      The glomerular zone seems to be concerned with controlling water and salts. *mineralcorticoids*
      The fasciculate zone appears to control protein and carbohydrate metabolism. *glucocorticoids*
      The reticular zone produces hormonal steroids of the male and female types. *steroids*
    Over-functioning manifests itself when cortical (adrenogenital) tumors develop.
      In women there is a masculinizing effect (appearance of beard, etc.).
        Or a premature appearance of male secondary sexual characters in children.
      Tumors that feminize males have also been reported.
The *medulla* is not essential to life, and not surely important to normal functioning.
  It produces the hormones *(epinephrine; norepinephrine)* located in the granules.
  The number of chromaffin granules in a cell is an index of its secretory state.
  Similar granules appear in the suprarenal vein after stimulating the splanchnic nerve.
    This is perhaps the only hormone identifiable in its cells of origin, and traceable and
      exactly measurable during discharge.
The medulla is said to be an emergency organ, normally storing most of its product.
    Ordinarily it discharges so little secretion that its effect is unimportant.
    Under emotional stress it discharges more hormonal secretion.
      This excess augments the action of sympathetic nerve endings on tissues.
        The tissues affected are smooth muscle, cardiac muscle and glands.
  Cells recover rapidly after stimulation, and refill with secretory granules.

V. THE PARAGANGLIA

These bodies consist of small masses of *chromaffin cells* that give the chromaffin reaction.

They lie retroperitoneally, mostly along the course of the sympathetic trunks.

Minor groups occur in relation to the gonads, liver and heart.

At birth there are some 40 of these masses, ranging from microscopic clusters to pea size.

They reach the height of their development in infancy and then regress.

The largest are the paired or joined *para-aortic bodies* (Zuckerkandl).

These lie behind the peritoneum, ventral to the dorsal aorta.

Each is about 1 cm. long, but by puberty they are no longer macroscopic.

A *paraganglion* may be isolated or closely associated with sympathetic nerves or ganglia.

It consists of cell strands, commonly penetrated by rich capillaries.

The cells resenble those of the suprarenal medulla and have a similar origin.

It is said that they secrete norepinephrine only.

There is a rich supply of autonomic nerve fibers.

The whole mass tends to be encapsulated.

VI. THE PINEAL BODY

It is also called, from its shape, the *epiphysis* or *conarium.*

Epiphysis means 'a sprout upon' (the brain); pineal and conarium refer to a pine cone.

A. STRUCTURAL PLAN:

The *pineal body* is a stalked outgrowth from the roof of the diencephalon.

It is an encapsulated, lobulated organ about 7 mm. long.

Internally it is densely packed with cells, and may contain calcareous concretions.

it calcifies

B. DETAILED STRUCTURE:

1. Framework.

A thin *capsule*, supplied by the pia mater, sends *septa* and vessels inward.

The septa are mostly composed of reticular fibers.

They enclose incompletely masses of cells that constitute *lobules.*

Neuroglia (astrocytes) provide a delicate support for the specific *pineal cells.*

2. Parenchyma.

The organ consists of *epithelioid* and *neuroglial cells*, arranged in plates.

Neither type shows to advantage without special silver techniques.

The epithelioid cells have long, branched processes with bulbous endings.

They are specific *pineal cells*, characteristic of the organ.

Several types have been described, based on cytoplasmic content.

These include homogeneous, granular and lipoidal cells.

The granular cells are acidophilic, basophilic or pigmented.

The neuroglial elements are less numerous and chiefly resemble *astrocytes.*

3. Vessels and nerves.

Blood vessels are confined almost exclusively to the capsule and septa.

The parenchyma is richly supplied with capillaries.

Lymphatics have not been demonstrated.

Many *nerve fibers* enter and supply both vessels and parenchyma.

Some (unmyelinated) are autonomic; others (myelinated) are from the brain.

C. INVOLUTION:

The pineal body reaches its fullest development (but not size) in middle childhood.

Later (after puberty) there are regressive changes, but the time of onset is variable.

These changes involve the fibrous stroma more than the parenchymal cells.
Connective tissue increases and the lobules are more plainly delimited.
The tissue ultimately undergoes hyaline degeneration.
The sharp demarcation between fibrous tissue and parenchyma is lost.
Concretions become more frequent; glial fibers thicken.
Acervuli are concretions ('brain sand'), located mostly in the septa and capsule.
They increase in number with age, and may become 1 mm. or more in diameter.
They are lamellated and are externally pimply or knobbed.
They consist of carbonates and phosphates of calcium and magnesium.

D. DIAGNOSTIC FEATURES:

Cellular masses are separated into imperfect lobules by septa.
The general appearance resembles somewhat a lymphoid organ.
In ordinary sections, the cells appear crowded and without clear boundaries.
The relatively large nuclei are lightly stippled; the cytoplasm is scanty and pale.
Between the cells there is a fine fibrillar mesh.
Darkly basophilic, lamellated 'brain sand' is a characteristic feature.
But even in adults these concretions are absent in one-fourth of all specimens.

E. FUNCTIONAL CORRELATIONS:

Functional relations are obscure, yet this organ is not a useless vestige.
It is known to exert an inhibitory influence on the development of gonads.
There is general agreement that it is a neuro-endocrine organ.
Yet histological evidence of hormonal secretion is lacking.
The only active extractive as yet identified is *melatonin,* synthesized from serotonin.
In experiments on amphibian melanophores it causes the pigment to retract about the
nucleus, thus reversing the effect of MSH (p. 180).
This organ seems to be involved actively in the regulation of the light-influenced reproductive
cycles of birds and rodents.

VII. THE PLACENTA

Among its other functions, the placenta synthesizes hormones important in pregnancy.
These products continue or supplement activities of the hypophysis and ovaries.
The tissue responsible for hormone production is developed by the fetal chorion (p. 288).
It consists of a double layer of *trophoblast,* clothing the chorionic villi.
The inner layer is *cellular trophoblast,* a simple sheet of cuboidal cells.
It elaborates a gonadotrope, much like LTH, that preserves the corpus luteum.
As this layer is used up (see below), the hormone production declines.
The outer layer is *syncytial trophoblast,* derived from cellular trophoblast.
The latter cells divide, and daughter cells merge into a common mass.
By the end of the third month of pregnancy, little cellular trophoblast remains.
This syncytial layer progressively replaces the ovary in hormone production.
Both estrogen and progesterone are secreted by it in large amounts.

Chapter XVII

The Integumentary System

The *integument* comprises the skin and certain specialized derivatives of it.
The latter are the nails, hair and several kinds of glands.

I. THE SKIN

The *skin* is an organ that provides an external covering to the body.
It weighs about 9 pounds, is 0.5 to 5.0 mm. thick, and has an area of some 18 sq. ft.
The *epidermis* is a specialized epithelium at the free surface.
The *dermis,* or corium, is the subjacent dense bed of vascular connective tissue.
This layer corresponds to the lamina propria of a mucous membrane.
Tanned commercially, this part of an animal skin is known as 'leather.'
The *subcutaneous layer* is a still deeper, looser, fibrous bed beneath the skin.
It is the 'superficial fascia' of gross anatomy.
This layer corresponds to the submucosa beneath a mucous membrane.
The boundary between epidermis and dermis is usually uneven, but abrupt.
There is a fairly even, smooth junction on the forehead, ear and scrotum.
Elsewhere there is interlocking between two systems of ridges.
The free surface of the skin is furrowed by criss-crossing systems of delicate creases.
These form small rhomboidal or rectangular areas.
The palmar and plantar surfaces bear parallel ridges (*cristae*) and furrows (*sulci*).
These are structural adaptations to meet heavy mechanical demands.
The patterns are individually specific in the details of their loops and whorls.

A. Epidermis:

The *epidermis* is a dry, stratified squamous epithelium, usually about 0.1 mm. thick.
On the palm and sole it may become 0.8 and 1.4 mm. thick, respectively.
Moreover, pressure or friction tends to increase the thickness still further.
Yet there is an hereditary factor, since it is already thick in the fetus.
This epithelium is characterized by having its superficial layers cornified.
Hence the entire body is encased within a dead husk.
The thickness of this husk is related to the mechanical contact encountered.
It also thickens markedly as an accompaniment of sun-tanning.
The epidermis is a nonvascular layer, but it is in close relation with the dermis.
Nutrition is achieved by fluids transuding from out the dermis.
The epidermis is most highly differentiated on the palmar and plantar surfaces.
The maximum layering and cellular differentiation occur there.
The layers are: (1) *germinative;* (2) *granular;* (3) *lucid;* and (4) *horny.*
As in all stratified epithelia, there is a continuous loss and replacement of cells.
Cells proliferate at low levels; daughter cells are pushed up by still younger ones.

1. Stratum germinativum.

This so-called *Malpighian layer* is irregularly ridged on its lower surface.
Regions over dermal papillae are much thinner than those between papillae.
The *basal cells* are columnar elements, comprising the *stratum basale.*

They constitute a single layer of deeply basophilic cells.
Tooth-like processes (and their basement membrane) are anchored in the dermis.
Next higher are the *prickle cells* of the stratified *stratum spinosum*.
These cells are polyhedrons, somewhat flattened at higher levels in the layer.
Shrinkage slightly separates them except at the so-called *intercellular bridges*.
A 'bridge' represents two cytoplasmic extensions meeting at a *desmosome* (p. 40).
Hence the cells, although in contact through 'prickles,' are independent entities.
Bundles of *tonofilaments* pass into the bridges and insert on the desmosome.
They are believed to give strength and elasticity to the cell.
The cytoplasm is decreasingly basophilic (*i.e.*, less RNA) at higher levels.
Mitoses occur in the basal and prickle cells, and mostly during sleep.
Daughter cells reach the surface in 4 to 14 weeks (depending on thickness).

2. *Stratum granulosum.*

The component cells are somewhat flattened, deeply staining elements.
In the thick epidermis of the palm or sole they are 3 to 5 cells deep.
Elsewhere this layer is thinner, or even lacking.
In vertical section the cells are diamond-shaped, with a thin cell membrane.
The nucleus becomes pale and indistinct; it shows degenerative changes.
The cytoplasm contains irregular-shaped granules of *keratohyalin*.
These refractile granules stain with some acid dyes and certain basic dyes.
Such granules are unrelated to melanin pigment in the germinative layer.
In man the 'granules' seen are deposits of keratohyalin on tonofibrils.
The synthesized material is laid down on the fibril and becomes a coating.
Intercellular bridges and tonofibrils are recognized with difficulty.

3. *Stratum lucidum.*

This is a clear, translucent layer, 3 to 5 cells deep.
It is a constituent only of especially thick epidermis (palm; sole).
The flattened, dying cells are compacted into a homogeneous, glassy plate.
Nevertheless, the individual cells can still be isolated by chemicals.
In vertical sections the lucid layer is a wavy stripe; its former granules have merged.
It is highly refractile and stains feebly with most dyes.
The nuclei are no longer visible; the cytoplasmic organelles have been lost.
The cells are dying or already dead.

4. *Stratum corneum.*

This is a layer of cornified (*i.e.*, keratinized) cells, progressively flattened and adherent.
On the palm and sole the layer becomes extremely thick.
The component cells are closely packed; each retains its thickened cell membrane.
The cell surfaces interlock, and desmosomes still bind them together.
Cytoplasm has been replaced with a homogeneous substance embedded with filaments.
This material is dry, shiny and highly refractile.
The dense, amorphous substance is held to be the end stage of keratohyalin.
The filaments are similarly interpreted as retained tonofibrils.
Chemically the final product is keratin, which is a fibrous protein.
It is a 'soft' type of keratin, low in sulfur; cells are not fused as in nails.
At the surface the dried, caked cells are sloughed off in scale-like aggregates.

5. *Regional differences.*

The thick epidermis of the palm and sole have all the layers just described.
These are the most highly differentiated regions of the total epidermal surface.
The epidermis of the general body surface is both thinner and simpler.
Only the germinative layer and a thin, horny layer are constantly present.
The granular layer is at best two cells thick, and is often lacking.
This is because keratinization is less marked and is intermittent.

A lucid layer cannot be demonstrated, except as a trace on the leg.

Toward the surface the cells become thin *keratin plates,* firmly joined.

The keratinized cells are not retained long, and hence the layer remains thin.

At the margin of the lip, nostril, anus and vulva there is a junctional region.

Here the epidermis is transitional into a mucous membrane.

The epithelium is thick and is moistened by mucus.

A thin stratum corneum permits the red blood color to show through plainly.

6. Pigmentation.

The color of skin itself is yellow; this is due to *carotene* in foods eaten.

Blood, showing through, gives the reddish tints.

Fine granules of *melanin pigment* are responsible for the yellow to black colors.

This substance is especially present in the basal cells.

It disappears in cells that have risen above the granular layer.

Pigment is said to be elaborated through the interaction of an oxidase (*tyrosinase*) with a chromogen precursor-substance (*tyrosine*).

Both the formation and fate of melanin need further investigation.

Pigment is practically absent from the palm and sole of all races.

In whites, pigment granules are almost always confined to the basal cells.

Certain regions (areola; circumanal area; etc.) are more richly pigmented.

Local spots with deep pigmentation are known as *pigmented moles.*

In the colored races, pigment may extend even into the stratum granulosum.

Epidermal pigment is elaborated in special cells derived from the neural crest.

These *melanocytes* migrate into the basal layer and become highly branched.

Here they elaborate pigment and turn it over to germinative cells.

Deep pigmentation reflects greater synthesis, not more melanocytes.

Melanocytes appear as 'clear cells' in ordinary stained sections.

Such cells have shrunken, so that they are surrounded by a clear halo.

Melanocytes blacken specifically with a special reagent called *dopa.*

This reaction indicates the presence of a precursor substance of melanin.

The synthesized pigment particles are contained within tiny *melanosomes.*

The particles are deposited upon the concentric layers of these structures.

Eventually the melanosome becomes stuffed with melanin.

'Sun-tanning' is a secondary pigmentation following exposure to ultraviolet light.

The initial pigmentation results from the darkening of melanin already present.

In a few days there is an actual increase in melanin synthesis.

Without further exposure to sun, this extra activity soon comes to an end.

The surplus degenerates, producing *melanoid,* which gradually disappears.

Freckles are local regions of intensified pigmentary activity.

B. DERMIS:

The *dermis*, or corium, underlies a thin *basement membrane.*

The presence of the latter is not manifest in ordinary preparations.

It is demonstrable with the PAS stain or with the electron microscope.

The thickness of the closely interwoven dermis varies between 0.3 and 4.0 mm.

A thin epidermis may have a thin dermis (eyelid) or a thick dermis (back).

The dermis can be subdivided for convenience into two strata, *papillary* and *reticular.*

1. Papillary layer.

This stratum includes ridges and papillae protruding into the epidermis.

There can be as many as 65,000 of these papillae to the square inch.

In the palm and sole the papillae are numerous and tall (50 to 200 μ).

They tend to occur in a double row and are often branched.

They are also tall in the lips, penis and nipple.

Such interlocking with the epidermis is mechanically advantageous.

Where mechanical demands are slight, there are few, low and irregular ridges.

Example: face; trunk.

Some papillae contain tactile sensory corpuscles; they are *tactile papillae*.
Other papillae contain only blood vessels; they are *vascular papillae*.
The fundamental tissue of the papillary layer is a closely interwoven mesh.
    It is composed of thin collagenous and elastic fibers and some reticular fibers.

2. *Reticular layer.*

This stratum comprises the main fibrous bed of the dermis.
It consists of coarse, rather densely interlacing fibers.
    Their preponderant direction is parallel to the surface.
    Elastic networks intermingle with collagenous fiber-bundles.
    Cells are relatively few, but are those typical for connective tissue.
Pigmented, branched connective-tissue cells (*chromatophores*) may occur superficially.
    They are numerous only in areas where the epidermis is heavily pigmented.
        Example: areola; circumanal region.
    They are also more abundant in individuals with darker skins.
    Such cells apparently do not elaborate pigment, but merely receive and store it.
True dermal *melanocytes* (dopa positive) are known also to occur locally.
    They are responsible for the *Mongolian spot* of the sacral region in infants of the yellow
        race, and for certain tumors (*blue nevi*).
Hairs, sweat glands, sebaceous glands and lamellar corpuscles are represented.
The perineum, scrotum, penis and nipple have smooth-muscle fibers in the dermis.
    This muscle content is responsible for the dartos reflex of the scrotum and for the
        erection of the nipple; it responds to local stimulation.
    Small bundles of fibers constitute the erector muscles of hair follicles.
In the face and neck, skeletal fibers terminate in the dermis.
    They provide the basis for skin movements (muscles of facial expression).
    Extensively developed in many mammals is the highly mobile *panniculus carnosus*.

C. Subcutaneous Layer:

This layer constitutes the so-called *superficial fascia*.
    It is not considered to be a part of the skin, yet blends (unsharply) into the dermis.
    It is a looser network of connective-tissue bands and septa.
The density and arrangement of the subcutaneous layer determine the mobility of the skin.
    Much of the skin can be displaced considerably, except on the palm and sole.
        Here mobility is greatly reduced and the fibers are thick and numerous.
    With aging, elasticity declines; the skin loses tone and becomes wrinkled.
The spaces of the subcutaneous mesh are occupied by lobules of fat.
    Where these are continuous, the subcutaneous layer is called a *panniculus adiposus*.
    On the abdomen the panniculus may reach a thickness of 1 inch, or more.
    Yet there are regions (eyelids; scrotum; penis) where fat never occurs.

D. Vessels and Nerves:

Arteries form networks beneath the reticular and papillary layers.
    They also send extensions into the papillae and form capillary loops there.
    The epidermis is nourished by tissue fluid that passes into the intercellular spaces.
Veins form a superficial plexus beneath the papillae, and also two deeper plexuses.
    There is still another plexus in the subcutaneous tissue.
Lymphatics begin as blind vessels or networks in the papillae and beneath them.
    These drain into a plexus at the junction of the dermis and subcutaneous layer.
Efferent nerves supply the smooth muscle of blood vessels, erector muscles of hairs, and the
        myoid elements and gland cells of sweat glands.
Afferent nerves connect with lamellar corpuscles, tactile corpuscles and hair follicles.
    They also form free nerve endings in the dermis and epidermis.

E. Regenerative Ability:

The capacity for regeneration and the repair of gross losses is highly developed.
Epidermal cells glide across small gaps in mass movement; hair follicles may supply cells.
   Restoration of thickness is achieved secondarily by mitoses.
   Larger gaps are bridged by combined movement and proliferation.
Intact connective tissue produces fibroblasts and a provisional fill of mucous tissue.
   The latter is converted into fibrous tissue, but elastic fibers are slow to re-form.
A graft from the same individual survives; one from a different person is rejected.

F. Diagnostic Features:

The *epidermis* is a stratified squamous epithelium; cornification produces matted scales.
   In ordinary skin of the body the cornified layers are few, but begin abruptly.
   In the palm and sole the cornified layers make a very thick stratum.
      Distinctive granular and lucid layers are plainly seen also.
      The epidermis usually is cut to show the scalloped, superficial ridging.
The *dermis* is composed of relatively dense connective tissue.
   Sweat glands, sebaceous glands and hairs are usually, but not always, encountered.
      On the palm and sole, hairs and sebaceous glands are lacking.
The *subcutaneous layer* is a looser connective tissue.
   It contains lobules of fat and the roots of hairs.

G. Functional Correlations:

The superficial layer of the epidermis is a practically impermeable coat of dead cells.
   It is primarily protective against trauma, bacteria, drying, water loss or absorption,
      noxious gases and fluids, ultraviolet light, etc.
Cornification (*i.e.,* keratinization) is kept in control by vitamin A.
The skin excretes water, fat and various catabolic wastes.
It is important in the regulation of body temperature (by insulation and sweating).
It is the most extensive receptor of tactile, thermal and painful impressions.
The skin is a storehouse for glycogen, cholesterol and water; it aids in water-balancing.
   In it ergosterol is activated by ultraviolet light to form vitamin D.
Subcutaneous tissue serves to bind the skin to the deep fascia or periosteum.
   It also affords mobility to the skin in accordance with local requirements.
Bursae occur between the skin and deeper prominences, such as the elbow and kneecap.
   Like bursae elsewhere, they are closed fibrous sacs containing a viscid fluid.
   They facilitate the play of skin over bony prominences and also provide cushioning.

II. THE NAILS

Nails are features present only in man and other primates.

A. Structural Plan:

A *nail* is a convex, rectangular specialization of the skin.
It consists of a horny *nail plate*, lying upon a less specialized *nail bed*.
   The plate is contained within a U-shaped *nail groove*, formed by the skin.
   The nail plate has a *free edge*, a *body* (mostly exposed, but attached beneath), and a *root*
      (covered, and attached beneath).
      At the base of the exposed plate a crescentic whitish zone, the *lunule,* may show.
         The lunule often is concealed by the skin fold, except on the thumb.
   The *nail groove* is bordered by a similarly coursing skin fold, the *nail wall.*
      The nail wall overlaps the nail plate where it lies in the groove.
      On each side the nail groove is shallow; proximally it is a deep pocket.
   The *nail bed,* underlying the nail plate, consists of the germinative layer of the epidermis,
      and the dermis beneath it.
      There is no subcutaneous layer beneath the nail bed.

B. **DETAILED STRUCTURE:**

1. Nail wall and groove.

The curved furrow of the *nail groove* is lined with epidermis.
Cells from the horny layer of the *nail wall* extend onto the nail plate.
This adherent material constitutes the *eponychium*, commonly called cuticle.
At the bottom of the groove the epidermis loses all but the germinative layer.
This layer turns back, continuing onto the undersurface of the nail plate.

2. Nail bed.

The *nail bed* underlies both the exposed and concealed portions of the nail plate.
It consists of the germinative layer of the epidermis and of dense dermis.
The germinative layer under the nail root is thicker than elsewhere.
This region, where nail growth chiefly occurs, is named the *matrix*.
Here keratinized cells are formed and added to the nail plate.
In this transformation granular and lucid layers are lacking.
There is no evidence of keratohyalin granules, but fibrils do occur.
The epidermis beneath the exposed nail plate is reduced to the germinative layer.
Irregular projections from the nail substance pass between the germinative cells.
This arrangement serves to attach the nail plate in this region.
The basal surface is longitudinally ridged, alternating with dermal ridges.
Beneath the exposed portion of the nail plate the dermis is longitudinally ridged.
Glands do not occur in the dense connective tissue of the nail bed.
The deepest part of the bed is fused to the periosteum of the terminal phalanx.
The epidermis of the fingertip extends under the free edge of the nail plate and becomes
continuous with the germinative layer of the nail bed.
Its specialized layers attach to the plate and extend slightly rootward.
This horny, cellular tissue is called the *hyponychium*.

3. Nail plate.

The *nail plate* consists of intimately fused, keratinized epidermal scales.
The component cells appear to merge into a homogeneous nail substance.
However, alkalies can make the individual cells swell and separate.
This treatment also discloses a shrunken nucleus in each cell.
Nail cells contain 'hard keratin,' like hair (p. 193); they do not desquamate.
The nail plate and its germinative layer may be viewed as a modified epidermis.
The component scaly cells of the nail plate are arranged in layers.
This gives a striated appearance when cut in vertical section.
In the root the layers are unequal in extent, and so overlap.
The superficial layer extends farthest back into the nail groove.
Deeper layers extend progressively shorter distances in this direction.
The deepest layer of all extends only to the distal margin of the *lunule*.
This is a whitish crescent, commonly exposed at the base of the nail plate.
Air spaces between cells cause the well known white spots in the nail plate.
The plate is thin proximally in the root but quickly reaches its maximum thickness
where the root passes into the exposed body of the nail.
In the finger this thickness is 0.5 mm.; in the toe, it is considerably thicker.
The body of the plate is translucent and transmits the pink color of the bed.
Here the plate tends to show longitudinal ridges.
The root is more opaque than the body; cornification and drying are incomplete.
Its distal margin may be exposed, showing as the crescentic, whitish lunule.
This region is often concealed by the skin fold, except on the thumb.

4. Vessels and nerves.

The vascular and nerve supply of a nail are like that in the skin (p. 189).
Arterio-venous anastomoses occur in the nail bed (and on the fingertips).

C. GROWTH AND REGENERATIVE ABILITY:

New nail substance is added from the matrix (under the root of the nail plate).
>   The most proximal cells of the matrix form the surface layer.
>   The most distal cells of the matrix (lunule margin) form the deepest layer.
Beyond the lunule the nail bed does not participate in growth appreciably.
>   The nail plate merely glides progressively over the germinative layer.
A fingernail grows nearly 1 mm. each week, and is renewed in about 6 months.
>   Unlike hair, nails grow continuously throughout life—fingernails faster than toenails.
Formation of a new nail will follow the forcible removal of an old one.
>   Only if the matrix is destroyed will this regeneration fail.

D. DIAGNOSTIC FEATURES:

Sections of the nail and fingertip show characteristic surroundings.
>   These are: nail groove and wall; free edge; epo- and hyponychium; terminal phalanx.
The *nail plate* lies on a typical germinative layer; more specialized layers are absent.
>   The transition in structure between the plate and its bed is exceedingly abrupt.
>   The plate is striated longitudinally, but gives little indication of its cellular origin.
The densely fibrous component of the *nail bed* lacks glands.
>   There is no subcutaneous tissue, since dermis and periosteum fuse.

E. FUNCTIONAL CORRELATIONS:

Nails, claws and hoofs are homologous epidermal products.
Nails are not only protective, but they also have utility as tools.
>   Small objects can be picked up, and various manipulations are performed by them.

III. THE HAIR

Hairs are elastic, tapering, horny threads; they are characteristic of mammals alone.
>   Their length varies from 1 mm., or less, to an extreme of 5 ft.
>   Their thickness ranges from 0.005 mm. (vellus) to 0.2 mm. (beard).
>   The distribution in man covers the entire skin, except for a few regions.
>   Example: palm; sole; neighborhood of anal and urogenital apertures.
>   Their frequency varies regionally; example: vertex, 1300 per sq. in.; chin, 140 per sq. in.

A. STRUCTURAL PLAN:

There is a free *shaft*, and a *root* which embeds in the skin.
>   The hairs are not set perpendicularly, but slope at an angle.
A tubular *hair follicle*, part epidermal and part fibrous (dermal), encloses the root.
>   Toward its deep end, the follicle swells and there is named the *hair bulb*.
>   Indenting the basal end of the bulb is a connective-tissue *papilla*.
Associated with the follicle are a *sebaceous gland* and *erector muscle*.

B. STRUCTURE OF SHAFT AND ROOT:

A hair consists of epidermal cells arranged about a cylindrical core (*medulla*).
>   Peripheral to the core, the cells are in two concentric layers (*cortex; cuticle*).
>   In the deep end of the root the cells are softer and less compacted.

1. Medulla.

The *medullary core* is a looser central axis, 2 or 3 cells in diameter.
>   It rarely extends the total length of any hair.
Hairs of the axilla, beard and eyebrows contain a medulla.
>   Hairs of the head may or may not possess this core.
>   A medulla is always absent in the fine, short hairs of the downy type.
The cells of the medulla are shrunken, keratinized cuboidal cells.
>   These are partly separated by air spaces.

The cells contain refractile droplets and, often, pigment.
The keratin of medullary cells is of the 'soft' type, as in epidermis (p. 187).

2. Cortex.

The main bulk of a hair, the *cortex*, appears compact and longitudinally striate.
It consists of spindle-shaped, flattened cells (keratinized and acidophilic).
Maceration can isolate them, and demonstrate nuclei and horny fibrils in them.
The fibrils are embedded in a dense substance, as in epidermal keratin.
Pigment granules occur, transferred to the cells by melanocytes.
Black hair has much pigment that represents well oxidized tyrosin.
Brown and blond hair contains pigment of the same quality, but less of it.
Red hair contains pigment that is the product of limited oxidation.
Air spaces, located between cells, probably can modify the hair color.

3. Cuticle.

Superficially there is a very thin, single layer of cells, known as the *cuticle*.
These are keratinized scales that have lost their nuclei.
The scales overlap, like shingles, with their free edges directed upward.
An interlock with cells lining the follicle aids in resisting detachment.
In surface view the scales are arranged in a wavy, mosaic pattern.

The keratin of the cortex and cuticle is of the 'hard' type, as in nails and feathers.
It does not pass through a keratohyalin stage; its compacted cells do not desquamate.
It is an albuminoid (with a large content of sulfur) that resists chemical change.
Keratin molecules are long polypeptide chains, parallel and connected by side chains.
These threads follow zig-zag courses, but when wet they stretch and bend easily.
Such properties are the basis on which wet hair can be 'set' temporarily in curls.
Permanent waving utilizes heat or chemicals to establish more lasting effects.
Old linkages, in and between molecules, are replaced by new alignments.

C. STRUCTURE OF FOLLICLE:

A hair follicle consists of a double sheath whose two components are wholly different.
Externally there is a *dermal root sheath*; internally, an *epidermal root sheath*.
Toward its deep end the follicle is expanded into a *hair bulb*.
Here the hair root and its sheaths blend in a mass of formative cells, the *matrix*.
The base of the bulb is indented by a prominent, connective-tissue *papilla*.
Around the lower half of the papilla, the hair root and its sheaths merge.
All layers of the follicle are not present at all levels.
They are represented best at some distance above the bulb.

1. Dermal root sheath.

This fibrous *sheath* exists only around the lower two-thirds of the follicle.
It is developed best in coarse hairs such as those of the scalp.
There are three layers, corresponding to similar strata of the corium.
A. OUTER LAYER.
This is a poorly defined layer of longitudinally directed fibers.
It corresponds to the deep (reticular) layer of the dermis.
B. MIDDLE LAYER.
This is a thicker, denser and more cellular layer of circular, fine fibers.
It corresponds to the papillary layer of the dermis.
The *hair papilla* is like an ordinary dermal papilla, but far larger.
It contains capillaries, nerve fibers and, sometimes, pigment cells.
Its shape is like an egg, expanded above a slender stalk.
C. INNER LAYER.
Most internally, next to the follicle, there is a homogeneous *glassy membrane*.
It corresponds to the basement membrane beneath the epidermis.
Similarly it consists of amorphous ground substance and reticular fibers.

2. Epidermal root sheath.

There are an outer and an inner *epidermal sheath*, each with subordinate strata.

The outer sheath corresponds to the less modified, deep epidermal layers.

The inner sheath corresponds to the more specialized, superficial layers.

A. OUTER ROOT SHEATH.

Above the outlet of the sebaceous gland, ordinary epidermis lines the follicle.

Below this level the germinative layer alone continues as the outer sheath.

It thins as it approaches the bulb, but can be traced even to its base.

This sheath has its two subordinate layers arranged as in the epidermis.

1. *Columnar layer.* A single layer of taller cells, next to the glassy membrane.

2. *Prickle-cell layer.* Several layers of cells, with intercellular bridges.

This layer is the more internal of the two in position.

B. INNER ROOT SHEATH.

This constitutes a keratinized, cellular sheath enveloping the growing root.

Like the hair, it is pushed up by additions from the bulb.

Advances in keratinization intensify from the bulb upward.

Unlike the hair, it gives out before reaching the outlet of the sebaceous gland.

It elaborates 'soft keratin,' with a keratohyalin stage, like epidermis.

Nuclei and discernible cells occur only at the deeper levels of the sheath.

There are three layers which may be likened to the specialized epidermal strata.

In epidermis these are the granular, lucid and keratinized layers.

1. *Henle's layer.*

This is an outer, single layer of elongate cells, connected by 'bridges.'

The clear cells, at the lower levels, contain acidophilic trichohyalin granules.

These correspond to keratohyalin granules in epidermis.

2. *Huxley's layer.*

This consists of several layers of transparent, prekeratinized cells.

They contain *trichohyalin granules,* but at somewhat higher levels.

3. *Cuticle.*

This is a single layer of thin, transparent, horny scales.

The cells overlap like shingles, with their free edges directed downward.

Interlocking with similar cells of the hair cuticle explains why the inner root sheath is also removed when a hair is extracted.

D. ASSOCIATED MUSCLE AND GLANDS:

1. Arrector pili muscle.

The *erector muscle* of a hair is a characteristic accessory.

It is a band of smooth muscle, 0.05 to 0.2 mm. wide.

Long or coarse hairs have thick bands, but there are exceptions (axilla; beard).

Some hairs lack an erector muscle (eyelashes; nasal hairs).

A muscle arises high in the dermis and, for a distance, is a single bundle.

It then subdivides, each division passing to a hair of a hair group.

Such a terminal bundle usually joins the follicle below the sebaceous gland.

However, the muscle may be perforated by a large, branched gland.

The muscle inserts on the dermal root sheath, slightly above its mid-level.

This is on the side that makes an obtuse angle with the epidermis.

Contraction, as by cold or fright, contracts the muscle, erects and lifts the hair, and depresses the adjacent skin; this is 'goose flesh.'

At the same time, sebum is expressed from the squeezed sebaceous gland.

2. Sebaceous glands.

One to several *sebaceous glands* always connect with a hair.

There is, however, no direct correlation between the sizes of the two.

On the contrary, some of the smallest hairs have the largest glands.

A gland usually is located in the angle between the follicle and its muscle.

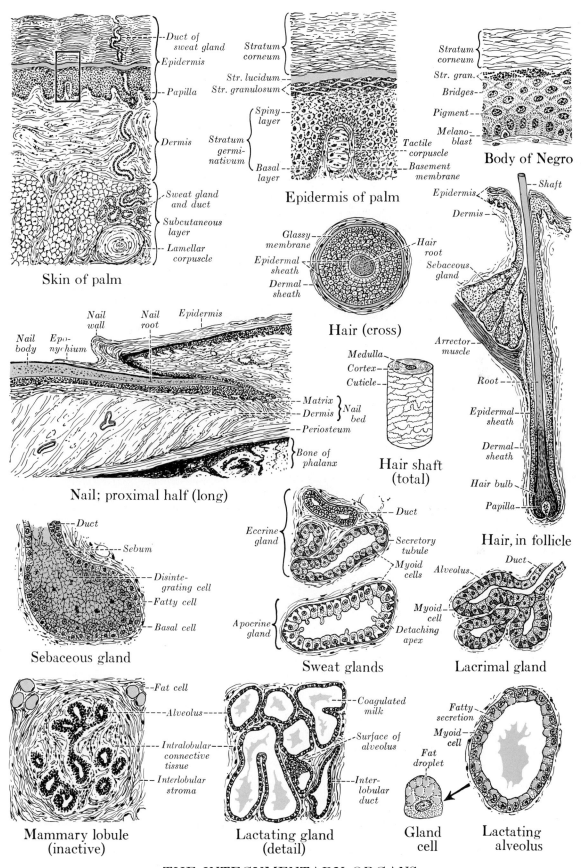

Duct of sweat gland
Epidermis
Papilla
Dermis
Sweat gland and duct
Subcutaneous layer
Lamellar corpuscle

Skin of palm

Stratum corneum
Str. lucidum
Str. granulosum
Spiny layer
Stratum germinativum
Basal layer
Tactile corpuscle
Basement membrane

Epidermis of palm

Stratum corneum
Str. gran.
Bridges
Pigment
Melano-blast

Body of Negro

Glassy membrane
Epidermal sheath
Dermal sheath
Hair root

Hair (cross)

Medulla
Cortex
Cuticle

Hair shaft (total)

Shaft
Epidermis
Dermis
Sebaceous gland
Arrector muscle
Root
Epidermal sheath
Dermal sheath
Hair bulb
Papilla

Hair, in follicle

Nail wall
Nail root
Epidermis
Nail body
Epo-nychium
Matrix
Dermis } Nail bed
Periosteum
Bone of phalanx

Nail; proximal half (long)

Duct
Sebum
Disinte-grating cell
Fatty cell
Basal cell

Sebaceous gland

Duct
Eccrine gland
Secretory tubule
Myoid cells
Apocrine gland
Detaching apex

Sweat glands

Alveolus
Duct
Myoid cell

Lacrimal gland

Fat cell
Alveolus
Intralobular connective tissue
Interlobular stroma

Mammary lobule (inactive)

Coagulated milk
Surface of alveolus
Inter-lobular duct

Lactating gland (detail)

Fatty secretion
Myoid cell
Fat droplet

Gland cell

Lactating alveolus

THE INTEGUMENTARY ORGANS

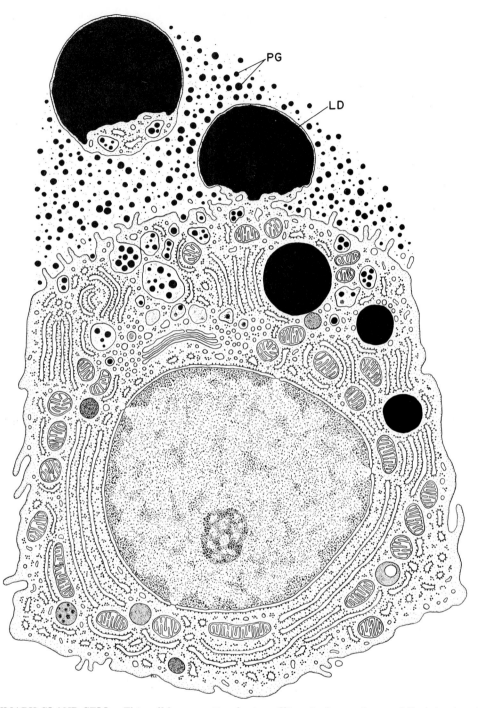

MAMMARY GLAND CELL.   This cell bears scattered microvilli on its free surface, and the lateral surfaces interlock irregularly with those of adjacent cells. Protein material (PG) is synthesized on the rough endoplasmic reticulum and is transported to the Golgi apparatus which concentrates and packages it into membrane-bounded vesicles. These merge at more apical levels into large vacuoles containing multiple, denser granules. Discharge is without gross rupture of the cell membrane, as in other mesocrine glands. Fat droplets (LD) arise free in the general cytoplasm throughout the cell and do not come into relation with the Golgi apparatus. They move toward the cell apex, enlarging by coalescence the while, and then pinch off encased in a thin sheath of cytoplasm; this mode of release is apocrine. Other cytoplasmic constituents are mitochondria, lysosomes and sparse smooth tubules and vesicles.

Its short duct empties into the follicle at a level three-fourths of the way up. (For the structure of sebaceous glands, see p. 197.)

E. GROWTH:

The hair root and its sheaths end in a bulbous enlargement which surrounds the papilla.
> This mass of syncytial-appearing cells is not organized into layers.
> Its nuclei are often seen in mitosis, and it is a proliferating matrix-tissue.

Cells about the apex and sides of the papilla move upward as new cells are produced.
> Cells at the apex form the medulla (when it is to be represented).
> Cells on the upper slope form the cortex; prior to keratinization they are basophilic.
> Cells on the sides form the cuticle.
> Gaining higher levels, these cells transform into definitive hair cells.
>> Prior to keratinization they are basophilic, because of sulfonic-acid groups.

Pigment is acquired from *melanocytes* in the same way as in epidermis (p. 188).

Cornification is gradual, as the hair cells are moved upward toward the surface.
> When about half the distance is gained, cornification is complete.
> The hair cells are dead; they have become acidophilic and doubly refractive.

Cells next to the lower papilla-third transform into the inner root sheath.
> Like the hair root this sheath grows upward, but it disintegrates before reaching the level of the sebaceous-gland duct.

Cells at the bottom of the follicle are continuous with those of the outer root sheath.
> It is possible that this sheath is pushed up from below, as is the inner sheath.
>> Yet most authorities think that it grows from mitoses in its outermost layers.

Weekly growth ranges from 1.5 mm. (leg) to 2.7 mm. (scalp).
> The final length attained in any region varies in different individuals.

F. SHEDDING AND REPLACEMENT:

Hair has a definite period of growth, after which it ceases growing, is retained for a time in its follicle, and then is lost and replaced.
> At any given time, about half of the hair follicles are active and half are inactive.
>> Growing and resting periods are about equal, except on the head and face.
> The life-span of an eyelash is 3 to 4 months; of a scalp hair, about 4 years.

In some mammals there is periodic shedding (winter and summer coats).

In other mammals, including man, hair loss is irregular and continuous.
> Each follicle has an independent and characteristic rhythmic cycle.

Cutting or shaving has no effect on the coarseness or rate of growth of hair.

1. Shedding.

When the growth period nears its end, proliferation slows and ceases.

The bulb then changes into a solid, keratinized, club-shaped mass.

This mass, including the cornified inner root sheath which fuses with it, detaches from the papilla but remains bound to the remainder of the hair-root.

Such a *club hair* is forced up to the level of the sebaceous duct.
> This results from the proliferation of indifferent matrix cells.
> (Here it remains until it is pulled out or is pushed out by a new hair.)

The papilla then atrophies and may even seem to disappear completely.

The outer root sheath collapses and becomes an epithelial cord.
> It extends from the atrophic papilla to the lower end of the elevated club hair.
> It shortens and draws the papilla-remnant upward.

2. Replacement.

After a rest period, the epithelial cord at the follicular base (outer epithelial sheath) proliferates and regains its former length and thickness.

Simultaneously, the papilla-remnant enlarges.
> It indents the mass of the epithelial sheath, and a new bulb is formed.

From the new cell matrix about the papilla an inner sheath and hair differentiate.
They grow progressively upward, through the follicle, toward the surface.
For a time the old hair may lie above, or at one side, of the new upgrowing one.

3. Regeneration after injury.

Forcible extraction of a growing hair results in only a temporary loss.
The outer sheath, and probably some matrix, remain; restoration soon follows.
Superficial injuries to skin are followed by a regeneration of follicles and hairs.
However, healing of wounds by scar tissue chokes and destroys any remnants of
follicles that survive a more severe injury.

G. AGE CHANGES:

Baldness is more frequent (6:1) in males than in females.
It is an hereditary and sex-controlled trait.
The genetic factors are effective only when male hormone is present in the body.
Follicles first show declining vigor by forming short hairs of the downy type.
Then they atrophy and disappear totally.
Whitening of the hair is due to the failure of pigment formation in replacement-hairs.
An additional factor is the presence of tiny air spaces between the cortical cells.
A prominent medulla, combined with pigment loss, makes hair 'silvery.'
Truly gray hair is rare; mingled white and dark hairs give the common gray effect.
Sudden blanching through fear is not proved; it is an irrational folk belief.

H. VESSELS AND NERVES:

Blood vessels of the dermis supply a rich capillary plexus to the papilla.
Other vessels vascularize the fibrous root sheath.
Lymphatic connections have not been demonstrated.
Nerve fibers encircle the follicle in a plexus and make sensory endings within it.
Vasomotor fibers enter the papilla; pilomotor nerves innervate the erector muscle.

I. DIAGNOSTIC FEATURES:

Hair follicles are to be expected in most sections containing skin.
Chief exceptions are the palmar and plantar surfaces.
The cylindrical follicle, with its bulb and papilla, is a unique structure.
In longitudinal section it is wholly distinctive.
The associated sebaceous gland and erector muscle are also unique features.
Transverse sections show a variety of concentric layers at different levels.
All layers are seen best at a level about two-thirds of the way down the follicle.
(Empty follicles, with the hair dropped out, are sometimes encountered.)

J. FUNCTIONAL CORRELATIONS:

Hair is primarily for protection, warmth and tactile reception.
The coarser hairs, appearing after childhood, are controlled by the sex hormones.
Some hairs (axillary; pubic) are common to both sexes.
Other hairs of the male (beard; chest) are a secondary sexual characteristic.
They also appear after puberty, but only when the male sex hormone is adequate.
Subsequently they are maintained by the hormone, supplied in proper amounts.
Hair follicles provide foci of epidermal regeneration after superficial loss of skin.
Curly hairs and their follicles are flatter (less cylindrical) than straight ones.

IV. THE CUTANEOUS GLANDS

Several kinds of glands differentiate from the epidermis, and some are highly specialized.
There are: *sebaceous glands; lacrimal glands; sweat glands; mammary glands.*

A. SEBACEOUS GLANDS:

These are holocrine glands in which secretory cells are lost along with the secretion.
In most instances they occur in company with a hair.
Usually several glands drain into a hair follicle; hence the total number is large.
Glands independent of hairs occur in a few locations.
The duct then opens onto the free surface of the skin.
Example: margin of lips; glans penis; inner surface of prepuce; labia minora; nipple; tarsal (Meibomian) glands of eyelids.
These glands are entirely lacking from the palm and sole.

1. Structural plan.

Sebaceous glands are located in the dermis of the skin.
The duct opens typically into the neck of a hair follicle.
Each gland is encapsulated by a thin layer of connective tissue.
The diameter of groups of glands ranges from 0.2 to 2.0 mm.
There is somewhat of an inverse relation between gland size and hair size.
The largest, as on the nose, are associated with a delicate hair.
Sebaceous glands belong to the saccular group of glands.
Some small glands consist of but one saccule.
Most glands have several saccules opening into a short, relatively wide duct.
The largest are compound glands, with a branching duct.
The saccules are pear-shaped and ordinarily appear filled with puffy cells.

2. Detailed structure.

A. SECRETORY PORTION.
The *saccule* consists of a stratified epithelium, supported by a delicate basement membrane and a thin layer of connective tissue.
Cells of the epithelium tend to fill the saccule completely.
The basal glandular cells are small, low, cuboidal elements.
They are continuous with the basal cells of the epidermis.
Toward the center of the sac the cells become progressively larger.
They are also more globular and have a greater lipid content.
A fatty metamorphosis of cytoplasm occurs, leaving only cytoplasmic strands.
These thin, basophilic strands separate the lipid droplets.
Cells crowded upward undergo further deterioration when near the duct.
The nuclei shrink, condense and disintegrate.
Finally, the whole cell breaks down into a fatty mass and cellular debris.
The lost cells are replaced by proliferation from the basal cells.
Glands are subject to change; new buds grow out from ducts or saccules.
B. EXCRETORY DUCT.
The short, wide *duct* of a gland is lined with stratified epithelium.
This lining is continuous with the epithelial sheath of the hair.
(Or with the germinative layer of the epidermis if the gland opens on skin.)
Toward the saccule the layering decreases progressively.
Finally it merges with the low basal cells of the saccule.
The mouth of a large, exposed duct is visible; it often shows as a 'blackhead.'
A retention cyst in the scalp is a 'wen.'
C. SEBUM AND ITS DISCHARGE.
The secretion, formed by fatty metamorphosis and cell-disintegration, is *sebum*.
It is an oily product, containing also cellular remnants.
It fluoresces in ultraviolet light; sebum in undischarged glands glows also.
Discharge is aided by contraction of the erector muscle and by general pressure.
D. VASCULAR SUPPLY.
Capillary basketworks closely invest the saccules.

3. Specialized sebaceous glands.

The *tarsal glands* (of Meibom) of the eyelids have an unusual arrangement.
There is one long, axial duct into which saccules open from all sides.
Tyson's glands are twisted tubes of undetermined status.
They occur inconstantly on the glans penis and inner surface of the prepuce.
Sebaceous cells have been described in them.

4. Diagnostic features.

Saccules, simple or branched, lie in the dermis; they open off a short duct.
Except for some special locations, they are always associated with hair follicles.
The peripheral cells of saccules are cuboidal and of the ordinary type.
The more central cells are large, puffy and pale.
Those pushed to the vicinity of the duct show signs of disintegration.
The cytoplasm appears frothy because of vacuoles left by dissolved lipid droplets.
The short duct usually opens into a hair follicle, not far below the epidermis.

5. Functional correlations.

Sebum is a grease that oils hair, lubricates the epidermis and combats drying.
It is mildly bactericidal and helps to protect epidermis against water penetration.

B. LACRIMAL GLAND:

This derivative of the modified skin of the conjunctiva is a *tear gland*; see p. 304.

C. SWEAT GLANDS:

The ordinary *sudoriparous glands* are unbranched, coiled tubular glands.
They are highly developed in man, but lack in some mammals.
They do not suffer cytoplasmic loss when secreting, and hence are *merocrine glands*.
This particular kind of sweat gland is also called *eccrine*.
They occur throughout the skin, except upon the nail bed, eardrum, glans penis, inner surface of the prepuce and margin of the lip. They occur independently of hairs.
The frequency of ordinary sweat glands varies regionally.
In general, they are more abundant than sebaceous glands or hairs.
On the palm and sole there are about 3000 per sq. in.; on the back, about 500.
The total for the human body is calculated to be several million.

1. Structural plan.

The *secretory tubule* lies mostly in the superficial subcutaneous tissue.
This portion is coiled into a mass about 0.4 mm. in diameter.
The tubule is about 3.0 mm. long and 0.06 mm. wide in ordinary sweat glands.
(Certain larger, specialized glands will be described separately on p. 199.)
The *duct* is a narrower, inactive continuation of the secretory tubule.
It rises through the dermis to the epidermis by a slightly tortuous course.
The duct joins the epidermis, and spirals through it to the free surface.
Its entrance is at the crest of a ridge projecting into the dermis.
Its opening, the *sweat pore*, is a minute pit on the epidermal surface.
They are best seen on the ridges of the palmar and plantar surfaces.
Here they are easily visible under a magnifying lens.

2. Detailed structure.

A. SECRETORY TUBULE.

This tubule consists of a simple epithelium, bordered by peculiar 'myoid cells.'
A basement membrane supports it, and connective tissue embeds it.

1. Gland cells.

The *main type* is a single layer of faintly basophilic pyramidal cells.
They border the lumen and their height varies with functional states.
Hence the easily seen lumen also varies in size correspondingly.

The cells bear *microvilli;* cell boundaries are usually not plain.

The cytoplasm contains vacuoles filled with polysaccharide secretion.

A *second type* is deeper lying pale cells, drained by typical *secretory canaliculi.*

They are assumed to secrete a watery fluid containing various solutes.

The glandular epithelium rests upon a prominent *basement membrane.*

2. *Myo-epithelial cells.*

At the periphery of the tubule there are peculiar spindle-shaped cells.

They lie mostly wedged between the bases of gland cells.

They wind in longitudinal spirals about the tubules.

These *myo-epithelial cells* are slender, flattened cells, 30 to 90 μ long.

The nucleus is elongate; the cytoplasm is fibrillar and acidophilic.

They are considered to be a specialized type of smooth-muscle fiber.

Their contractions presumably help to empty the gland.

The origin (ectodermal) is unlike that of ordinary smooth muscle.

B. EXCRETORY DUCT.

The secretory tubule suddenly narrows into a slenderer *excretory duct.*

This tube consists of two layers of dark-staining, cuboidal cells.

Cells bordering the lumen have apically a refractile *terminal web* (p. 221).

Myo-epithelial cells are lacking in this type of duct.

The duct joins the germinative layer at a thicker region, where it dips between connective-tissue papillae; here its own epithelium ceases.

A spiral duct then continues through the epidermis to the free surface.

This part of the duct is merely a cleft-like tunnel.

It is bordered by concentrically arranged epidermal cells.

The ridges of palmar and plantar surfaces bear rows of funnel-like openings.

C. VESSELS AND NERVES.

Blood vessels and capillaries fashion plexuses about the gland tubules.

Nerve fibers form periglandular networks, from which fibers enter the tubules.

These end on the myo-epithelial cells and between the gland cells.

3. *Specialized sweat glands.*

Certain large, branched sweat glands have a distinctive method of secretion.

Apical bits of the gland cells, with contained secretory products, pinch off.

In this way the secretion is liberated within a thin shell of cytoplasm.

Such glands are known as *apocrine glands.*

This group is less coiled than are ordinary sweat glands.

The lumen of the secretory tubule is conspicuously wider.

Also the myo-epithelial cells are larger and more numerous.

The secretion is thicker, more pigmented and contains larger lipid droplets.

A. CERUMINOUS GLANDS.

These glands occur in the external auditory canal (p. 306).

The secretion is a yellow, pigmented, fatty fluid.

It is a constituent of *cerumen,* or earwax.

B. CILIARY GLANDS (OF MOLL).

These glands of the eyelids are twisted, spiraling tubes.

They sometimes branch.

C. RUDIMENTARY MAMMARY GLANDS.

This group occurs along the course of the mammary ridge of the embryo.

Representatives are found in the axilla, mammary areola, mons pubis, labia majora, scrotum and circumanal region.

The coiled tube may reach a length of 30 mm. and make a mass 5 mm. in diameter.

Its duct opens into a hair follicle, as do sweat glands of lower mammals.

Some ducts, however, become separate secondarily and open independently.

The *axillary glands,* for example, acquire their large size at puberty.

At this time they begin to secrete a fluid, apocrine style.

Its characteristic odor results secondarily from bacterial action.
Periodic changes, paralleling the menstrual cycle, have been claimed.

4. Regenerative ability.

Sweat glands can regenerate if their deeper ends escape destruction.

5. Diagnostic features.

Sweat glands can be expected in almost every section of the skin.
The coiled, secretory portion lies at about the dermal-subcutaneous junction.
Its coils, sectioned in various planes, make a characteristic group.
The secretory cells are low columnar; peripherally there are myoid cells.
The duct passes vertically to the epidermis and channels through it in a spiral.
It is relatively long; its double layering in the free portion is distinctive.

6. Functional correlations.

The sweat glands, in excreting sweat, act as accessory excretory organs.
The secretion contains many of the ingredients of urine.
It is an oily fluid that becomes watery on nervous stimulation of the gland.
These glands are also important in the regulation of body temperature.
Evaporation of sweat from the skin surface has a cooling effect.
The utility of ceruminous glands is obvious, but not that of the axillary type.

D. MAMMARY GLAND:

The *mammary gland* is a specialized, cutaneous gland located in the subcutaneous tissue.
It resembles and exaggerates the modified sweat glands of the apocrine type.
Development and structural conditions in lower mammals support this conclusion.
Glands are represented in both sexes, and they progress slightly during childhood.
At puberty they advance rapidly in the female, but very slowly in the male.
At 20 years the male glands stabilize in a feebly developed state.
They then correspond to the female glands in early puberty.
Moreover, the female glands remain imperfectly developed until pregnancy occurs.
Full differentiation and function are attained only after childbirth.

1. Structural plan.

The mammary tissue comprises the *corpus mammae,* covered by skin.
The skin-cover is capped by a circular, pigmented area, the *areola.*
At the center of the wrinkled, pebbly areola lies the elevated *nipple.*
The glandular substance comprises 15 to 20 *lobes.*
Actually each is an independent gland with its own duct system.
A *lobe* is surrounded by interlobar connective tissue and much fat.
The fatty and fibrous tissue also subdivides a lobe into many *lobules.*
The epithelial parenchyma is embedded in loose, delicate connective tissue.
The *intralobular ducts* drain into *interlobular ducts,* and these into a main duct.
This single excretory duct from each lobe is a *lactiferous duct.*
It dilates, near its end, into a *lactiferous sinus.*
The duct then narrows again and opens at the summit of the nipple.
The functioning mammary gland is typical of the compound saccular type of gland.
It then differs greatly from its relatively undeveloped, inactive state.

2. Detailed structure.

A. AREOLA AND NIPPLE.

The *areolar region*, including the nipple, has a thin, pigmented epidermis.

Pigmentation is deeper in brunettes and during pregnancy.

The dermis contains tall papillae and smooth-muscle fibers.

The muscle is arranged both circularly and radially.

In the nipple it is mostly circular, but some fibers follow the ducts.

Contraction of the muscle elevates and hardens the nipple.

The *areola* contains special *areolar glands* which open on surface elevations.

These glands (of Montgomery) are large, branched apocrine glands.

They are regarded as transitions between sweat glands and mammary glands.

The areola also contains ordinary sweat glands and large sebaceous glands.

The columnar *nipple* is traversed by *lactiferous ducts*, 2 to 4 mm. in diameter.

Ducts have a 1- to 2-layered columnar epithelium until near the outlet.

A duct opens by a pore, about 0.5 mm. in diameter, at the top of the nipple.

There are fewer pores (8 to 15) than main ducts, owing to fusions.

At the base of the nipple, each main duct bears a local dilatation.

This spindle-shaped *lactiferous sinus* attains a diameter of 5 to 8 mm.

During lactation it is supposed to serve as a little reservoir for milk.

B. INACTIVE GLAND.

The *ducts* are the chief epithelial tissue seen, both inside and outside lobules.

The lining advances from simple cuboidal to a two-layered epithelium.

Peripheral to the lactiferous sinus, the epithelium stratifies progressively.

At the pore, it becomes continuous with the epidermis.

Between epithelium and basement membrane are stellate *myo-epithelial cells.*

They enclose the ducts (and alveoli, if present) in a loose basketwork.

The glandular *lobules* are small and have a rudimentary appearance.

The *intralobular ducts* appear narrow or collapsed.

Alveoli at best are mere buds, as in a sprouting embryonic gland.

Many believe that alveoli are lacking prior to the first pregnancy.

Intralobular connective tissue is loose and fine in texture.

It is cellular and vascular, but contains no fat.

It furnishes a nutritive and expansible bed for future, functional alveoli.

This territory of the potentially active lobule is plainly recognizable.

Interlobular connective tissue is relatively abundant, dense and coarse.

Cells are few, but fat is present and sometimes plentiful.

Here also course the *interlobular ducts.*

C. ACTIVE GLAND.

The gland arouses during pregnancy and becomes functional after childbirth.

The cessation of nursing is followed by marked retrogression.

1. *During pregnancy.*

In the first half of pregnancy, *secretory ducts* extend and *alveoli* become plain.

These result from rapid budding-off at the ends of existing ducts.

Their lumina hollow out by the middle of pregnancy.

The lining epithelium is of the simple cuboidal type.

Interlobular fat disappears to make room for lobular expansion.

The 15 to 20 lobes become plainly recognizable entities.

In the second half of pregnancy the proliferation and budding decline.

The alveoli, however, enlarge and elaborate secretion-precursors.

Some fluid (*colostrum*, p. 202) is secreted, and the alveoli dilate.

Lobules fill out internally, expand grossly and become well demarcated.

This is partly at the expense of the abundant intralobular stroma.

Yet even at the end of pregnancy some lobules are still laggard.

2. *During lactation.*

The prominent *alveoli* are closely packed within well demarcated *lobules.*

They become *saccules* and comprise most of the tissue of the breast.

Conversely, the interlobular stroma is reduced to thin septa.
The secretory end-pieces show regional differences in appearance.
That is, not all parts of the gland, or even of the same lobule, are in the same functional state at the same time.
Many saccules are dilated by milk and have a thin epithelial wall.
Others are resting; they have a relatively thick wall and small lumen.
The basophilic *gland cells* have indistinct cell boundaries.
Between them and a delicate basement membrane are stellate *basket cells.*
These are *myo-epithelial cells,* demonstrably contractile.
Gland-cell shapes range from low cuboidal to columnar in active saccules.
The taller cells often have rounded tops; cells develop microvilli.
The nucleus is rounded to oval, and centrally situated.
Synthesized protein granules move from the Golgi area to the cell apex.
Lipid is also synthesized, and small droplets appear in the cytoplasm.
Larger, coalesced fat globules then collect at the free, bulging apex.
Secretion is a double process, partly merocrine and partly apocrine.
Protein droplets are discharged without cytoplasmic loss.
Fat droplets leave the cells through the detachment of bits of cell apex.
Secretion and storage occur intermittently, interrupted by nursing.
Intralobular ducts are much like alveoli in structure and function.
Hence they are true *secretory ducts* (as in some salivary glands).
They contain cuboidal cells and elongate myo-epithelial elements.
The latter are believed to express milk from the ducts.
Interlobular ducts of all sizes are purely excretory in function.
They change but little during pregnancy and lactation.

3. *After lactation.*
When milk is no longer removed from the glands, secretion ceases.
Milk in the lumina of saccules is then resorbed.
Secretory residues in the ducts may be retained for a long time.
Regressive changes return the gland to the resting state.
Intralobular connective tissue becomes plainly less cellular.
The saccules dwindle, lose their obvious lumina, and some disappear.
However, the gland does not quite return to the nulliparous state.
After the first pregnancy, many alveoli remain recognizable as such.
Connective tissue apparently increases, and again infiltrates with fat.

D. MILK.
The secretion discharged during the first few days after delivery is *colostrum.*
It also follows the termination of lactation.
Similar to it is the *witch's milk* of the newborn of both sexes.
Colostrum is a watery milk, containing protein but little fat.
Colostrum contains a characteristic component known as the *colostrum corpuscle.*
These are large, globular cells that contain numerous lipid droplets.
Such corpuscles have often been interpreted as detached gland cells.
More probably they are outwandered lymphoid cells, capable of amebism.
They are said to acquire fat globules from the lumen by phagocytosis.
Within a few days after childbirth, the colostrum is replaced by *milk.*
Milk is a complex solution and emulsion.
It contains casein, lactose and inorganic salts in solution.
It also contains fat globules (mostly 2 to 5 μ) in suspension.
Each droplet is enclosed in an all albuminous envelope.
This prevents ready coalescence of the droplets.
Free nuclei and some cellular fragments can be found in milk.

E. VESSELS AND NERVES.
The *vascular supply* becomes much richer in the active gland.
Blood vessels ramify in the stroma and terminate in capillary plexuses about saccules and intralobular ducts.

Lymphatic networks surround the secretory portions of the gland.

They drain chiefly to the axillary lymph nodes.

Efferent nerves supply the smooth-muscle of vessels and of the areolar region.

Secretory fibers also innervate the glandular epithelium.

Afferent nerve fibers supply numerous sensory endings in the nipple.

Some of these endings resemble those on the genitalia.

3. Involution.

After the menopause the mammary gland undergoes regressive development.

The secretory epithelium atrophies, as do the excretory ducts to a less degree.

Only a few scattered remnants (mostly of the duct system) persist.

The stroma becomes less cellular and the collagenous fibers decrease in number.

The fibers appear as if 'melted down' into a more homogeneous mass.

Elastic fibers increase in amount.

4. Diagnostic features.

Intralobular ducts are poorly distinguished from alveoli, or not at all.

Interlobular ducts lie in the coarse fibrous stroma between lobules.

In the active gland they occur in the compressed septa between lobules.

The *inactive gland* consists of scattered groups of epithelial cords or tubules.

These appear like a sprouting, fetal stage of a gland.

Such groups of rudiments occur within a loose, cellular, connective-tissue bed.

These unit areas (lobules) are embedded in a coarse, fibrous and fatty stroma.

The *lactating gland* shows sharply demarcated, crowded lobules.

The interlobular connective tissue is compressed into thin septa.

Secretory end-pieces often differ in appearance regionally.

The larger ones are very closely packed saccules with wide lumina.

The cell-tops tend to bulge and appear vacuolate (or ragged, if discharged).

Milk in the lumen appears as a granular mass.

(There is a superficial resemblance to the lung, thyroid and prostate.)

During pregnancy, conditions are intermediate between inactivity and lactation.

After the menopause, conditions are simpler than before the first pregnancy.

The appearance is one of wasting; epithelial strands and ducts persist variably.

5. Functional correlations.

The mammary gland is controlled by ovarian and hypophyseal hormones.

Details, gained solely from lower mammals, are somewhat conflicting.

For this reason, statements concerning the human are partly inferential.

The growth of the duct system, at puberty, is induced by ovarian *estrogen*.

At the same time an accumulation of fat swells the breasts.

Some periodic swelling of the breasts accompanies the subsequent menstrual cycles.

This is due largely to engorgement of blood vessels and to stromal edema.

Some epithelial increase, nevertheless, does occur cyclically in the monkey.

Similar evidence from precisely timed human biopsies is lacking.

The growth occurring in pregnancy is induced by an increased supply of *estrogen*.

Progesterone apparently aids in this completion, especially in alveolar development.

Somatotropin, the growth hormone, also plays a role.

The initiation of secretion is induced by the hormone *prolactin.*

This is another name for the luteotropic hormone, LTH.

Another hormone, *oxytocin,* contracts myo-epithelial cells and expresses milk.

This response is initiated by reflexes set off by stimulation through sucking.

Lactation may continue for several years if milk is removed regularly.

Milk production ceases when undrained milk collects and distends saccules.

Chapter XVIII

The Mouth and Pharynx

The *digestive system* comprises the mouth, pharynx, and digestive tube (or alimentary canal).
 In addition, it includes the salivary glands, pancreas and liver which open into these parts.
The hollow passage, from mouth to anus, can be called the *digestive tract*.
 It exhibits regional specializations at various levels along its course.
 These modifications are correlated with the different functions performed locally.
  The primary functional component in each instance is the lining of the hollow canal.
  This lining is a *mucous membrane*, adapted at each level to its specific purpose.
   Chief in importance is the epithelium and its glandular derivatives.

I. STRUCTURAL PLAN OF THE MOUTH AND PHARYNX

The lining is a mucous membrane connected to firmer supporting structures.
 Teeth project through the epithelium, and glands open onto it.

1. Mucosa.

 The *epithelium* is moist and mostly of the stratified squamous type.
  It is not so highly flattened as epidermis, and is incompletely keratinized.
  Its superficial cells desquamate into the saliva.
 A *basement membrane* serves for the basal attachment of the epithelium.
 The fibrous *lamina propria* bears vascular papillae that indent the epithelium.
  In the pharynx, lymphocytes collect massively in this layer.
 A *lamina muscularis mucosae* is lacking throughout the mouth and pharynx.
  In the pharynx an elastic network substitutes in the same position.

2. Submucosa.

 This stratum is present in certain regions as a lax layer, but is not delimited sharply.
  Where existent as an entity, it permits the mucosa to be lifted as a fold.
  It serves to attach the mucosa to the underlying muscles or bone.
 A submucosa is absent in the hard palate (in part), gums and dorsum of the tongue.

3. Glands.

 These are compound, tubulo-alveolar elements, not present in all regions.
  They may be serous, mucous or mixed sero-mucous.
 They lie in the submucosa, wherever this stratum is recognizable, or even deeper.

4. Supporting wall.

 In all regions the superficial tissues attach to deep-lying skeletal muscle or bone.

5. Vessels and nerves.

 Blood vessels, lymphatics and nerves form coarse plexuses in the submucosa.
  Finer subdivisions pass into the mucosa and extend into the papillae.
  The mucosa is a well vascularized, highly sensitive membrane.

II. THE VESTIBULE

This is a sort of anteroom to the oral cavity proper.

Superficially it is bounded by fleshy folds that constitute the lips and cheeks.

Internally it is separated from the mouth by the gums, alveolar bone and teeth.

Ducts of the parotid gland and of numerous local glands open into the vestibule (p. 230).

1. Lip.

On the outer side is typical *skin*, with a thin keratinized epidermis.

Hair follicles, sebaceous glands and sweat glands are conspicuous features.

Centrally within the lip is a plate of skeletal muscle (mostly the *orbicularis oris*).

Slips of muscle insert among the fibers of the dermis, so that the skin is mobile.

These constitute the *mimetic muscles* (*i.e.*, of expression) of this region.

On the inner side is a typical *mucous membrane* and a less definite *submucosa*.

The stratified (but unkeratinized) epithelium is markedly thicker than epidermis.

The lamina propria indents the epithelium with moderately prominent papillae.

Rounded groups of *labial glands* lie deep in what can be termed a *submucosa*.

They are mixed sero-mucous, but are preponderantly mucous.

Their ducts open onto the surface epithelium of the vestibule.

There is a *transitional zone* at the red, marginal region of the lip.

Here the thick epithelium contains translucent prekeratin.

Tall vascular papillae indent the epithelium far toward the surface.

Blood in the capillaries shows through, and the lip appears red.

The virtual absence of glands in this region favors drying.

Hence the lip margins have to be moistened by wiping with the tongue.

The lips, like the cheeks, are regions that possess marked mobility.

They aid in eating, drinking, phonation and facial expression.

They restrict the opening of the mouth to a convenient size.

2. Cheek.

The general plan and composition of the lips continue into the cheek (bucca).

Even the transitional zone of the lips extends outward from the angles of the lips.

In this strip of buccal mucosa the papillae are very tall; glands lack completely.

As a whole, the epithelium lacks even prekeratin.

In general, the *mucosa* has short papillae; elastic fibers are abundant (unlike the lips).

The rather compact lamina propria is bound down at intervals to the muscle layer.

This prevents large folds and lessens the opportunity of injury when biting.

The *submucosa* is definitely a looser, fat-containing layer.

Buccal glands occur and even invade the stratum of muscle (the buccinator).

Although these are mixed sero-mucous glands, their cells are mostly mucous.

3. Gum.

It comprises that part of the oral mucosa attached to the alveolar bone of the jaw.

At the gum margins, the surface epithelium turns inward for a distance of about 2 mm.

It is separated from the surface of the tooth by a groove (*gingival sulcus*).

At the bottom of the groove there is an *epithelial attachment* to the teeth.

As the gum recedes in later years, this zone of attachment undergoes a shifting.

The shift is from the enamel to enamel and cementum, and finally to cementum.

The *epithelium* resembles that of the labial mucosa, but is keratinized apically.

The *lamina propria* is dense fibrous tissue.

It binds the gum to the cementum and to the alveolar bone.

Near the free margins, surrounding teeth, the papillae are very tall and vascular.

By contrast, the vicinity of the epithelial attachment is devoid of papillae.

It is suspected that the lamina propria may be unusually active metabolically.

Neither glands nor submucosa are represented in the gum.

4. Teeth.

Teeth, gums and alveolar bone provide a wall between the vestibule and mouth proper.
Since the teeth are complicated structurally, they will be treated as a major topic.

III. THE TEETH

The *teeth* are modified, soft papillae, covered by peculiar, hard substances.
The exposed part of the hard coating develops from an ectodermal epithelium.
All concealed portions of a tooth (in its natural position) are mesenchymal in origin.
Teeth are unique among organs by having the childhood set replaced by a permanent set.

A. STRUCTURAL PLAN:

A *tooth* consists of a free *crown* and one to three buried *roots*.
Crown and root meet at the *neck*, which is surrounded by the *gum margin*.
The root of a tooth occupies an *alveolus*, or socket, in the bone of the jaw.
A *periodontal membrane* attaches the root of the tooth to the bone of the alveolar wall.
The hollow *pulp chamber* of the crown extends into *root canals*.
At the tip of each root, the canal opens by an *apical foramen*.
The entire cavity is occupied by a soft core of *dental pulp*.
The hard wall of the tooth consists of three different kinds of specialized substance.
Dentin borders all the pulp and furnishes the body of the entire tooth.
It is interrupted only at the apical foramen.
Enamel covers the crown, becoming thinner at the neck.
Cementum encrusts the root; it is thinner at the neck.

B. DETAILED STRUCTURE:

1. Dentin.

Like bone, it consists of a collagenous mesh and calcified ground substance.
Unlike bone, it contains neither vessels nor total cells.
Dentin is harder than ordinary bone; it is 72 per cent inorganic.
In the crown, uncalcified areas produce the so-called *interglobular spaces*.
Next to the cementum, similar spaces constitute the *granular layer* (of Tomes).
Dentin appears radially striate because of countless *dentinal tubules*.
These tubules pursue S-shaped courses with many minor twists.
Each is a tiny tubule, 1 to 3 μ in diameter and up to 4 mm. long.
It branches and tapers peripherally; side branches may anastomose with other sets.
Each canal is lined with a dark-staining, uncalcified *dentinal sheath* (of Neumann).
The sheath is dense, refractile and resistant to chemicals.
The lumen of the tubule is occupied by a *dentinal fiber* (of Tomes).
It belongs to a specialized osteoblast (*i.e., odontoblast*) in the pulp cavity.
Hence this canal is a type of bone-canaliculus, with its peculiar capsule.
In old age these tubules are often obliterated by advancing calcification.
Incremental lines (of Owen and of Ebner) represent layered deposits of dentin.
In transverse sections they resemble the growth rings of a tree.
Dentin is deposited slowly throughout life, reducing the size of the pulp chamber.
Abrasion or irritation can stimulate the deposit of *secondary dentin*.
This irregularly arranged dentin may even obliterate the pulp cavity.

2. Enamel.

This highly specialized epithelial product is the hardest tissue of the body.
It is composed almost totally (97 per cent) of inorganic salts.
The chief component (90 per cent) is calcium phosphate.
The structural unit is a rod-like *enamel prism*, radially arranged.

Each is bordered by a thin *prism sheath*, richer in organic matter.
Union is by a scanty, cementing *interprismatic substance* that also calcifies.
Each prism was formed by a separate cell; it extends from dentin to surface.
The diameter varies from 3 to 6 μ; it thickens progressively toward the surface.
As many as 12 million prisms occur in a molar tooth.
In surface view a prism is evenly cross-banded and often slightly beaded.
The banding presumably reflects periodic rhythms in lengthwise growth.
In transverse section a prism is rounded on the surface facing dentin.
Most of them appear scale-shaped, with two notches on the side opposite dentin.
The arrangement resembles the pattern made by the scales in fish skin.
The prisms are grouped in bundles that may cross at acute angles.
The enamel as a whole is arranged in series of arching, superposed layers.
These layers represent periods of rhythmic growth.
Successive layers are demarcated by the *incremental lines* (of Retzius).

3. Cementum.

A thin layer of bone invests the dentin of the root.
It contains some bone cells (*cementocytes*) occupying lacunae within a typical matrix.
There is irregular and inconstant lamellation, but vessels are usually lacking.
In old age, Haversian systems may appear, as the cementum continues to thicken.
Cementum resists resorption better than bone; this permits teeth to be moved.

4. Dental pulp.

The main *pulp chamber* and *root canals* together comprise the *pulp cavity*.
This cavity is filled with a soft, gelatinous core which is the *pulp*.
The pulp is popularly called the 'nerve' of the tooth.
Its cells are fusiform and stellate; most of them are much like mesenchyme.
Some macrophages and lymphocytes are also present.
Reticular fibers are interspersed in a viscid ground substance.
At the periphery occurs an epithelioid layer of columnar cells, the *odontoblasts*.
These are peculiar, specialized osteoblasts, of mesenchymal origin.
From each cell a long process extends into an adjacent dentinal tubule.
These slender, branching processes are the *dentinal fibers* (of Tomes).
Vessels and nerves are described beyond under a separate heading.

5. Periodontal membrane.

This is a kind of periosteum that lies between the alveolar bone and the root.
It also supports the gum, with which it merges in the region of the tooth-neck.
At this level it helps to form the so-called *circular dental ligament*.
The membrane consists of densely arranged, coarse collagenous fibers.
It contains fibroblasts and osteoblasts; elastic fibers are lacking.
Sharpey's fibers extend away from both surfaces and bind the membrane to the alveolar wall in one direction, and to the cementum in the other direction.
The membrane also serves as a suspensory ligament for a tooth.

6. Vessels and nerves.

Usually a single *arteriole* enters each root-tip and ascends into the pulp chamber.
Capillary loops supply the odontoblasts and then open into thin-walled venules.
These *venules*, located more centrally, retrace the course of entering arterioles.
The presence of *lymphatics* within the pulp is still a subject of dispute.
Myelinated nerves accompany the arterioles and branch with them.
Nearing the periphery of the pulp, the fibers lose their sheaths.
Naked twigs pass between odontoblasts, but do not enter dentinal tubules.
The dentinal fibers apparently serve as pain receptors.
These intermediaries transmit sensory stimulations to the free nerve endings.
Unmyelinated nerve fibers also enter the pulp; they are vasomotor in function.

C. Diagnostic Features:

Enamel and dentin are distinctive histological tissues that specifically characterize teeth.
The spatial relations of enamel, cementum, dentin and pulp are diagnostic.
The relation of the tooth to its alveolus is also unique.

D. Functional Correlations:

The teeth serve to bite and grind food to proper size.
They are of considerable use in speech.
Experiments with radioactive tracers show mineral turn-overs in both dentin and enamel.
Active interchanges of calcium and phosphorus occur between teeth and the blood.

IV. THE TONGUE

The *tongue* is an organ that belongs partly to the mouth and partly to the pharynx.
It rises above the floor of these regions as a mobile organ.

A. Structural Plan:

A mass of *skeletal muscle* is largely contained within a covering of *mucous membrane*.
The under-surface of the tongue is smooth, and in places there is a *submucosa*.
The top-surface is uneven, with a tightly adherent *mucosa* (but no submucosa).
A longitudinal, *median sulcus* over-lies a deeper *lingual septum*.
The anterior two-thirds and posterior one-third are separated by a V-shaped boundary.
The angle opens forward and has the *foramen cecum* at its apex.
The larger oral portion is the *body;* the smaller pharyngeal portion is the *root.*
The dorsum of the tip and the body of the tongue bears numerous *lingual papillae.*
This area includes two-thirds of the entire top surface.
The dorsum of the root presents irregular bulgings, containing the *lingual tonsils.*
The floor of the mouth has a loose *submucosa;* it contains fat and the *sublingual glands.*

B. Detailed Structure:

1. Mucosa.

The fairly thick *epithelium* is of the stratified squamous type, mostly unkeratinized.
The epithelium is tightly bound down (except the under surface of the tongue).
The *lamina propria* is compact and intimately united to deeper muscle bundles.
The superficial portion, throughout the dorsum, bears vertical projections.
Over-draped with epithelium, they constitute the *lingual papillae.*
These gross elevations are quite different from the ordinary connective-tissue
papillae, also present, which merely indent the epithelium.
Lingual papillae are of four types: *filiform; fungiform; vallate;* and *foliate.*
A. Filiform Papillae.
These are so numerous as to constitute the 'plush' of the tongue.
They are arranged in parallel rows, diverging from the median sulcus.
A typical papilla begins as a primary columnar elevation of the lamina propria.
This bears 5 to 30 tall, secondary, connective-tissue *papillae.*
Epithelium clothes these papillary tufts and ends in tapered points.
The whole papilla resembles a 'cat of nine tails,' about 2 to 3 mm. long.
The surface of the epithelium is hyaline and scaly, but not fully keratinized.
B. Fungiform Papillae.
These are knob-like projections, scattered singly among filiform papillae.
Many vessels and a thin, translucent epithelium give them a red color.
They are larger than the filiform papillae, but much less numerous.
They have a columnar stalk and a broader, rounded top.
The shape resembles a button-mushroom (whence their name, 'fungiform').
The largest papillae are as much as 1.8 mm. high and 1 mm. wide.
The primary connective-tissue core bears many secondary papillae.

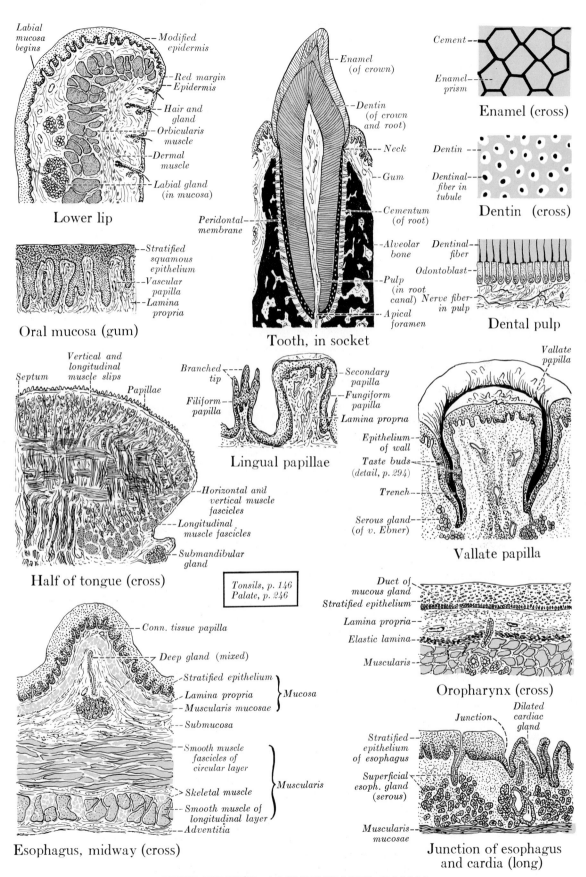

Lower lip

Labial mucosa begins
Modified epidermis
Red margin
Epidermis
Hair and gland
Orbicularis muscle
Dermal muscle
Labial gland (in mucosa)

Oral mucosa (gum)

Stratified squamous epithelium
Vascular papilla
Lamina propria

Tooth, in socket

Enamel (of crown)
Dentin (of crown and root)
Neck
Gum
Cementum (of root)
Alveolar bone
Pulp (in root canal)
Apical foramen
Peridontal membrane

Enamel (cross)

Cement
Enamel prism

Dentin (cross)

Dentin
Dentinal fiber in tubule

Dental pulp

Dentinal fiber
Odontoblast
Nerve fiber in pulp

Half of tongue (cross)

Septum
Vertical and longitudinal muscle slips
Papillae
Horizontal and vertical muscle fascicles
Longitudinal muscle fascicles
Submandibular gland

Lingual papillae

Branched tip
Filiform papilla
Secondary papilla
Fungiform papilla
Lamina propria

Vallate papilla

Vallate papilla
Epithelium of wall
Taste buds (detail, p. 294)
Trench
Serous gland (of v. Ebner)

Tonsils, p. 146
Palate, p. 246

Esophagus, midway (cross)

Conn. tissue papilla
Deep gland (mixed)
Stratified epithelium
Lamina propria } *Mucosa*
Muscularis mucosae
Submucosa
Smooth muscle fascicles of circular layer
Skeletal muscle } *Muscularis*
Smooth muscle of longitudinal layer
Adventitia

Oropharynx (cross)

Duct of mucous gland
Stratified epithelium
Lamina propria
Elastic lamina
Muscularis

Junction of esophagus and cardia (long)

Junction
Dilated cardiac gland
Stratified epithelium of esophagus
Superficial esoph. gland (serous)
Muscularis mucosae

THE UPPER ALIMENTARY CANAL

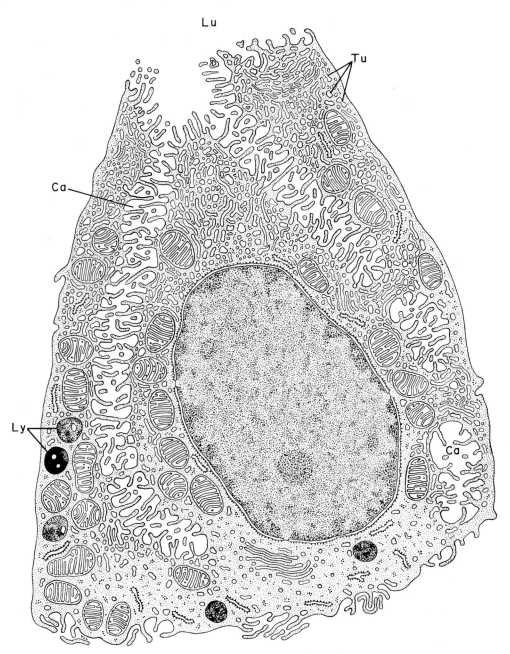

GASTRIC PARIETAL CELL.   Apically there are microvilli and basally there are projecting folds. The cytoplasm contains sparse rough endoplasmic reticulum and free ribosomes, extensive small tubules (Tu), numerous mitochondria with closely set cristae, lysosomes (Ly), and a basally located Golgi complex. Secretory granules are lacking. A conspicuous feature is secretory canaliculi (Ca), flanking the nucleus and opening apically into a common outlet that is continuous with the gland lumen (Lu). Long microvilli throughout may partially occlude the canalicular lumen; they are continuous with those of the outlet and gland lumen.

They merely indent the epithelium, however; the free surface is smooth.

Some fungiform papillae bear one to several *taste buds.*

Large, *conical papillae,* up to 3 mm. long, occur sparingly.

They are considered to be a modified, fungiform type.

C. VALLATE PAPILLAE.

This type makes a V-shaped row that demarcates the body and root of the tongue.

The total number is usually 7 to 11.

These papillae are much larger than any other type.

Their height ranges from 0.5 to 1.5 mm.; their width, from 1 to 3 mm.

These papillae do not extend much above the lingual surface.

On the other hand, they are counter-sunk beneath the surface level.

Each papilla is encircled by a deep *trench;* beyond this is a facing *wall.*

A papilla has the shape of an inverted, truncated cone with a nearly flat top.

It resembles the fungiform type in shape, but it is larger and flatter.

The connective-tissue core forms secondary papillae on its top surface alone.

The covering epithelium is indented by them, yet has a smooth free-surface.

The sides of a vallate papilla contain many *taste buds* (about 200).

The opposite wall, across the trench, has fewer buds (about 50).

These totals are highly variable; the numbers decrease greatly in old age.

Von Ebner's glands, purely serous, are associated with each papilla.

They intermingle with the muscle, and some 30 ducts empty into the trench.

D. FOLIATE PAPILLAE.

These are parallel mucosal folds on the lateral margins of the tongue.

They are located at the junction of its body and root.

In adult man, foliate papillae are regressive or rudimentary.

Infants may have 4 to 8 well developed, vertical folds on each side of the tongue.

These bear *taste buds* along the middle region of their side surfaces.

Von Ebner's glands, purely serous, open into the bottom of the trenches.

In some mammals (*e.g.,* rabbit), foliate papillae are highly developed.

E. TASTE BUDS.

These prominent, ovoid bodies embed in the epithelium of some lingual papillae.

As the receptor organs of taste, they are described on p. 297.

2. Lingual tonsil.

Its multiple, lymphoid units in the root of the tongue cause surface bulgings.

These tonsillar structures are described on p. 147.

3. Glands.

The *lingual glands* lie deep in the lamina propria and extend into the muscle.

A. ANTERIOR LINGUAL GLANDS.

These are located under the apex of the tongue, at each side of the median line.

They are mixed sero-mucous glands, with several ducts.

B. GLANDS OF VON EBNER.

This group is limited to the region of the vallate and foliate papillae.

All the alveoli are purely serous.

Numerous ducts (4 to 38) can be traced to the trench of each vallate papilla.

C. MUCOUS GLANDS OF THE ROOT.

These occur in the lymphoid area, but encroach slightly onto the body-region.

They are pure mucous glands, whose ducts open onto the dorsum of the tongue.

Some of the ducts empty into the pits of the lingual tonsils.

None, however, open into the trenches of the vallate papillae.

The submandibular and sublingual glands open alongside the tongue.

Both types will be described with similar major glands (p. 231).

4. Muscle.

The muscle mass is halved incompletely by the median, fibrous *lingual septum.*
The skeletal muscle fibers belong to two general groups.
　　Intrinsic fibers of the m. lingualis lie wholly within the tongue limits.
　　Extrinsic fibers enter from without and serve also to anchor the tongue.
　　　　These include the hyo-, genio-, stylo-, palato- and chondroglossus muscles.
The muscle fibers are arranged in definite bundles, interlacing at right angles.
　　Some bundles are longitudinal in direction; others, vertical or transverse.
　　The muscle fibers are embedded in loose, fatty areolar tissue (endomysium).
　　The fibers insert onto the perimysial connective tissue which surrounds bundles.
　　　　Some of the fibers branch near their insertions.

5. Vessels and nerves.

Blood vessels supply the lingual muscles and form a plexus in the lamina propria.
　　From the latter, capillaries extend to the papillae.
Lymphatics drain the papillae and produce plexuses in the lamina propria.
Efferent nerve fibers distribute to the muscles, glands and blood vessels.
Some *afferent nerve fibers* end freely and mediate general sensibility.
　　Others terminate within taste buds and are gustatory in function.

C. DIAGNOSTIC FEATURES:

Bundles of skeletal muscle interlace in three different planes; this is a unique feature.
　　They are divided incompletely by a fibrous median septum.
Stratified squamous epithelium provides an external covering.
　　Lingual papillae project from the mucosa of the dorsal surface of the body.
　　Tonsillar units, with pits, characterize the mucosa of the dorsal surface of the root.
Small glands occur constantly in sections through the root.
　　They may be present or absent in sections through the body.
Taste buds occur dependably only about the trench of each vallate papilla.
　　They are ovoid bodies, prominent and pale-staining, set in the epithelium.
　　The component cells are elongate, and most of them extend the length of a bud.

D. FUNCTIONAL CORRELATIONS:

The tongue is of use in selecting food, and in directing it to the teeth and pharynx.
　　Chewing and swallowing are thus furthered; the tongue also aids in speech.
The receptors of taste reside in taste buds whose cells respond to substances in solution.
　　Distinctive taste-bud types have not been correlated with taste discrimination.
General chemical sensibility (nongustatory) exists where taste buds do not occur.

V. THE PALATE

The *palate* furnishes a roof, separating the mouth from the nasal passages and nasopharynx.
The oral side bears the oral type of mucosa.
The nasal side bears the respiratory type of mucosa.
Between the two mucosae is a middle lamina of bone (in front) or of muscle (in rear).

1. Hard palate.

The *oral side* bears a mucosa, covered with a stratified squamous epithelium.
　　Its epithelium is the best keratinized in the mouth.
　　It is indented with tall papillae extending from a densely fibrous lamina propria.
　　　　The lamina is also elevated into a series of gross transverse ridges.
　　A submucosa exists except in a midline seam (the *raphe*) and near the gum.
　　　　The anterior one-third contains fat.
　　　　The posterior two-thirds contains pure *mucous glands.*
The *middle layer* is supplied by horizontal parts of the maxillary and palate bones.

The *nasal side* bears a mucosa with a pseudostratified, ciliated epithelium.
There are mixed *sero-mucous glands* and a deep layer of elastic fibers.

2. Soft palate.

This is a backward continuation of the palate, ending in a conical, free *uvula.*
The *oral side* continues the covering of stratified squamous epithelium.
The lamina propria bears tall papillae and is infiltrated with lymphocytes.
Mucosa and submucosa are separated by a dense network of elastic fibers.
The loose submucosa contains pure *mucous glands.*
The *middle layer* is a sheet containing bundles of the palatine skeletal muscles.
The *nasal side* continues the components from the hard palate, as already described.
Near the free posterior margin, however, there is stratified epithelium.
(This is reflected for a distance from the under-surface onto the upper-surface.)

3. Diagnostic features.

The palate is a plate bearing two mucous membranes, back to back.
On the oral side the mucosa has stratified squamous epithelium.
The submucosa contains mucous glands.
On the nasal side the mucosa has a pseudostratified, ciliated epithelium.
The mucosa has sero-mucous glands; there is no recognizable submucosa.
The middle support is either bone (hard palate) or skeletal muscle (soft palate).

4. Functional correlations.

The palate, in general, was developed to separate nasal passages from mouth.
The *hard palate* is firm, as an adaptation to the action of the tongue against it.
It withstands the force applied in crushing, mixing and swallowing food.
The transverse elevations aid mechanically in these maneuvers.
The mucosa as a whole is firmly attached to prevent slippage.
The *soft palate* is movable during the act of swallowing.
It is then drawn upward, thereby closing off the naso-pharynx.

VI. THE PHARYNX

The *pharynx* is a somewhat flattened conical chamber, through which air and food pass.
It is partly divided at the level of the soft palate into a superior and inferior region.
The superior part, respiratory in function, is called the *naso-pharynx.*
Its mucosa continues the general structure of the nasal passages, farther in front.
The inferior part consists of an *oro-pharynx* (behind the palatine arches) and of a *laryngo-pharynx* (behind the larynx).
This region progressively approaches the structural plan of the digestive tube proper.
A group of *tonsils* encircles the beginning of the pharynx.

A. MUCOSA:

1. Epithelium.

The *naso-pharynx* is lined chiefly by a pseudostratified epithelium.
The columnar cells are ciliated; some are specialized as goblet cells.
Lower levels have first stratified columnar epithelium, then stratified squamous.
This is a result correlated with the circumstance that the soft palate comes frequently in contact with the posterior pharyngeal wall.
The *oro-* and *laryngo-pharynx* are lined with a soft, stratified squamous epithelium.
Here the opposed surfaces come into contact, and are rubbed by passing food.

2. Lamina propria.

Only the naso-pharynx has a distinct *basement membrane* beneath its epithelium.
Small connective-tissue papillae indent the stratified epithelium.

The lamina, composed of fibro-elastic tissue, contains *lymphoid infiltrations.*

On the posterior surface of the naso-pharynx is the *pharyngeal tonsil* (p. 147).

Laterally, at the junction of mouth and oro-pharynx, are *palatine tonsils* (p. 145).

Basally, in the root of the tongue, is the *lingual tonsil* (p. 147).

In the oro- and laryngo-pharynx are scattered, solitary lymph nodules.

Regions associated with pseudostratified epithelium have small *sero-mucous glands.*

Regions associated with stratified epithelium have small *mucous glands.*

The deepest stratum of the lamina is occupied by fibers of a thick *elastic layer.*

This takes the place of the muscularis mucosae of the digestive tube proper.

B. Accessory Coats:

1. Submucosa.

This tunic is well developed in two localities only.

These are laterally in the naso-pharynx and in the approach to the esophagus.

Elsewhere the elastic stratum of the lamina propria abuts against the muscle.

Regions of the pharynx having stratified epithelium have small *mucous glands.*

These may even extend deep into the muscular layer.

2. Muscularis.

The muscular tunic consists of two layers of *skeletal muscle.*

The inner layer is longitudinal; the outer layer is oblique or circular.

3. Adventitia.

A thin, fibrous sheath occurs in most regions.

In other regions the muscles attach directly to the skull.

C. Diagnostic Features:

The general *naso-pharynx* resembles the respiratory nasal cavities in structure.

The absence of a venous plexus and the presence of a muscular coat are differences.

The *oro-* and *laryngo-pharynx* increasingly resemble the esophagus as they near it.

The presence of an elastic layer (instead of a muscularis mucosae) is distinctive.

The submucous glands are purely mucous, not mixed.

The muscle layers are reversed from the order in the digestive tube.

The several types of tonsils are distinctive features of their regions (pp. 145-147).

D. Functional Correlations:

The pharynx is a common passageway for air and food; their pathways cross.

Air, reaching it, has been warmed and filtered; food has been prepared for digestion.

The phase of swallowing performed by the pharynx is a complicated, involuntary act.

Stimulation by food or drink sets off a reflex involving the skeletal muscles.

Chapter XIX

The Digestive Tube

The *digestive tube*, or *alimentary canal*, begins with the esophagus and ends with the anus.
It is a typical example of the hollow organs of the body.

I. THE STRUCTURAL PLAN OF HOLLOW ORGANS

Most tubular and saccular organs are constructed according to a common plan.
Typically there are four concentric coats, named *tunics.*
 In certain organs there is a reduction within a coat or even the elimination of a coat.
 There are also minor structural variations to meet local requirements.
The appearance of the wall differs when the lumen is empty or distended.
 It is customary to describe only the empty, unstretched condition.

1. Tunica mucosa.

 The innermost tunic, commonly called a *mucous membrane*, has four component layers.
 A. EPITHELIUM.
  This may be of any type, correlated with the particular function performed.
  The *epithelium* faces the cavity of a hollow organ, which is called the *lumen.*
  In the relaxed condition an actual cavity does not exist to any degree.
   The folded epithelial surfaces are then in contact; the lumen is potential only.
  A lumen exists wherever fluid or solid material is passing, or is retained.
   In special situations the lumen is kept open by a reinforced outer wall.
    Example: trachea; auditory tube.
 B. MEMBRANA PROPRIA.
  The epithelium usually attaches to a sheet-like support of firm consistency.
   This is the membrana propria, or *basement membrane* as ordinarily named.
  It consists of a structureless ground substance and reticular fibers.
   If thin, its presence may be unnoticed in sections stained in a routine manner.
   The thickness is not always correlated with the amount of stress encountered.
 C. LAMINA PROPRIA MUCOSAE.
  Areolar tissue, reticular tissue, or both, form the basis of the *lamina propria.*
  There may be a *lymphoid infiltration*, and even *lymph nodules.*
  The superficial portion may be elevated into papillae, villi or folds.
  Smaller vessels and nerves invade the lamina propria throughout.
  Simple or compound *glands* are abundant in some organs.
 D. LAMINA MUSCULARIS MUCOSAE.
  When present, this layer consists of smooth muscle; usually there are two layers.
   An inner layer is circular; the outer is longitudinal.
  Where present, an exact boundary is established between mucosa and submucosa.
  The muscular layers aid in mixing and transporting the contents of the tube.
   In the small intestine dislocated slips of muscle wave and contract villi.

2. Tunica (or tela) submucosa.

 Coarse areolar tissue comprises this web-like membrane, usually called the *submucosa.*
  Its considerable laxity and elasticity provides mobility to the mucosa.

The submucosa also supports the larger blood vessels, lymphatics and nerves.

It contains a vascular plexus, nerve plexus and, commonly, small autonomic ganglia.

In a few organs there are compound *glands* in the submucosa.

3. Tunica muscularis.

The *muscular tunic* is often relatively thick; in a few tubes (*e.g.,* trachea) it is omitted.

Almost without exception, it is composed of smooth muscle.

The commonest arrangement is 2 concentric tubes (rarely 3 or 1).

The inner layer is usually circular in arrangement; the outer, longitudinal.

Knowing the arrangement of these layers in a given organ, the plane of a section taken from that organ can be determined by the way its fibers are cut.

A vascular plexus, nerve plexus and small ganglia commonly lie between the two layers.

The muscularis maintains tonus in a tube and also propels its contents onward.

The circular layer is able to control the size of the lumen.

By its action the contents are churned or propelled in a wave.

Contraction of the longitudinal layer shortens the tube locally.

This raises the pressure on the local contents in the lumen.

It can dilate the wall and pull it over the local mass being pushed along.

4. Tunica adventitia or serosa.

The outermost coat is primarily fibrous—an *adventitia,* or *fibrosa.*

In a few organs the adventitia becomes strengthened with cartilage.

Hollow organs contained within the peritoneal cavity, or projecting into it, are surfaced with a reflection of the peritoneum.

This outer tunic is then known as a *serosa.*

Through the adventitia or serosa, vessels and nerves pass to deeper levels of the wall.

II. THE ESOPHAGUS

This simple tube, the *esophagus* or gullet, is 10 in. long; it connects pharynx with stomach.

There is a fairly gradual transition from the structure of the pharynx into the esophagus.

In effecting this, a muscularis mucosae replaces the elastic layer of the pharynx.

Also the tunica muscularis becomes more regularly arranged.

A. MUCOSA:

1. Surface epithelium.

The stratified squamous epithelium is continued from the pharynx unchanged.

There is, however, an abrupt transition into the simple epithelium of the stomach.

Only the basal cells of the esophagus continue into the stomach.

The line of junction of the two epithelia follows a jagged, circular course.

The *epithelium* is highly stratified (about 25 cell-layers).

It is indented by tall connective-tissue papillae of the lamina propria.

In man it is not keratinized or highly flattened, as in some mammals.

2. Lamina propria.

This layer consists of areolar tissue, poor in elasticity and not highly cellular.

Tall *papillae* indent the epithelium (even for two-thirds of its thickness).

A few solitary *lymph nodules* occur mostly in relation to the ducts of mucous glands.

Superficial glands occur at the extreme upper and lower ends of the esophagus.

They are variable in number and sometimes fail (especially the upper set).

These are compound tubular glands that sometimes take a weak mucin stain.

Each duct opens at the summit of a connective-tissue papilla.

They resemble the cardiac glands of the stomach, and the lower set joins them.

For this reason, they are sometimes called 'cardiac glands' (*cf.,* p. 216).

3. *Muscularis mucosae.*

This layer of smooth-muscle is thicker than anywhere else in the body.
> At the upper end it occurs as bundles that do not make a complete layer.
> Toward the stomach it is complete and increasingly robust (0.2 to 0.4 mm. thick).
Its muscle fibers are arranged longitudinally; a circular layer is lacking.

B. ACCESSORY COATS:

1. *Submucosa.*

This fibro-elastic layer is lax; its thickness decreases when food is swallowed.
> When the esophagus is empty, 7 to 10 prominent longitudinal folds are formed.
> These involve both the mucosa and submucosa and give the lumen a star-shape.
> A squeezing force, resulting from constant muscular tone, produces the folds.
Deep glands, which are the *esophageal glands* proper, lie within the submucosa.
> Their number is variable (60 to 740); more occur in the upper half of the tube.
> Each is a small, compound tubular gland; it produces typical mucus.
>> The chief duct of each gland, in passage, pierces the muscularis mucosae.
>> A duct enters the epithelium where the latter dips downward between papillae.

2. *Muscularis.*

Two thick layers of muscle are conspicuous features.
> The inner layer is circular; the outer layer is longitudinal.
The composition of the muscle coat varies at different levels.
> The upper quarter consists of skeletal muscle; some oblique bundles occur.
> A middle segment contains a mixture of skeletal- and smooth muscle.
> The lower third consists of smooth muscle, whose layers are arranged regularly.
> (The smooth- and skeletal-muscle extents are subject to individual variation.)

3. *Adventitia.*

The most external tunic is a typical, loose, fibrous investment.
> It connects with surrounding structures and conducts many vessels and nerves.
The short segment of esophagus below the diaphragm is invested with a serosa.

C. VESSELS AND NERVES:

The distribution of blood vessels, lymphatics and nerves within the entire digestive tube
> follows a similar, fundamental pattern.
These features will be summarized at the end of this chapter (p. 228).

D. DIAGNOSTIC FEATURES:

The esophagus is a tube with a stratified squamous epithelium, robust muscularis mucosae
> and strong, two-layered muscular coat.
The mucosa and submucosa tend to be thrown into alternate major and minor folds.
> In transverse section they produce a characteristically branched, stellate lumen.
The muscularis mucosae is by far the thickest present in any organ.
Mucosal glands are too local in extent to be dependable as a general diagnostic aid.
> When present they indicate an extreme upper or lower level of section.
> (Whether upper or lower can be told by the composition of the muscularis.)
Submucosal glands are commonly encountered in sections, but may be lacking.
The composition of the muscularis establishes the general level of the section.
> If skeletal muscle only is present, the upper quarter of the tube can be assumed.
>> No other organ contains skeletal muscle and a muscularis mucosae.
> If mixed skeletal and smooth-muscle are present, the middle third can be assumed.
>> No other organ has a muscularis of this sort.
> If smooth-muscle only is present, the lower third can be assumed.

E. FUNCTIONAL CORRELATIONS:

The esophagus is a conducting tube that completes the warming or cooling of food to an appropriate temperature for reception into the stomach.
Food and drink are carried downward rapidly by muscular contractions and gravity.
Glandular secretions are mucoid and solely for lubricative purposes.

III. THE STOMACH

The *stomach* is a tube that became dilated and distorted into a potentially capacious sac.
To aid description, the stomach is divided into cardia, fundus, corpus and a pyloric region.
Fundus and corpus are similar structurally; hence the histological regions are but three.

A. MUCOSA:

The thickness varies from about 0.3 mm. at the cardia to 1.5 mm. at the pylorus.
The *mucosa* (and submucosa) is thrown into mostly longitudinal folds, the *rugae*.
The height and number of these depend on the degree of gastric distention.
Also there is a finer system of furrows, marking off *gastric areas* (1 to 5 mm. across).
On these bulging mounds open the *foveolae*, also known as *gastric pits*.
The foveolae range from 17 (in fundus) to 9 (in pylorus) per sq. mm.
In all, there are some 3,500,000 foveolae in the gastric mucosa.
Several gastric glands empty into the bottom of each foveola, which serves as a duct.

1. Surface epithelium.

Tall columnar cells, with basal nuclei, are regularly arranged in a simple *epithelium*.
At the cardia they continue into the basal layer of the esophageal epithelium.
The transition from simple to stratified epithelium is abruptly precipitous.
All the cells secrete mucus constantly; none assumes a goblet shape.
The mucus, however, is peculiar since not all 'specific' mucus stains color it.
In life, mucigen fills the cytoplasm above the level of the depressed nucleus.
These globules are preserved with great difficulty.
As a result, routinely stained sections show clear, pale cells.
Terminal bars encircle the cell-tops; electron micrographs demonstrate microvilli.
This cell-type also lines foveolae; here they are shorter and produce less mucigen.

2. Glands.

The *gastric glands* are of the simple, branched tubular type.
They extend more or less vertically through the full thickness of the mucosa.
Each foveola serves as a short duct to several glands.
The total number of glands is estimated at 15,000,000.
Most of these are said to differentiate after birth; one-half, after 10 years.
The total secreting area of the glands is large (30 sq. ft.).
There are three regional types of gland in the stomach: *cardiac; fundic; pyloric*.
A. CARDIAC GLANDS.
This type occupies a narrow band next to the cardio-esophageal junction.
The zone varies in width between 5 and 40 mm.
They are essentially like the superficial glands of the lower esophagus.
Both make a continuous series of small, sometimes compound, tubular glands.
The foveola (about equal to the gland-length) receives several glands.
The secreting portions are tortuous; their component cells are mucous elements.
These cells are much like the mucous cells of fundic and pyloric glands.
The gland-lumen is of fair diameter; some become cystically dilated.
At caudal levels within the zone there are transitions into the fundic type.
The significance of cardiac glands is obscure, although some hydrolytic enzymes occur.

B. FUNDIC GLANDS.

This type is poorly named, since it occurs in both the fundus and corpus.

The term *gastric gland* is also used to designate this particular type.

It is obviously an inappropriate name for glands of a limited region.

Each is a fairly straight, tubular gland that may branch somewhat.

Buds occur from the sides, and bifurcation at the end.

Several regional segments are recognized in a total gland.

There are: a short, constricted *neck*; a long *body*; and a slightly dilated and bent blind end, or *fundus*.

Three to seven glands open into each *foveola*, a short functional duct.

Gland length ranges from 0.3 mm. (fundus) to 1.5 mm. (corpus).

The ratio of foveola length to gland length is about 1:4.

The lumen of the secretory portion is narrow and often scarcely noticeable.

The component cells of the secretory portion show four cytological types.

Cell-types 1 to 3, below, bear inconspicuous microvilli on their free surface.

1. *Mucous neck-cells.*

This type is characteristic of the neck region of fundic glands.

Here they are interspersed with parietal cells (type 3, below).

They become progressively abundant in glands nearer the pyloric region.

In routine preparations these low columnar cells stain paler than chief cells, but resemble them.

But they differ in having basally located nuclei, usually flattened.

Specific mucus stains reveal a content of mucigen in them.

Nevertheless, the expelled mucus is watery and of a special nature.

2. *Chief cells.*

This type is progressively abundant in glands nearer the cardiac region.

They constitute most of the tubule below the level of the gland neck.

Such cells are pyramidal, granular elements, with basophilic cytoplasm.

Basally in the cell there is striate, basophilic *ergastoplasm* (p. 21).

The spherical nucleus is located not far below the center of the cell.

After a period of rest, a cell contains coarse *presecretion granules.*

After activity, the cells are smaller and the granules fewer.

Good preservation is difficult, since postmortem disintegration is prompt.

In ordinary preparations much of the cytoplasm is clear and vacuolate.

With proper fixation and staining, the *zymogen granules* (corresponding to these vacuolate spaces) can be demonstrated.

They consist of *pepsinogen*, the precursor of pepsin.

3. *Parietal cells.*

This cell type is progressively abundant in glands nearer the pyloric region.

Parietal cells are interspersed between the mucous neck-cells, where they are most common, and wedge in singly between the chief cells.

For this reason, they tend to occupy a peripheral position in the tubule.

Especially is this true toward the basal end of the gland.

Here they may even bulge prominently (when chief cells are depleted).

The cell shape is wedge-like to spheroidal; they are the largest gland cell.

The nucleus (sometimes two or more) is spherical and centrally located.

The finely granular cytoplasm stains strongly with acid aniline dyes.

Mitochondria are abundant; the Golgi complex is located basally.

There are, however, no distinctive secretory granules.

No cytological changes during functional activity are demonstrable.

Infoldings of the plasma membrane occur at the apices of parietal cells.

These produce intracellular channels, bearing microvilli.

A tubular groove between chief cells may serve as a stem channel.

The whole is a *secretory canaliculus*, opening into the gland lumen.

Only the electron microscope demonstrates best such tiny channels.

The function of parietal cells is to 'secrete' hydrochloric acid (pH is less than 2).

Free acid occurs in secretory canaliculi, but not in the cytoplasm.
The actual mode of acid formation is not surely established.
This is the only cell in the human body known to produce acid.
4. *Argentaffin cells.*
These *enterochromaffin cells* occur scatteringly in fundic glands.
They lie between the basement membrane and the chief cells.
A slender extension often reaches the gland lumen.
Granules in the broad cell-base stain with chrome salts or silver.
They are precursors of *serotonin,* a potent vasoconstrictive hormone.
C. PYLORIC GLANDS.
This type occupies one-seventh, or more, of the gastric area.
An *intermediate zone,* between fundic and pyloric areas, can be recognized.
Here the glands combine certain features of both types.
The *pyloric glands* are simple, branched, convoluted-tubular glands.
They are more branched than the fundic type, and their foveolae are deeper.
Their foveolae are at least as long as the secretory tubules themselves.
Several glands open into each foveola.
The body of the gland is short, tortuous and contains a prominent lumen.
Only one cell-type is found in the body (except for a few argentaffin cells).
This cell may be identical with the mucous neck-cell of fundic glands and the
secretory cell of the cardiac glands.
It stains palely in routine preparations, but colors with mucigen stains.
The secretion-antecedent is definitely mucoid in nature.
The nucleus is often flattened against the cell base.
Pyloric glands are intermediate in sequence and composition between the fundic
type and the duodenal glands (of Brunner).
They are usually said to function solely as slime-producing glands.
Yet there is demonstrable evidence of some hydrolytic enzymes.

3. Lamina propria.

The surface and glandular epithelium rest upon a *basement membrane.*
The connective tissue of the *lamina* is scanty because the glands are so numerous.
Especially is this true of the region supplied with crowded fundic glands.
Here it merely fills-in the narrow spaces between the glands proper.
The most abundant tissue is located high in the lamina, between foveolae.
The basic tissue is a delicate network of collagenous and reticular fibers.
There is a diffuse infiltration of lymphocytes among some other cell-types.
Solitary lymph nodules occasionally are seen.
They are more abundant in the cardiac and pyloric regions.
The *muscularis mucosae* is mostly thin, yet it is arranged in layers.
The inner layer consists of circular fibers.
Delicate strands of muscle pass from this sheet upward between the glands.
The outer layer consists of longitudinal fibers.
In some regions there is still another layer; this outermost one is circular.

B. ACCESSORY COATS:
1. Submucosa.

This coat is a loose, fibrous and vascular layer, with considerable elasticity.
It participates in producing the folds that comprise the *rugae.*
These folds (and the rugae) are effaced as the stomach distends with food.

2. Muscularis.

There are three thick layers of smooth muscle, arranged somewhat irregularly.
The *inner layer* consists of oblique fibers.

It occurs on the front and back surfaces in the fundus-corpus region.

The *middle layer* consists of circular fibers.

It is the best developed and most regular of the three.

At the pyloric orifice it forms the thick *pyloric sphincter*.

The *outer layer* consists of longitudinal fibers.

It is best represented along the inner and outer curvatures.

3. Serosa.

There is the usual connective-tissue layer, surfaced with mesothelium.

This investment is continuous with the gastric mesenteries (here called *omenta*).

C. REGENERATIVE ABILITY:

Surface replacements come from the deeper parts of foveolae where mitoses are frequent.

Cells are pushed up to replace those lost in cardiac, fundic and pyloric regions.

Deep cells, labeled with a radioactive substance, reach the surface within four days.

In the secretory tubule of the fundic type of gland, infrequent replacements occur also.

New mucous neck-cells probably are recruited downward from foveolae.

Chief cells, in turn, seem to be recruited from proliferating mucous neck-cells.

These cells presumably transform and move downward to deeper levels.

Parietal cells exhibit mitoses; neck-cells and chief cells are not known to divide.

In the glands of the cardia and pylorus, mitoses occur at levels below foveolae.

These are among the mucous cells of the gland-tubules proper.

Regeneration of the mucosa, even to restore total losses locally, is also successful.

Cells resembling foveolar cells migrate from the wound margin.

Moving in a centripetal direction, they cover the denuded area.

Presently new foveolae appear and glands bud from them.

In the fundus and corpus, glands soon consist entirely of mucous neck-cells.

Mucous neck-cells then differentiate into both chief and parietal cells.

D. DIAGNOSTIC FEATURES:

The stomach is thick-walled and heavily musculatured.

Local variations in the number and arrangement of muscular layers are to be expected.

Sections usually are cut from randomly oriented blocks of stomach-wall.

This adds confusion to the normally skewed arrangement of muscle.

The free surface and foveolae are covered with pale columnar cells, all alike.

This epithelium is subject to prompt autolysis after death.

It results in poor preservation, or even surface erosion in many instances.

The mucosa between foveolae, when cut vertically, resembles intestinal villi somewhat.

The epithelium, however, lacks the obvious striate border that characterizes villi.

It also lacks goblet cells, scattered among ordinary columnar cells.

Fundic glands are nearly straight and are several times longer than their foveolae.

The gland lumen is unusually inconspicuous.

Most of the gland cells (chief cells) are pale in routinely stained specimens.

In addition there are parietal cells (usually wedged in) farther from the lumen.

These stain brightly with acid dyes and are most numerous near the gland neck.

Pyloric glands are somewhat shorter than their very long, prominent foveolae.

The glands are tortuous and are never cut to include their full length.

Instead, short segments are seen; many are cut transversely or slantingly.

All the cells are alike—clear and pale-staining; the lumen is conspicuous.

Cardiac glands are mucoid, the gland cells resembling the pyloric type.

The foveolae, however, are much shorter than those of pyloric glands.

The secretory tubules tend to disorderly arrangement; some show local dilatations.

E. Functional Correlations:

1. Mechanical.

The muscular coat churns food, mixes it with secretions and empties the stomach.
>The upper half of the stomach is a reservoir; peristaltic movements are slight.
>The pyloric sphincter controls the intermittent escape of food into the duodenum.

The muscularis mucosae produces independent mucosal movements.
>It is able to orient objects that have been swallowed (fish bones; pins; etc.).
>Contraction of the muscular strands lying between glands compresses the mucosa.
>>This presumably helps to empty the glands of their secretion.

The lax submucosa allows the mucosa to shift position independently of the muscularis.
>It also accommodates marked changes in the volume of stomach contents.

The mucus lubricates, moistens and, perhaps, protects against autodigestion.

2. Chemical.

The 1.0 to 1.5 liters of gastric juice, secreted daily, contain various products.

Hydrochloric acid is supplied by the parietal cells of the fundus and corpus.
>The amount of acid present regionally varies with the abundance of these cells.
>Consequently, the pyloric region, which lacks such cells, is alkaline.

Pepsin is elaborated by the chief cells, as various facts attest.
>The content of pepsinogen in the gastric mucosa varies regionally.
>>The local amount is proportional to the abundance and fullness of chief cells.
>It is discharged continuously, but chiefly on neural and hormonal stimulation.
>It splits proteins, in an acid medium, into proteoses and peptones.
>Why the surface epithelium is not digested in life is not well explained.
>>Possibly the mucosa protects itself by producing an antienzyme or by mucus.

Chief cells produce a substance necessary to normal erythrocyte production.

Rennin is an enzyme that curdles milk; it is apparently a product of chief cells.

Unlike the peptic glands, the pyloric glands secrete continuously at a significant rate.
>Slight enzymic secretion occurs, but not in significant amounts.
>A hormone, *gastrin* (formed elsewhere, p. 234), is extractable from the mucosa.

Some absorption takes place in the stomach, but it is relatively slight.
>Substances absorbed include water, salts, sugar, and alcohol (and some other drugs).

IV. THE INTESTINE (GENERAL FEATURES)

The *intestine* is a tube, much longer than the cavity that contains it.
>Hence it follows a coiled and irregular course between the pylorus and anus.

It is composed of a long, slender portion and a shorter, but thicker, portion.
>These divisions are named the *small intestine* and *large intestine*, respectively.

Both segments are typical, tubular organs that have many features in common.
>Yet both the small and large intestine possess important, distinctive characteristics.

It will be simplest to discuss first those features shared by the entire intestine.
>Subsequently the individual peculiarities of the subdivisions can be made clear.

A. Mucosa:

1. Epithelial cell-types.

A layer of simple epithelium constitutes the innermost lining of the intestine.
>It covers the general surface, drapes over finger-like villi, and dips into glands.

Its component cell-types are the same throughout the entire intestine.
>(An exception is the local epithelium comprising the special duodenal glands.)

Four types of epithelial cells can be recognized at all levels of the tube.
>Their frequencies, however, are not uniform at the various levels.

A. Simple Columnar Cells.
>There are some 5 trillion of these cells in the small intestine alone.
>Each is tall, plastic and quite elastic; its components take polarized positions.

The cytoplasm is finely granular; the ovoid nucleus is somewhat basal.

At the free surface it elaborates a prominent (1.0 to 1.4 μ.) vertically *striate border*.

The striation is produced by closely packed, prominent microvilli.

Up to 3000 microvilli project from a single columnar cell.

They bear an enzyme-resistant, *fuzzy coat* (p. 39).

The border is best developed on epithelium that is exposed to the main lumen.

It thins progressively on cells extending into tubular intestinal glands.

Just beneath the border there is a felt-like ectoplasm, the *terminal web*.

This ectoplasm lacks all cell organelles; it anchors microvilli.

Its fine, horizontal filaments insert on an encircling terminal bar.

Organelles include, among others, smooth and rough endoplasmic reticulum.

B. GOBLET CELLS.

These cells are typical unicellular mucous glands (p. 164).

They occur on villi, on the general surface and in glands.

All stages of the secretory cycle (filling; discharge; recovery) can be seen.

They bear short, sparse microvilli; mucus extrudes from the cell-apex.

The number of goblet cells increases progressively from duodenum to rectum.

This increase is accompanied by a compensatory decrease in columnar cells.

Since mitoses almost never occur, these cells are not self-perpetuating.

Replacement is believed to be through the transformation of columnar cells.

C. PANETH CELLS.

These prominent, pyramidal cells occur at the bottom of the simple intestinal glands.

They are most numerous in the small intestine and appendix.

They are serous, zymogenic cells — labile and often not well preserved.

The base of the cell contains dark-staining and striated *ergastoplasm* (p. 21).

It consists of basophilic, iron-containing ribonucleoprotein.

Above the nucleus are large, round, refractile, *acidophilic granules*.

These accumulate during fasting and disappear during digestion.

Although this is a special secretory cell, its exact function is in doubt.

D. ARGENTAFFIN CELLS.

These cells are also known as *enterochromaffin cells*.

They occur chiefly in the intestinal glands; rarely, on villi.

Present in moderate numbers, they are scattered basally throughout a gland.

They are most numerous in the duodenum and appendix.

The flask-shaped cell has small granules beneath its nucleus.

These granules are yellow when fresh; they are acidophilic.

They brown with chromates and blacken with silver.

The function of these cells, whose granules are not discharged, was long unknown.

Now their granules are identified with *serotonin* production (p. 228).

2. Surface epithelium.

The epithelium covering the general surface of the mucosa is limited in area.

It occupies the intervals between the myriads of glands (and villi, when present).

Its components are the columnar cells and goblet cells.

3. Intestinal glands.

Another name for this pit-like gland is the *intestinal crypt* (of Lieberkühn).

There are about 180,000,000 glands in all; each resembles a glove finger.

A gland is a simple epithelial tube that dips below the general surface.

It extends vertically through the lamina propria to a distance of 0.1 to 0.7 mm.

The base of a gland almost reaches the muscularis mucosae.

The epithelium contains columnar, goblet, Paneth and argentaffin cells.

The striate border is reduced progressively toward the fundus of the gland.

In the fundic region its microvilli are short and sparse stubs.

Goblet cells are more numerous in the upper half of a gland.

Paneth and argentaffin cells occur, the former at the base of the gland.

4. Membrana propria.

A delicate *basement membrane* underlies the intestinal epithelium everywhere.

5. Lamina propria.

Its substance fills-in between the glands and forms cores to the finger-like villi.
It is mostly a reticular-tissue framework, infiltrated with free cells.
In addition, there are elastic fibers and delicate collagenous fibers.
The components are somewhat different from those of ordinary lymphoid tissue.
Besides abundant lymphocytes, there are many other kinds of cells.
These include plasma cells, eosinophils and mast cells.
Many lymphocytes pass between the epithelial cells; both slough and die (p. 227).
Solitary lymph nodules occur frequently (some 30,000 in all).
They are conspicuous features that push aside the neighboring glands.
They often encroach on the submucosa, and become large and pear-shaped.
Aggregate nodules, or Peyer's patches (p. 144), are commonest in the lower ileum.
The *muscularis mucosae* is thin, yet contains two layers of smooth muscle.
The inner layer is circular; the outer layer, longitudinal.
Fibers, derived from the inner layer, extend into the villi.
These layers are often broken by large, solitary nodules and by Peyer's patches.

B. ACCESSORY COATS:

1. Submucosa.

This layer is composed of loose areolar tissue, which contains some fat cells.
It bears the customary plexuses of vessels and nerves.
In the small intestine it is elevated into ring-like folds, the *plicae circulares.*
The submucosa of the duodenum harbors the specific *duodenal glands.*

2. Muscularis.

The inner coat of smooth muscle is arranged circularly.
The outer coat of smooth muscle is arranged longitudinally.
In most of the large intestine it thickens into three equally spaced bands.

3. Serosa.

The typical serosa is continuous with the mesentery of the free intestine.
Some regions of both the small and large intestine have an incomplete serous coat.
That is, these 'bare' portions are pressed against the body walls.

V. THE SMALL INTESTINE

This division of the intestine is about 23 feet long, and hence is thrown into coils.
Such ample length provides a large internal expanse for absorptive activities.
For descriptive purposes the small intestine is divided, without sharp limits, into three portions.
The *duodenum* is short, the *jejunum* much longer, and the *ileum* still longer.
The jejunum and ileum have no important structural differences.
Both the small and large intestine are characterized by having simple *intestinal glands.*
These dip into the lamina propria like so many tubular pits.
The entire small intestine is distinctive because it alone possesses *villi.*
These elevations give a velvety appearance to the mucosal lining.
The duodenum is further distinguished by special *duodenal glands* in its submucosa.

A. MUCOSA:

1. Surface epithelium.

The epithelium of the general surface (between villi and glands) is limited in extent.
This is because the villi and glands are numerous and crowded.

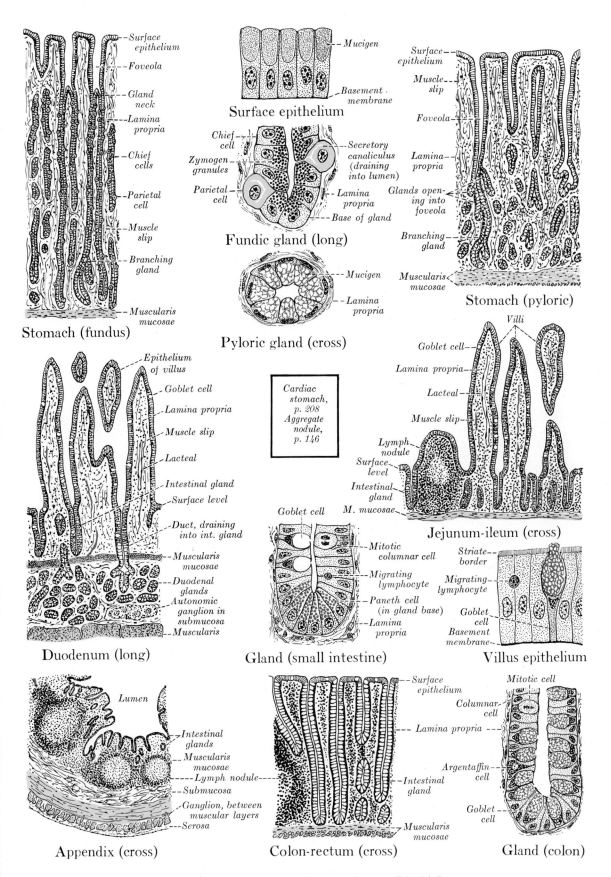

Surface epithelium

Foveola

Gland neck

Lamina propria

Chief cells

Parietal cell

Muscle slip

Branching gland

Muscularis mucosae

Stomach (fundus)

Mucigen

Basement membrane

Surface epithelium

Chief cell

Zymogen granules

Parietal cell

Secretory canaliculus (draining into lumen)

Lamina propria

Base of gland

Fundic gland (long)

Mucigen

Lamina propria

Pyloric gland (cross)

Surface epithelium

Muscle slip

Foveola

Lamina propria

Glands opening into foveola

Branching gland

Muscularis mucosae

Stomach (pyloric)

Epithelium of villus

Goblet cell

Lamina propria

Muscle slip

Lacteal

Intestinal gland

Surface level

Duct, draining into int. gland

Muscularis mucosae

Duodenal glands

Autonomic ganglion in submucosa

Muscularis

Duodenum (long)

Cardiac stomach, p. 208
Aggregate nodule, p. 146

Villi

Goblet cell

Lamina propria

Lacteal

Muscle slip

Lymph nodule

Surface level

Intestinal gland

M. mucosae

Jejunum-ileum (cross)

Goblet cell

Mitotic columnar cell

Migrating lymphocyte

Paneth cell (in gland base)

Lamina propria

Gland (small intestine)

Striate border

Migrating lymphocyte

Goblet cell

Basement membrane

Villus epithelium

Lumen

Intestinal glands

Muscularis mucosae

Lymph nodule

Submucosa

Ganglion, between muscular layers

Serosa

Appendix (cross)

Surface epithelium

Lamina propria

Intestinal gland

Muscularis mucosae

Colon-rectum (cross)

Mitotic cell

Columnar cell

Argentaffin cell

Goblet cell

Gland (colon)

THE LOWER ALIMENTARY CANAL

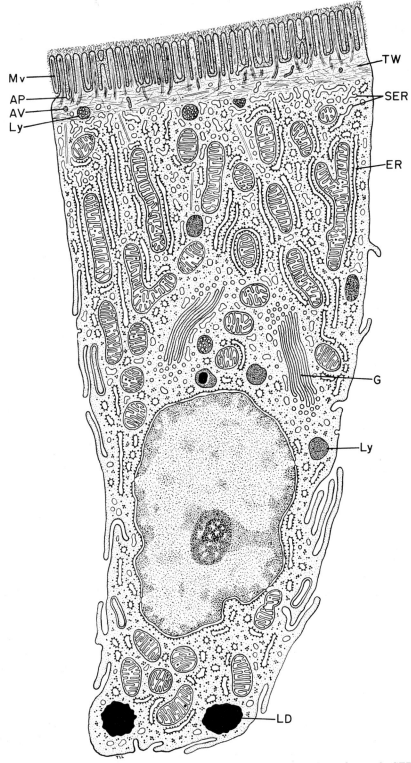

Mv —
AP —
AV —
Ly —

TW —
SER —
ER —
G —
Ly —
LD —

INTESTINAL EPITHELIAL CELL. The cytoplasm contains both rough (ER) and smooth (SER) endoplasmic reticulum, free ribosomes, a large Golgi complex (G), lysosomes (Ly), lipid droplets (LD), microtubules and mitochondria. At the apex of the cell lies the filamentous terminal web (TW), from which bundles of filaments extend as cores into the long, closely packed microvilli (MV). The latter are covered with a filamentous surface-coat. The plasma membrane dips inward as apical pits (AP); nearby are apical vesicles (AV). The nucleolus is prominent.

The general surface is seen best in the ileum, and especially toward its end.

Here the glands and villi are spaced farthest apart.

2. *Intestinal glands.*

These test-tube-shaped *glands*, or *crypts*, are only 0.1 to 0.3 mm. long.

Due to crowding, glands often look in sections like mere intervals between villi.

Actually, villi are local projections of the mucosa, while glands are wholly separate, tubular invaginations into its substance.

Paneth and argentaffin cells are relatively abundant.

3. *Villi.*

These structures are local elevations of the mucosa, 0.2 to 1.0 mm. tall.

Each is a projection above the level of the general surface.

Their abundance varies with the absorptive work done at any level.

(Duodenum, up to 40 per sq. mm.; ileum, as few as 18 per sq. mm.)

The total for the small intestine is about 4,000,000.

The main purpose of villi is to enhance the absorptive area of the epithelium.

They increase this area at least five times in man.

In the small intestine the total surface expanse thereby becomes about 60 sq. ft.

The shape of the villi varies in different mammals, and also at different levels.

In the human duodenum they are leaf-shaped plates, and shortest.

In the human jejunum they are still compressed and have clubbed ends.

In the human ileum they are finger-shaped and tallest.

Structurally, a villus has a core of lamina propria, covered with epithelium.

The axis of a villus is a blind lacteal, set in a bed of lamina-propria tissue.

An arteriole and venule course nearby and supply a capillary net.

The embedding stroma contains slips of smooth-muscle, longitudinally oriented.

The epithelium is composed mostly of the ordinary columnar-type cells.

There are some goblet cells and, rarely, argentaffin cells.

Goblet cells become progressively more numerous at lower levels of the tube.

Epithelial cells of the villi are shed abundantly from the tips of villi.

With mucus, they constitute the feces of starving individuals.

In preserved specimens, especially at the tips of villi, the epithelium tends to separate from the basement membrane and lamina propria.

This is an artifact produced by the agonal contraction of local muscle fibers.

B. ACCESSORY COATS:

1. *Submucosa.*

The only special features of the submucosa are the *plicae* and *duodenal glands*.

A. PLICAE CIRCULARES.

Elevations of the submucosa produce about 800 incomplete ring-like ridges.

These permanent laminae, the *plicae circulares*, are covered with mucosal folds.

Plicae appear near the pylorus and are tallest (8 mm.) in the jejunum.

They become less abundant in the ileum, and largely disappear at its middle.

Plicae are not effaced by distention or stretching of the bowel.

In this they differ from the impermanent rugae of the stomach.

B. DUODENAL GLANDS.

These mucous glands (of Brunner) are continuous with the pyloric glands.

Once in the duodenum, however, they promptly descend into the submucosa.

Here they become distinctive glands of this region.

The *duodenal glands* occur in lobules; they are carried up into the plical folds.

In the upper duodenum they are abundant and crowded.

In the lower two-thirds of the duodenum they decrease in size and frequency.

They disappear entirely before the duodenum comes to an end.

The glands are compound tubular in type; the tubules have a prominent lumen.

The *secretory cells* are low, columnar elements that secrete an alkaline mucin.

Yet they stain weakly with some specific dyes for mucin.
They resemble somewhat the mucous neck-cells or pyloric glands.
The *ducts* are mucoid in nature, much like the long secretory tubules.
They pass through the muscularis mucosae and open into intestinal glands.
Rarely they terminate on the surface, between glands and villi.

2. *Muscularis and serosa.*

There are no unusual features in these tunics.
Wherever the intestine is free, its serosa continues into a suspending mesentery.

C. MESENTERIES:

A *mesentery* arises when the serosa leaves the abdominal wall to reflect around the gut.
This peritoneum, from each side, unites into a double sheet.
As a result, the mesentery contains an internal sheet of connective tissue.
Also on each exposed, flat surface there is a layer of mesothelium.
The connective tissue carries blood vessels, lymphatics and nerves to the intestine.
It also contains lymph nodes and, usually, considerable fat.
Where the mesentery meets the intestine it splits into its component halves.
These continue as the *serosal coat* which envelops the tube.
The dorsal and ventral mesentery of the stomach are called by a special name, *omenta.*
The omenta, and associated 'ligaments,' are similar to the intestinal mesentery.
The omental bursa is perforated in places by many holes, net-like.

D. DIAGNOSTIC FEATURES:

Columnar cells of the general surface and villi possess a well developed striate border.
This feature and goblet cells distinguish intestinal mucosa from stomach.
Otherwise pyloric mucosa is sometimes confused with that of the small intestine.
This is because the interspaces between pyloric foveolae are mistaken for villi.
Simple tubular glands in the mucosa identify the intestine throughout its length.
Villi are specific features that are diagnostic of the small intestine alone.
Submucosal plicae are characteristic of the small intestine alone.
Nevertheless, plicae are lacking near the pylorus and in the lower ileum.
Also, they are seen to advantage only in longitudinal sections.
Lengthwise sections through villi and glands are readily distinguishable from each other.
Their position in the intestinal lumen or lamina propria, respectively, suffices.
Transverse sections through villi and glands can also be distinguished easily.
Both show bands of epithelium facing on a free space.
The glands are smaller, are almost perfectly circular and surround a small lumen.
Villi are much larger, are mostly elliptical and are surrounded by free space.
In villi, the epithelial bands border on a voluminous space (intestinal lumen).
(This space, however, may contain mucus or food debris.)
A prominent striate border caps the free ends of the component, columnar cells.
The sizable interior of the villus is filled with lymphoid tissue and vessels.
Nuclei of the epithelial cells lie nearer this central core.
In glands, the epithelial circular bands lie in a bed of solid lymphoid tissue.
A striate border is thin or not seen, depending on the level of section.
The interior is a small open space (the lumen), often containing mucus.
Epithelial nuclei lie nearer the periphery of the circular band.
The *duodenum* is recognized by the compound mucous glands in its submucosa.
Only the esophagus, among tubular organs, also possesses submucosal glands.
But its stratified squamous epithelium is an obvious differential feature.
The *jejunum* and *ileum* are structurally similar and are mostly indistinguishable.
The lower ileum has its villi spaced slightly farther apart.
Plicae are absent (determinable only in longitudinal sections).
Aggregate follicles are highly characteristic of the ileum, but not exclusively so.
However, their presence in sections cannot be depended upon.

E. Functional Correlations:

The activities of the entire intestine are treated as a unit on p. 227.

VI. THE LARGE INTESTINE

This tube is about 5 ft. long, and about double the width of the small intestine.
It includes the *cecum, appendix, colon, rectum* and *anal canal.*
The lining lacks the villi and transverse plicae that characterize the small intestine.
  Consequently, the epithelium that covers the general surface is plainly seen.
Intestinal glands are longer and lie closer together than do those of the small intestine.
  Although more conspicuous than the latter, their only differences are quantitative.
Epithelial cell-types are identical with those in the small intestine.

A. Ileo-cecal Valve and Cecum:

The *ileo-cecal valve* is formed by two apposed folds of the mucosa and submucosa.
  Each fold is supported by a central plate of smooth muscle.
    This is supplied by the circular muscle layer.
  The parallel free-edges of the two folds guard a slit-like orifice into the cecum.
The blind sac known as the *cecum* is like the rest of the colon in structure.
  At the ileo-cecal junction there is an abrupt change in some structural features.

B. Vermiform Appendix:

This is a blind, finger-like extension of the cecum, once called the *vermiform process.*
Its wall is relatively very thick, and its lumen proportionately small.
  Deep pockets between mucosal folds give the lumen an irregular, often angular, form.
    In adults the lumen tends to become more rounded.
  The lumen frequently contains detritus; sometimes it is even obliterated.

1. Mucosa.

The simple tubular *glands* decrease in number and length in middle age and later.
  They contain many goblet cells and occasional Paneth cells.
  Argentaffin cells are perhaps more numerous than elsewhere in the intestine.
Lymphoid tissue in the lamina propria constitutes a conspicuous layer.
  It is responsible for the relatively great thickness of the total wall.
  It contains closely spaced, solitary *lymph nodules* (except in old age).
    These often show in sections as a fairly complete, confluent lymphoid ring.
    Germinal (or reaction) centers tend to be very large, like those of the tonsil.
The *muscularis mucosae* is poorly represented.
  It is often interrupted and broken by the large lymph nodules.
  These nodules, pushing far into the submucosa, make the boundary between mucosa
    and submucosa indefinite and hard to follow.

2. Accessory coats.

  A. Submucosa.
    This layer is of the ordinary type and quite thick.
      It usually contains fat cells and is encroached on by the lymphoid tissue.
    After middle age the mucosa, and the submucosa (in part), may fibrose.
  B. Muscularis.
    The muscular coat is somewhat thin, but contains the two typical layers.
    Thick bands (teniae), such as characterize the cecum and colon, are lacking.
  C. Serosa.
    The serous coat is like that of the intestine in general.
      A rudimentary mesentery is continuous with it.
    In some instances, the appendix lies partly or wholly behind the peritoneum.

C. Colon:

1. Mucosa.

The mucous membrane is smooth and not involved in forming plicae or villi.
The *surface epithelium* consists chiefly of simple columnar cells.
  Each has a thin, striate border.
  There are scattering goblet cells, as well.
The *glands* are longer (0.4 to 0.6 mm.) than in the small intestine.
  Hence the mucous membrane, as a whole, is thicker.
  The glands are arranged as regular vertical columns, set close together.
  They are characterized by an abundance of goblet cells.
    Often the glands appear as if almost composed of these cells alone.
  Argentaffin cells occur occasionally, but Paneth cells are rare.
The *lamina propria* is small in amount because the glands are closely spaced.
  It is organized as in the small intestine.
    Eosinophils are numerous among the other cell types.
  Solitary *lymph nodules* are larger and more numerous than in the small intestine.
    As many as 21,000 nodules have been estimated as a total number.
    They commonly intrude well into the submucosa.
The *muscularis mucosae* has the two typical layers of smooth muscle.

2. Accessory coats.

A. Submucosa.
  There are no peculiarities in this tunic.
B. Muscularis.
  The internal, circular coat of smooth muscle is typical.
  The external, longitudinal coat is peculiar and unique.
    It contains three longitudinal, ribbon-like thickenings, named *teniae*.
    These narrow bands are spaced equally from each other.
    Between the bands the longitudinal coat is thin, yet usually complete.
  Since teniae are shorter than the rest of the wall, sacculations are produced.
    These *haustra* disappear when the teniae are cut or stripped off.
  Between sacculations the wall is thrown into crescentic *plicae semilunares*.
    These crescentic folds include the entire wall and project into the lumen.
C. Serosa.
  The peritoneal reflection does not surround most of the colon completely.
    This is because the colon tends to be pressed against the body wall.
    Here in these 'bare areas' the outermost coat is an *adventitia*.
  Attached scatteringly to the colonic serosa are small sacs or fringes.
    These structures, usually containing fat, are named *appendices epiploicae*.
    They represent a redundant serosa that balloons away from the wall proper.

D. Rectum:

For the most part the *rectum* differs from the colon only quantitatively.
The *intestinal glands* are the longest (up to 0.7 mm.) of the entire intestine.
  They become small, sparse and then cease at the beginning of the anal canal.
Lymphoid tissue is less abundant than in the upper colon.
The *muscularis* has the typical two layers, which are thick; it lacks teniae.
A *serosa* is replaced, at progressively lower levels, by an *adventitia*.

E. Anal Canal:

This short tube is quite different structurally from the rest of the intestine.
The mucosa is folded into about 8 longitudinal *anal columns*.
  The ends of these folds, nearing the anal orifice, join one another.
    Thus pocket-like *anal valves* are created, whose recesses are *anal sinuses*.
  Above the valves the epithelium has changed into a stratified cuboidal type.
    At the level of the valves the epithelium becomes stratified squamous.

Also, the muscularis mucosae, which has suffered fragmentation, disappears.
The moist, unkeratinized epithelium of the canal changes into *epidermis* at the anal orifice.
Here hairs and cutaneous glands make their appearance.
Some of the sweat glands resemble the specialized sweat glands of the axilla.
These apocrine glands are named *circumanal glands* (*cf.*, p. 199).
The submucosa is notable for its rich plexus of hemorrhoidal vessels.
The circular layer of smooth muscle thickens terminally as the *internal anal sphincter*.
More superficially the nearby skeletal muscle forms the *external anal sphincter*.

F. DIAGNOSTIC FEATURES:

The *large intestine* is characterized by its prominent, closely packed intestinal glands.
A negative feature is its smooth internal surface, owing to the lack of villi.
Goblet cells are extremely plentiful in the glands.
A tenia, if included in a section, is a specific characteristic feature.
The *appendix* is a 'miniature colon,' but with certain identifying features.
The wall is very thick in comparison to the size of the lumen.
The lumen is often angular in shape, and may contain compacted material.
Intestinal glands are less numerous and often show an altered condition.
There is an abundance of lymph nodules, usually forming a lymphoid ring.
The germinal centers (or reaction centers) tend to be very large.
The muscular coat lacks the tenial thickenings that occur in the colon.
The *colon* and *rectum* are, for the most part, only quantitatively different.
On the whole, the rectal glands are somewhat longer than in the colon.
Yet the increase to this maximal length is gradual in the lower colon.
The colon has teniae, whereas the rectum lacks them.
The inclusion of a tenia in a section, however, cannot be relied on.
The longitudinal muscle coat of the rectum is thick.
In the colon, except for teniae, it is thin.
(Yet a longitudinal section along a tenia would show a thick outer layer.)
The *anal canal* undergoes transitions at different levels.
Its epithelium changes from simple columnar, to unkeratinized stratified, to epidermis.
Intestinal glands are lacking.

VII. REGENERATIVE ABILITY

Mitoses occur abundantly in the intestinal glands, and occasionally in duodenal glands.
Rather undifferentiated cells lie in a zone above the bottom of intestinal glands.
Their daughter cells differentiate into typical columnar and goblet cells.
These pass progressively upward in the gland and gain the free surface.
Continuing up the villi, they slough off at their tips; losses also occur in the colon.
Such a course has been traced by tagging nuclei with a radioactive substance.
A complete transit and replacement of cells is accomplished every few days.
Other daughter cells presumably replace Paneth and argentaffin cells.
Removal of an area of duodenal mucosa and submucosa imitates local destruction by ulcer.
Cell migration and mitosis take place from duodenal glands at the wound margin.
After resurfacing is completed, villi and duodenal-type glands differentiate.
The glands occupy the position of intestinal glands; the latter do not regenerate.
In the colon, however, intestinal glands do differentiate following local mucosal loss.

VIII. FUNCTIONS OF THE INTESTINE

1. Motility.

The muscular coat causes local segmental movements and propulsive peristalsis.
Peristaltic movements are the only ones that occur in the large intestine.

The muscularis mucosae produces ridging, grooving and pitting of the mucosa.

Displaced fibers in the villi are responsible for shortening and waving movements.

2. Secretion.

Goblet cells, throughout the intestine, produce lubricative mucus for the lining.

In the large intestine, the abundant mucus also binds the contents into a semifluid, progressively dehydrating fecal mass and lubricates its progress.

The duodenal glands secrete a mucous, alkaline fluid continuously.

This viscous secretion probably does not contain enzymes.

The intestinal glands secrete the yellowish, alkaline *intestinal juice.*

Those of the small intestine presumably produce the various enzymes.

It is not known which cells elaborate the different constituents.

Glands of the large intestine secrete much mucus, and little else.

There are several enzymes in the intestinal juice.

Erepsin reduces partly digested proteins to amino acids.

Several enzymes (*maltase; lactase; invertase*) split carbohydrates into simple sugars.

Lipase splits fats into glycerol and fatty acids.

Nuclease breaks down nucleic acid.

Enterokinase activates trypsinogen into trypsin.

Certain hormones are passed into the blood from the small intestine.

The exact cellular source of these secretions is unknown.

Secretin activates the pancreas; *cholecystokinin,* the gall bladder; *enterocrinin,* the intestinal glands.

Serotonin, a product of argentaffin cells, is an effective vasodilator.

3. Absorption.

This is a vital phenomenon performed by the ordinary columnar epithelial cells.

The great length of the intestine, its plicae and its villi expedite absorption.

But it is the microvilli that are primarily concerned in absorptive activities.

Large quantities of *water* are taken up, especially in the large intestine.

Inorganic salts in solution are absorbed readily by the epithelial cells.

Iron, fed as compounds, can be followed through the striate border.

Proteins are broken down into amino acids and absorbed as such.

Their entrance and segregation into vesicles have been traced by labelings.

Carbohydrates are admitted as glucose and other simple sugars.

Their course has not been followed in satisfactory detail.

Yet, like amino acids, they enter the capillaries and leave by the portal vein.

Digested fat, as fatty acids and glycerol, gains ready entrance into the epithelial cells.

In the cytoplasm they are resynthesized into droplets of neutral fat and protein.

Some *neutral fat,* in emulsified droplets, may also enter by pinocytosis.

The course of fat droplets, stained with osmic acid, can be followed easily: supranuclear cytoplasm → lateral cell membrane → intercellular space → basement membrane → lamina propria.

Lacteals of villi then take up fat droplets; they eventually reach the blood stream.

Bile salts and excreted lipids are largely recaptured and re-utilized.

IX. VESSELS AND NERVES OF THE DIGESTIVE TUBE

Blood vessels, lymphatics and nerves enter the tube, and by way of its mesentery when present.

1. Blood vessels.

Arteries and veins form a prominent plexus in the submucosa.

Branches from this plexus extend into both the mucosa and the muscularis.

Capillary networks supply the coats of the gut-wall, and their special components.

In the small intestine, additional branches supply the villi.

One (or more) arterioles pass up the villus, breaking down into a capillary plexus.

This superficial network is drained by one (or two) venules.

The venule usually takes a position opposite to the arteriole.

2. *Lymphatics.*

The mucosa has lymphatic loops or blindly ending vessels.

Each villus has a blind, axial *lacteal*, which collects fatty lymph (*chyle*).

Their total absorptive surface equals 34 sq. ft.

The submucosa and muscularis have typical plexuses.

The free lymphatic vessels, leaving the wall, drain into lymph nodes.

3. *Nerves.*

The innervating fibers come from the vagus nerves and from autonomic ganglia.

There is a *myenteric plexus* (of Auerbach) and a *submucous plexus* (of Meissner).

Included in these intramural plexuses are small autonomic ganglia.

In the myenteric plexus some neurons are interconnecting, or associative, units.

Terminal nerve fibers end in muscles and vessels; these are efferent in function.

Sensory endings in the epithelium have also been claimed, but are usually denied.

Parasympathetic fibers are those from the vagi, and also from the sacral outflow.

They terminate on cells of the intrinsic ganglia of the gut wall.

Axons from such ganglion cells pass to the muscle cells of the wall and its vessels.

They excite muscular activity, vascularity and secretion.

Sympathetic fibers arise in the ganglia of autonomic plexuses external to the gut wall.

They pass directly to their endings upon muscle of the wall and of vessels.

Their action is inhibitory, and hence antagonistic to the parasympathetics.

Chapter XX

The Major Glands of Digestion

The small glands, located in the wall of the digestive tract, have already been described.

These include the intrinsic glands of the mouth, pharynx and digestive tube.

In addition, there are extrinsic glands: the larger *salivary glands, pancreas* and *liver.*

These constitute the major gland-masses related to digestion.

I. THE MAJOR SALIVARY GLANDS

The extrinsic *salivary glands* occur in three paired sets.

Each is a merocrine gland of the branching tubular or tubulo-alveolar type.

Each compound, lobulated gland opens into the oral cavity by an excretory duct.

Saliva is a viscid fluid containing a mixture of all the oral secretions.

The daily amount for man is about 1.5 quarts; for the cow, 65 quarts.

Saliva contains mucus, proteins, salts and the enzyme *ptyalin.*

Desquamated epithelial cells and lymphocytes are characteristic constituents also.

Swollen, degenerating lymphocytes were long ago named *salivary corpuscles.*

The details of merocrine-gland structure are described on pp. 166-169.

Here will be presented only the distinctive features of the large salivary glands.

A. PAROTID GLAND:

Each gland is situated below and somewhat in front of the closely associated ear.

Its main *excretory duct* (of Stenson) opens into the vestibule of the mouth.

The parotid is *purely serous* in man, but this is not true of all mammals.

Also in infants and a few adults there are some cells that respond to stains for mucus.

The glandular mass is enclosed within a fibrous sheath, or *capsule.*

Septa pass inward to divide the organ into *lobes* and *lobules.*

A fine connective-tissue *stroma* embeds the alveoli and smaller ducts.

This tissue often contains many fat cells.

The *alveoli* are somewhat elongate and often exhibit branching.

Their pyramidal cells are typical serous elements with granular cytoplasm.

Secretory canaliculi extend from the inconspicuous lumen between alveolar cells.

Clasping *basket cells* are numerous, lying between the basement membrane and alveoli.

Intercalated ducts are slender and relatively long tubules, attached to the alveoli.

Their component cells are flat and elongate.

Secretory ducts, intermediate in position, likewise are relatively long.

They are a type of duct that is peculiar to the salivary glands.

Their columnar cells, bright-staining and basal striations make them conspicuous.

Excretory ducts begin as a simple columnar epithelium, and then become pseudostratified.

They finally gain true stratification near the main outlet.

A similar epithelial gradation is found also in the other large salivary glands.

B. Submandibular Gland:

Each gland is situated in the floor of the mouth, under shelter of the mandible.
It is a *mixed gland* in man and most other mammals.
In man purely serous alveoli outnumber the remaining (mixed) alveoli about 5:1.
A typical connective-tissue *capsule, septa* and *stroma* are present.
The *parenchyma* is divided by septa into *lobules.*
Most of the secretory end-pieces are *serous alveoli,* tending to be somewhat elongate.
All other end-pieces are *mixed tubules* of sero-mucous composition.
All such tubules have clusters of cells (*demilunes*) at their distal ends.
Most of the serous cells border on the general gland lumen.
They do not wholly over-lie mucous cells as a complete cap.
Secretory canaliculi occur between the serous components of the gland.
Stellate *basket cells* lie between gland cells and the basement membrane.
The *duct system* includes representatives of all three component types.
Most of the *intercalated ducts* are short, but some equal those of the parotid gland.
On the other hand, the *secretory ducts* tend to be longer than those of the parotid.
Hence these ducts are conspicuous features within the lobules.
The main *excretory duct* (of Wharton) opens at the frenulum of the tongue.

C. Sublingual Gland:

This is a composite organ, situated in the floor of the mouth, near the midplane.
There are one *major gland* and several *minor glands* on each side of the tongue.
Each glandular mass has its individual excretory duct opening on a separate papilla.
The *major duct* of the major gland opens near the frenulum of the tongue.
The sublingual gland is a *mixed gland* in man and various other mammals.
It is more variable in composition than the other salivary glands.
The several compound glands are not identical in composition.
Neither is any one gland uniform among different individuals.
Yet the minor glands are always highly mucous.
The secretory *end-pieces* are tortuous, branching tubules.
In man their mucous cells are much more numerous than serous cells.
Secretory tubules are either *purely mucous* or *mixed* (with demilunes).
The existence of purely serous alveoli is an exceptional local phenomenon.
It is noteworthy that even the serous cells have semimucoid characteristics.
Basket cells are present, as in other salivary glands.
There is no definite, common capsule, but *septa* and *lobules* are prominent.
The duct system is distinctive in a negative way.
Intercalated ducts, of the ordinary sort, are mostly lacking.
They are largely replaced by *mucous tubules*, continuous with the 'end-pieces.'
In fact, the two are indistinguishable.
Some *secretory ducts* occur, but they are very short segments that escape attention.
They bear only a patch of basally striated cells.
Hence sections show very few obvious ducts within a lobule.
Extralobular ducts are ordinary *excretory ducts.*

D. Vessels and Nerves:

See the general account on p. 169.

E. Regenerative Ability:

Removal of portions of glands can be followed by some successful regeneration.
But the replacement of lost tissue is never complete.
Restoration is accomplished by proliferation from ducts and secretory cells.

F. Diagnostic Features:

The distinguishing characteristics of serous and mucous cells are given on pp. 166-167.
The *parotid gland* has serous alveoli only.

Both the submandibular and sublingual glands are mixed (serous and mucous) glands.

The *submandibular* is preponderantly serous.

The *sublingual* is preponderantly mucous.

The parotid and submandibular glands have numerous secretory ducts within each lobule.

These stain brightly acidophilic, and hence are conspicuous.

The parotid and submandibular glands also have numerous slender, intercalated ducts.

These, however, are not conspicuous features.

The sublingual gland has but few obvious ducts of any kind within its lobules.

It is the only one to lack a distinct external sheath or capsule.

G. FUNCTIONAL CORRELATIONS:

Saliva moistens the oral mucosa, cleanses the teeth and lubricates food.

Food is prepared for taste, for salivary digestion, and for swallowing.

Saliva is chemically active, producing an enzyme and making salivary digestion possible.

Ptyalin is elaborated by serous cells; it converts starch into glucose.

The quality of saliva varies since the several glands may participate differently.

The *small oral glands* probably serve mostly to moisten and lubricate the mucosa.

In doing this they seemingly secrete continuously.

The *major salivary glands* secrete, following reflex stimulation of the secretory nerves.

Such stimulation is brought about especially by the presence of food in the mouth.

An infolded basal plasma membrane in secretory ducts is an adaptation.

Its presence is correlated with a copious transport of water.

II. THE PANCREAS

The *pancreas* is primarily a large digestive gland (9 inches long), connected to the duodenum. It also contains endocrine tissue in the form of tiny, scattered islets.

A. STRUCTURAL PLAN:

The connective-tissue *framework* is like that of the salivary glands.

A sheath of areolar tissue, which is not a typical *capsule*, invests the organ.

In some regions it is surfaced with peritoneal mesothelium.

Thin, fibrous *septa* continue into the pancreas and subdivide it.

In this way many distinct *lobules* and less complete *sublobules* are formed.

These lobules are loosely connected, but their interiors are quite compact.

Delicate fibrous tissue (*reticular tissue*) embeds the individual alveoli.

The *parenchyma* is glandular epithelium of two quite different sorts.

The *exocrine part* is organized as a compound, tubulo-alveolar gland.

It has purely *serous alveoli*, resembling those of the parotid gland.

This tissue makes up the greatest bulk of the organ, by far.

Its *duct system* drains into the duodenum by a main excretory duct.

The *endocrine part* consists of many, scattered, epithelial masses (*pancreatic islets*).

These islets elaborate a hormone that regulates carbohydrate metabolism.

This secretion is carried away by intimate capillary channels.

B. EXOCRINE PANCREAS:

1. Alveoli.

The secretory end-pieces, or *alveoli*, vary between a pear shape and short tubules.

Each is surrounded by a *basement membrane*, but *basket cells* apparently lack.

The component *gland cells* are pyramidal in shape and serous in quality.

A rounded nucleus lies basally; microvilli extend into the alveolar lumen.

A distinction between basal and apical halves of the gland cells is plain.

The *basal cell-half* contains very finely granular cytoplasm, often striated.

This is strongly basophilic *ergastoplasm*, rich in RNA granules.

It is better developed and darker staining than in salivary glands.

Ergastoplasm consists of abundant endoplasmic reticulum, rich in ribosomes.
Here vertically oriented mitochondria sometimes produce a striated pattern.
The *apical cell-half*, bordering the lumen, contains numerous *zymogen granules*.
When fresh they are highly refractile, semifluid globules.
When preserved and stained, they appear as acidophilic 'granules.'
The apex of the cell bears a few, short microvilli.
The breadths of the two 'halves' vary reciprocally before and after discharge.
The *Golgi apparatus* is a prominent feature, located above the nucleus.
It receives, concentrates and packages the developing zymogen granules.
These granules are synthesized by the basal ribosomes, and then transported.
The lateral boundaries between individual cells are indistinct.

2. Ducts.

A. SECRETORY CANALICULI.

Tiny *canaliculi* occur between gland cells, as in other serous glands (p. 166).
Such tubules drain between centro-alveolar cells into the central lumen.

B. CENTRO-ALVEOLAR CELLS.

These elements do not occur with any frequency except in the pancreas.
The gland cells of a pancreatic alveolus usually do not become directly continuous
with an intercalated duct in the manner typical of exocrine glands.
Instead, the gland cells tend to surround the beginning of the duct on all sides.
They may also overlap the duct along one side, or replace the duct-wall along
one side and overlap it on the other side.
The appearance is as if the customary lumen were clogged with pale cells.
Hence the name *centro-alveolar* or centro-acinar.
Wherever the gland cells overlie duct cells, secretory canaliculi exist.

C. INTERCALATED DUCTS.

These ducts are more extensively developed than in any other digestive gland.
This is because typical secretory ducts are wanting in the pancreas.
Hence the largest intercalated ducts exceed the size limit in salivary glands.
The component epithelial cells are somewhat flattened to cuboidal in shape.
They rest upon a basement membrane and reticular fibers.

D. EXCRETORY DUCTS.

These ducts course in the interlobular connective tissue.
The size of a duct is correlated with the amount of tissue served.
Short ducts drain the lobules and open at right angles into the axial main duct.
This main excretory tube then discharges into the duodenum.
Such a penniform arrangement of ducts is unique among the digestive glands.
The epithelial lining is composed of columnar cells (and some goblet cells).

C. ENDOCRINE PANCREAS:

This tissue is scattered unevenly as the *pancreatic islets* (of Langerhans).
Each islet is an epithelial mass, tunneled by labyrinthine capillaries.
The position of islets is mostly within lobules rather than between them.
The total number for man varies widely, but averages about 1 million.
The size ranges from a few clustered cells to aggregates 3 mm. in diameter.
About each spheroidal islet is a thin, delimiting membrane of reticulum.
Islets are sometimes connected to exocrine ducts by slender epithelial tubules or cords.
These strands are remnants, indicative of the manner of island origin.
Such connections do not serve as functional ducts and are rarely seen.
The islet tissue is arranged in irregular, anastomosing cellular *plates*.
These epithelial 'cords' are separated by closely applied, tortuous *blood capillaries*.
A sphincter controls the supply of blood.
Only delicate reticular tissue occurs within the islet and about its periphery.
In routine preparations the component, polyhedral cells appear paler than alveoli.
They also look as if they were syncytial, homogeneous and all of one type.

Special techniques demonstrate distinctive cytoplasmic granules.
Several cell types can be distinguished on the basis of staining, solubility, etc.
Alpha cells, or A-cells, are only fairly numerous in most islands.
Their large granules have a spherical core and are soluble in water.
Beta cells, or B-cells, are smaller and usually more numerous than A-cells.
Their smaller granules contain variable crystals and are alcohol soluble.
Delta cells, or D-cells, are large elements and the rarest by far.
Their granules are somewhat larger and much less dense than A-granules.
All types have the minute structure of gland cells, but are quite unlike alveolar cells.

D. VESSELS AND NERVES:

The arrangements follow the patterns that are typical for exocrine glands (p. 169).
The islets have a far richer blood supply than does the alveolar tissue.
Small *autonomic ganglia* and lamellar corpuscles occur in the interlobular tissue.

E. REGENERATIVE ABILITY:

The pancreas is able to differentiate a few alveoli and even whole islets after injury.
The restoration may follow duct ligation, surgical excision or disease.
This regeneration comes from proliferating duct tissue.

F. DIAGNOSTIC FEATURES:

The exocrine pancreas is a *purely serous* gland; it resembles the parotid.
The following features are, however, distinctive of the pancreas:
Scattered *pancreatic islets* occur throughout the exocrine parenchyma.
There are *no conspicuous ducts* within the lobules.
Any alveolar cell, cut through its full length, shows two *distinct zones.*
With ordinary stains the basal zone is dark; the apical zone, light.
With special stains for zymogen granules, these appearances may be reversed.
Alveoli cut lengthwise tend toward a short *tubular shape.*
Centro-alveolar cells are seen within alveoli cut along or across their main axes.

G. FUNCTIONAL CORRELATIONS:

1. External secretion.

About 2 to 3 pints of alkaline pancreatic juice are secreted daily.
A number of digestive pro-enzymes are elaborated by the alveoli.
The chief derivatives are *trypsin, amylase, lipase* and an enzyme-like *rennin.*
Yet all the alveolar cells are apparently cytologically alike.
Secretion is induced by two hormones, *secretin* and *pancreozymin.*
These are elaborated in the duodenal mucosa and released on the arrival of chyme.
Secretion also can be stimulated directly through the vagal nerve supply.

2. Internal secretion.

B-cell tumors oversecrete, and thereby decrease the content of blood sugar.
Without it carbohydrates cannot be fully utilized by the body (diabetes).
They are lost as sugar in the urine.
Various facts implicate the B-cells as the sole source of insulin.
In natural or experimentally induced diabetes it is B-cells that are injured.
An alcoholic extract, which dissolves the B-cell granules, is given to diabetics.
Its content (insulin) makes carbohydrates oxidizable and muscle-storable.
B-cell tumors oversecrete, and thereby decrease the content of blood sugar.
Insulin is surely localized in the B-cells by the fluorescent antibody technique.
The A-cells produce a hormone, *glucagon,* that offsets the influence of insulin.
It affects sugar metabolism so that the level of blood glucose is increased.
Such counterbalancing would serve to maintain a better controlled functioning.
The D-cells produce *gastrin* which increases the flow of gastric juice, mostly HCL.

III. THE LIVER

The *liver* lies beneath the diaphragm and is attached to it.

It is the largest gland of the body and weighs about 3.5 lbs.

The liver is basically a compound tubular *serous gland*, but it is highly modified in mammals.

The tubules are replaced by *cellular plates* that branch and anastomose.

Embryos of various lower vertebrates initially possess obvious glandular tubules.

Internal *lobulation* is realized only in adult birds and mammals.

A remodeling of the parenchyma into lobular units has paralleled changes that occurred simultaneously in the program of vascularization.

That is, an originally exocrine organ reorganized its structural plan in order to perfect activities that are primarily related to the blood stream.

A. STRUCTURAL PLAN:

The liver contains four incompletely separated *lobes*.

These are surrounded by a thick *capsule*, mostly overlaid with reflected peritoneum.

There is a definite *hilus* where vessels enter and ducts leave.

The *parenchyma*, in the interior, is subdivided into myriads of small *lobules*.

Each lobule is incompletely isolated by connective tissue named *Glisson's capsule*.

The interior of a lobule consists of radially arranged plates of liver cells.

These *hepatic plates* (often called cords) are separated by *hepatic sinusoids*.

The axis of a lobule is the *central venule*, which drains into a *sublobular vein*.

Sublobular veins unite and produce branches of the *hepatic veins*.

Connective tissue, at the edges of a lobule, embeds the so-called *portal canals*.

Each canal contains a branch of a *hepatic artery, portal vein* and *bile duct*.

This lobular arrangement is repeated hundreds of thousands of times.

To understand the liver, therefore, one needs to know well only a single lobule.

B. LOBULATION:

The hepatic parenchyma is subdivided into obvious anatomical units, called *lobules*.

Each is an irregular prism, measuring about 1×2 mm.

It is partially bounded and contained within its incomplete *Glisson's capsule*.

The total number of lobules is approximately one million.

The arrangement of lobules, except close to the surface of the liver, is irregular.

Each lobular unit consists of two chief components.

One is a *parenchyma*, composed of closely packed glandular epithelium.

It is arranged in *plates* radiating from an axis, which is the central venule.

The other is a system of *sinusoids* that converge radially into the central venule.

In their radial courses they tunneled the parenchyma into plate-like 'cords.'

Such channels communicate with both the central vein and vessels at the periphery.

The *hepatic lobule*, just described, is quite unlike lobules of ordinary glands.

That is, its central axis is a venule instead of the customary duct.

This sort of lobulation is an adaptation to certain activities (glycogenic, etc.).

Such lobules are organized with respect to the flow and drainage of blood.

In addition, a different kind of lobule can be recognized; this is the *portal lobule*.

It is arranged with reference to exocrine function (bile secretion).

This unit is formed from parts of the three hepatic lobules that adjoin a portal canal.

It is the territory drained by an interlobular bile duct in a portal canal.

The functional boundary of such a portal lobule runs from one central venule to another.

Its axis is a bile duct, located in the common portal canal servicing this territory.

In the seal the portal lobule, as a visible unit, is seen at its best.

Human livers show no physical demarcation into such recognizable units.

C. DETAILED STRUCTURE:

1. *Framework.*

The finest division of the supporting tissue is a *reticulum* of delicate fibrils.
  This makes a close network about the plates of glandular tissue.
  It serves to hold the plates in place and to keep the sinusoids open.
At the periphery of each lobule there is some ordinary, loose *connective tissue.*
  Reticulum of the lobule and such ordinary fibrous tissue merge in this region.
  A complete encapsulation of the lobule occurs in the hog, camel and polar bear.
  A similar connective-tissue sheath is incomplete in man and most other mammals.
    It is largely limited to the edges of lobules, where it acts as a bed (the so-called
      portal canal) for the vessels and bile duct serving adjoining lobules.
    All this perilobular tissue in the liver comprises *Glisson's capsule.*
      It should be understood that such a tissue-mass in any local region serves
        the contiguous lobules that abut against it.
The entire liver is encased within a fibro-elastic *hepatic capsule.*
  In most regions it is overlaid by a *serosa* that represents reflected peritoneum.
  At the hilus this external capsule is continuous with Glisson's capsule internally.

2. *Portal canals.*

This term refers to *portals* through which blood reaches the liver and bile leaves.
The basis of a 'canal' is the fibrous tissue of Glisson's capsule.
  It is located mostly along the edges where the sides of adjoining lobules meet.
This connective-tissue bed of a *portal canal* contains several functional components.
  A. PORTAL VEIN.
    This vessel is the largest component, but it is very thin-walled.
      Muscle fibers are present only in the larger branches.
    Its venous blood has already passed through capillary beds of splanchnic organs.
  B. HEPATIC ARTERY.
    Although rather thick-walled, it tends to be smaller than the vein or bile duct.
    There is a recognizable muscular coat and a distinct internal elastic membrane.
  C. BILE DUCT.
    Its size is commonly intermediate between that of the two blood vessels.
    The pale epithelium of this ductule is low cuboidal to columnar in shape.
    A connective-tissue investment surrounds the epithelium.
    Due to branching, more than one duct is often seen in a canal.
  D. OTHER COMPONENTS.
    Several delicate *lymphatic vessels* can usually be observed.
      They are mere endothelium-lined clefts.
    Nerves are present, but they are not conspicuous in routine preparations.

3. *Hepatic cells.*

The *hepatic plates* (commonly called hepatic cords) branch and anastomose.
The center of the system is the axially situated central venule.
  From here the plates radiate peripherally in a branching, spoke-like manner.
A plate is mostly one cell thick, except at regions of branching or union.
  Between the component cells pass microscopic *bile capillaries.*
    These drain toward the periphery and thence into a bile duct in a portal canal.
  The plates are interrupted by frequent perforations of considerable size.
The component *cells* of the parenchyma are large and polyhedral in shape.
  They measure about $22 \times 30 \ \mu$, but vary with storage and secretory activity.
The *nucleus* is rounded and vesicular, with one or more prominent nucleoli.
  Certain large cells have a large nucleus, or two or four of ordinary size.
    Such cells have multiples of the ordinary diploid number of chromosomes.
A clear, homogenous layer of ectoplasm comprises the periphery of the cell.
The granular endoplasm contains the cell organelles and stored substances.
  Many of the 'granules' are *glycogen droplets*, specifically stainable.

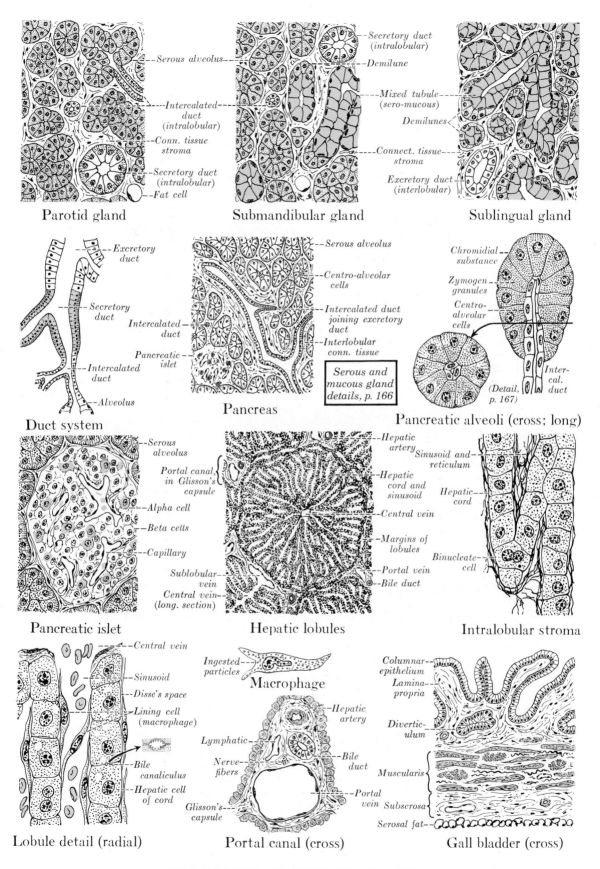

Parotid gland

- Serous alveolus
- Intercalated duct (intralobular)
- Conn. tissue stroma
- Secretory duct (intralobular)
- Fat cell

Submandibular gland

- Secretory duct (intralobular)
- Demilune
- Mixed tubule (sero-mucous)

Sublingual gland

- Demilunes
- Connect. tissue stroma
- Excretory duct (interlobular)

Duct system

- Excretory duct
- Secretory duct
- Intercalated duct
- Alveolus

Pancreas

- Serous alveolus
- Centro-alveolar cells
- Intercalated duct joining excretory duct
- Interlobular conn. tissue
- Intercalated duct
- Pancreatic islet

Serous and mucous gland details, p. 166

Pancreatic alveoli (cross; long)

- Chromidial substance
- Zymogen granules
- Centro-alveolar cells
- Inter-cal. duct

(Detail, p. 167)

Pancreatic islet

- Serous alveolus
- Alpha cell
- Beta cells
- Capillary

Hepatic lobules

- Hepatic artery
- Portal canal, in Glisson's capsule
- Hepatic cord and sinusoid
- Central vein
- Margins of lobules
- Sublobular vein
- Central vein (long. section)
- Portal vein
- Bile duct

Intralobular stroma

- Sinusoid and reticulum
- Hepatic cord
- Binucleate cell

Lobule detail (radial)

- Central vein
- Sinusoid
- Disse's space
- Lining cell (macrophage)
- Bile canaliculus
- Hepatic cell of cord

Macrophage

- Ingested particles

Portal canal (cross)

- Hepatic artery
- Lymphatic
- Nerve fibers
- Glisson's capsule
- Bile duct
- Portal vein

Gall bladder (cross)

- Columnar epithelium
- Lamina propria
- Diverticulum
- Muscularis
- Subserosa
- Serosal fat

THE MAJOR DIGESTIVE GLANDS

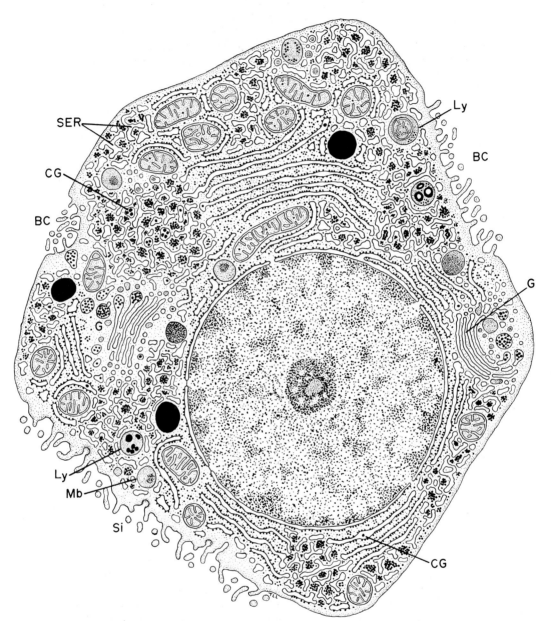

LIVER CELL. Both rough and smooth (SER) endoplasmic reticulum are represented. Both types may contain dense cisternal granules (CG), while aggregations of smaller glycogen granules occur between the smooth cisternae. Large elements are lysosomes (Ly), microbodies (Mb), lipid droplets, Golgi complexes (G) and mitochondria. Cell surfaces facing sinusoids (Si) bear microvilli, as do regions that form a half of a bile canaliculus (BC). The nucleolus is prominent, the nuclear membrane is fenestrated and at one point its outer, granular layer becomes continuous with rough endoplasmic reticulum.

Also there are *protein granules, fat droplets*, salts and pigments.

(In ordinary sections the glycogen and fat have usually been dissolved out.)

Each cell surface that borders a sinusoid bears microvilli.

Disse's space lies between the sinusoidal lining and hepatic-cell surfaces.

There is no basement membrane on which the cells rest.

However, the cell-plates are supported by a meshwork of reticulum.

Apparently dying cells are common in normal liver, yet mitoses are rare.

Probably increase in cell-size compensates largely for cell losses.

4. Bile passages.

A. BILE CANALICULAE.

No lumen is seen in the ordinary examination of hepatic plates.

Yet one exists, and the electron microscope demonstrates it plainly.

Also silver treatment or certain dyes (excreted with bile) reveal it.

It consists of a system of microscopic tubules called *bile canaliculi.*

A canaliculus is a tubule coursing between the apposed faces of hepatic cells.

It develops as a matched pair of grooves on facing cell membranes.

These combine and produce a canal with a tiny lumen.

The grooves bear microvilli and their lines of union have tight junctions.

Each canaliculus lies one-half of a cell-breadth from the adjacent sinusoids.

In an hepatic plate the total system looks like chick netting.

A bile canaliculus is a true secretory ductule, as in other serous glands.

Bile, leaving the cells, passes through it toward the periphery of a lobule.

B. INTRAHEPATIC BILE DUCTS.

At the periphery of a lobule the bile canaliculi open into tributaries of *bile ducts.*

The smallest of these twigs are called *cholangioles* or *canals of Hering.*

In this region there is a transition from the epithelium of the liver plate to that of a bile duct, the lumina of the two becoming continuous.

The cholangioles continue directly into branches of interlobular ducts.

An *interlobular bile duct* is a characteristic component of a portal canal.

Its epithelium varies according to the size of the duct.

The range is from low cuboidal to low columnar epithelium.

The component cells are distinct and have a clear cytoplasm.

The duct is embedded in fibrous tissue; the larger ones become ensheathed.

5. Vessels.

A. HEPATIC SINUSOIDS.

The *sinusoids* are tortuous channels that form a labyrinth of spaces 9 to 12 μ wide.

They receive blood from vessels at the periphery of the lobule.

They discharge blood into a central venule in the axis of the lobule.

A sinusoid is lined by two kinds of cells, but this lining has tiny gaps in it.

One cell-type is a thin '*endothelial cell*' that lies close to the hepatic cells.

It has a dark, flattened nucleus, and its cytoplasm is a thin film.

The other type is a larger cell with a large, vesicular, bulging nucleus.

It has an irregular shape and prominent cytoplasmic processes.

For many years it has been called the *stellate cell* of von Kupffer.

It is intensely phagocytic and belongs to that group of fixed macrophages called the macrophage system or reticulo-endothelial system.

When stuffed with foreign matter it detaches and enters the blood stream.

Cells may overlap and firm junctions are not demonstrable; gaps also occur.

Such cells overlie the microvilli that project from hepatic cells.

A space and a network of reticular fibers occur between lining and hepatic cells.

There is no basement membrane underlying the sinusoidal lining.

Some have thought that the two cell-types are distinct entities.

However, transitional forms are seen, and the ordinary 'endothelial' cells can, on occasion, become phagocytic.

The two are probably variations of the same general cell-type.

That is, they are like the primitive reticular cells and fixed macrophages of reticulo-endothelium elsewhere in the body.

B. BLOOD VESSELS.

The blood-flow through the liver makes it one of the richest vascularized organs.

The vessels of the liver are important since their arrangement is intimately related to function, both normal and abnormal.

There are two supplies of blood entering the liver; there is but one path out.

The large, entering vessels first follow the connective tissue between lobes.

They are *interlobar blood vessels* (hepatic artery; portal vein).

From them arise dwindling *interlobular branches* which follow portal canals.

The liver is drained by *hepatic veins* and their tributaries.

1. *Portal veins.*

Their venous blood is the primary supply (75 per cent) of hepatic lobules.

Small interlobular branches pass between the lobules and break down into pre-capillaries which connect directly with intralobular sinusoids.

2. *Hepatic arteries.*

These vessels supply, on the average, some 25 per cent of the total blood.

Such blood is distributed primarily to the connective tissue of the liver.

(It also nourishes the extrahepatic bile ducts and gall bladder.)

This blood returns from the capillary bed in the tissue of Glisson's capsule.

It feeds into small branches of the portal vein.

In this way it ultimately (and indirectly) reaches the hepatic sinusoids.

Some terminal arterial twigs connect directly with the sinusoids of a lobule.

Such local regions of a lobule may receive arterial blood only.

3. *Hepatic veins.*

This system begins with a *central venule*, which is axial within the lobule.

It is about 45 μ wide and drains the converging sinusoids of the lobule.

It lacks muscle but is ensheathed with some reticular fibers.

Each central venule connects at right angles with a *sublobular vein.*

This stouter, collecting vessel courses alone along the base of a lobule.

A solitary, isolated position is a specific characteristic of these veins.

Sublobular veins are tributary to branches of the *hepatic veins* proper.

The latter, also solitary, open eventually into the inferior vena cava.

4. *Intermittence of flow.*

It is said that three out of four lobules have inactive sinusoids at any time.

Inactive lobules may have their sinusoids packed with blood, or be empty.

Flow control exists at both the periphery and center of a lobule.

Yet muscle fibers are not demonstrable in these regions.

C. LYMPHATIC VESSELS.

Definite lymphatics are first seen within the smallest portal canals.

These increase steadily in size until main vessels emerge at the hilus.

More lymph arises in the liver than in any other organ of the body.

For this reason a source within the lobule has long been suspected.

Experiments suggest that lymph spaces do exist within the lobule.

These are the spaces of Disse, parallelling the sinusoids proper.

They occur between the sinusoidal lining and the hepatic cell plates.

The direction of lymph drainage is toward the periphery of a lobule.

6. *Nerves.*

The fibers are chiefly unmyelinated, from the autonomic system.

They accompany the blood vessels and bile ducts, and supply them.

Extensions from these plexuses into lobules, often asserted, are subject to doubt.

D. Structural Peculiarities:

The liver shows marked divergences from other compound tubular glands.

All hepatic cells are alike, in spite of a wide diversity in functions performed.

The ordinary secretory 'end tubule' of typical glands is replaced by a continuous system of thin cellular plates, drained by tiny canaliculi.

A lumen (*i.e.*, bile canaliculus) is usually in contact with two cells only.

On the other hand, a single cell abuts against more than one bile canaliculus.

The structural unit (lobule) is based on a relation to blood vessels, not to a glandular duct.

The interdigitation of hepatic and portal veins governs lobule formation.

The axis of the lobule is a central venule; in an ordinary gland the axis is a duct.

The relation of hepatic cells to sinusoids is unusually extensive and intimate.

Almost every cell is bathed on two surfaces by blood.

In this regard the liver resembles various endocrine glands.

Hepatic cells release substances both into the duct system and into the blood stream.

The afferent blood supply to the parenchyma is double, but mostly venous.

That is, most of the blood has already passed through capillary plexuses elsewhere.

The course within a lobule is from periphery to center, rather than the reverse.

The efferent veins take courses independent of the afferents, rather than following them.

The ducts are at the periphery of the obvious lobules, rather than at their centers.

The path of secretion within a lobule is from center to periphery, not the reverse.

Connective tissue within the lobule is lacking, except for a reticulum.

Interlobular connective tissue is restricted in extent in man and most other mammals.

It does not enclose lobules, but is largely limited to the angles of lobules.

Yet this tissue receives most of the arterial blood delivered to the liver.

E. Regenerative Ability:

Hepatic cells are replaced rarely in the normal, adult liver.

Yet the liver has a marked capacity for repairing even extensive tissue losses.

Such losses from toxic agents or surgery are recouped (as to liver weight) promptly.

New lobules bud out of old ones, hepatic cells enlarging and increasing by mitosis.

Bile ducts also proliferate and probably also form some new hepatic cells.

F. Diagnostic Features:

The *parenchyma* is arranged in polygonal areas; these are *hepatic lobules.*

The axis of a lobule is an endothelium-lined tube (central venule).

Sections cutting across this axis reveal a radiate arrangement.

Slender, branching cell rows alternate with sinusoidal spaces.

No other structures are seen within a lobule in routine examination.

Sections cutting along this axis show a finger-shaped central venule.

Cell rows pass horizontally from each side of this vertical vessel.

Connective tissue separates lobules at their angles, where *portal canals* occur.

Within the canal are the conspicuous components of the *hepatic triad.*

These are an artery, a vein and a bile duct (with pale cuboidal epithelium).

These three structures, in association, are specifically diagnostic of the liver.

G. Functional Correlations:

The liver is essential to life; death promptly follows its total removal.

Yet only a fraction of the parenchyma is necessary; 9 per cent is sufficient (dog).

The exocrine product of this gland is *bile*, a complex fluid.

Included are bile acids, bile pigment, cholesterol, lecithin, fats, urea, etc.

Bile is apparently secreted continuously; a pint or more is the daily output.

Functionally three concentric zones can be recognized within an hepatic lobule.

The periphery is the most actively functional region.

Here are the first deposit of glycogen and the first loss of bile precursors.

An intermediate zone is progressively less active, but loses glycogen first.

The central 'zone of repose' is called on only when demands are excessive.
Here fat and pigment may accumulate and become visible.

1. Secretion.

Bile acids are believed to arise as a synthesis by the liver cells.
As salts they aid in the emulsification of fats during intestinal digestion.
The fat is thereby made vulnerable to the action of lipase.
Some proteins of the blood plasma are synthesized by liver cells.

2. Excretion.

Bile pigment is derived from hemoglobin through the activity of reticulo-endothelium.
The macrophages of this system occur in the liver, spleen and lymph nodes.
The pigment is not reabsorbed, but is eliminated in the feces.
Urea is formed, at least mainly, in the liver from the break-down of amino acids.
It is a by-product of protein metabolism.
Cholesterol, lecithin and fats also are eliminated into the bile.

3. Storage.

An intermittent blood flow makes the liver a major storehouse for blood.
The liver cells store *glycogen* and release it to the blood, when needed, as glucose.
This constitutes the so-called endocrine function of the liver.
In this way the blood-sugar level is maintained under diverse dietary conditions.
Vitamins (particularly A and B) are stored in the liver, as are *enzymes* and *hormones*.
Fat exists in the liver cells, mostly in a masked form.
It can arise from carbohydrates and can be transformed into carbohydrates.
The liver maintains the proper lipid-level in the blood.

4. Extractives.

Heparin is an anticoagulant that is stored in the liver, but not exclusively so.
It originates in mast cells which are abundant in the liver, among other sites.
Fibrinogen is formed in the liver and is given off to the passing blood plasma.
It occurs as a dispersed protein that is instrumental in blood clotting.
An *anti-anemic substance* incites the regeneration of red corpuscles.
It is useful in combating pernicious anemia.

5. Phagocytosis.

The Kupffer cells act like the macrophages of reticulo-endothelium in general.
There is both a filtering action and a tendency to build up immunities.
Conditions in the sinusoids are favorable for phagocytosis.
The current is sluggish and the blood pressure is low.
The Kupffer cells remove particulate matter from the blood stream.
Bacteria, worn-out blood elements and foreign particles are phagocytosed.

IV. THE EXTRAHEPATIC PASSAGES

A main-line duct connects the liver with the duodenum.
The upper part is the *hepatic duct*; the lower part is the *common bile duct*.
The *gall bladder* and its *cystic duct* represent an offshoot from the main conduit.
The union of cystic and hepatic ducts produces a common drain, the *common bile duct*.

A. GALL BLADDER:

This simple organ is a pear-shaped sac, about 4 × 1.5 inches in size.
It consists of a blind *fundus*, a *body* and a *neck*.

1. Mucosa.

The *mucosal lining* is markedly folded, so that the surface appears honeycombed.
This appearance is largely effaced when the gall bladder is distended.

The *epithelium* consists of tall, palely staining cells with ovoid basal nuclei.
They contain some mucigen that responds feebly to the usual specific stains.
A very thin *striate border* can be demonstrated on the exposed surface.
This border is composed of short microvilli, bearing a filamentous *buffy coat*.
It is usually overlooked, because it is destroyed by routine fixation.
Terminal bars seal cell junctions at the top.
A *basement membrane* exists but cannot be identified with the light microscope.
The epithelium disintegrates rapidly after death, if still bathed in bile.
Glands do not occur, except for a few mucous glands at the neck of the organ.
However, far-outpouching diverticula (*Rokitansky-Aschoff sinuses*) are common.
These are said to result from prolonged distention of a weakened wall.
Such mucosal invasions may extend through the muscular coat.
The *lamina propria* consists of delicate, richly vascular connective tissue.
Some smooth-muscle fibers occur in it, and solitary lymph nodules also.

2. Submucosa.

This layer is not represented in the gall bladder.

3. Muscularis.

Interlacing bundles of smooth muscle form a thin, irregular *muscular coat*.
Most of the fibers are circularly or obliquely disposed.
Fibro-elastic tissue is interspersed between the flat bundles of muscle.

4. Serosa.

This tunic becomes an adventitia where contact is made with the liver.
It lies on a thick, loose, vascular layer which is a *subserosa* or *perimuscular layer*.
Luschka ducts are peculiar tubular structures sometimes occurring here.
They connect with bile ducts belonging to the liver itself.
They are probably aberrant bile ducts, formed during development.

5. Vessels and nerves.

Blood vessels form plexuses in the serosa and lamina propria.
Lymphatics are abundant, and are distributed much like the blood vessels.
Nerve fibers come from the vagus and the sympathetic system.
They are distributed to the muscular wall and blood vessels.

6. Diagnostic features.

The *mucosa* is highly folded in an irregular manner.
The *epithelium* consists of very tall, pale cells, with a weakly specialized border.
Glands are lacking, but epithelial diverticula may extend well into the wall.
The thin *muscularis* consists of bundles, separated by layers of connective tissue.
The outermost layer is either a *serosa* or *adventitia*, depending on the region viewed.
Between it and the muscle is a thick, loose, vascular layer.

7. Functional correlations.

Some mammals normally lack a gall bladder.
Example: rat; horse; certain ruminants; etc.
Removal of the human gall bladder does not cause serious functional disturbance.
There is commonly a compensatory dilatation of the biliary passages.
The gall bladder is a highly distensible reservoir for *bile storage* between meals.
Its capacity ranges from 15 to 90 ml.
It absorbs water and inorganic salts from the bile, concentrating bile greatly.
Evidence of secretion is small (except mucus from glands at the neck).
The gall bladder empties its contents on the entry of chyme into the duodenum.
Discharge is controlled by a hormone (*cholecystokinin*) produced in the duodenum.

B. Extrahepatic Ducts:

There are three large ducts outside the liver.

The *hepatic duct* receives the smaller ducts that converge from within the liver.

The *cystic duct* drains the gall bladder.

The *common bile duct* is the main tube that continues downward to the duodenum.

1. Structure.

The *mucosa* has a tall columnar *epithelium*, resembling that in the gall bladder.

The apices of the cells contain a slight amount of mucigen.

Mucous glands occur in the lamina propria and drain into the duct lumen.

The mucosal lining of the ducts is thrown into many folds.

Near the neck of the gall bladder it makes the *spiral valve* (of Heister).

These folds contain smooth-muscle.

A *fibro-muscular coat* constitutes the rest of the wall.

For the most part this sheath is fibro-elastic tissue.

Smooth-muscle is present only to a slight degree, mingled with the fibrous sheath.

In the cystic duct it is almost wholly lacking.

The hepatic duct has longitudinal bundles in occasional specimens.

The common bile duct usually contains muscle, especially in its lower portions.

These longitudinal bundles, however, do not form a complete sheath.

A *sphincter muscle* (of Oddi) encircles the outlet into the duodenum.

2. Diagnostic features.

The extrahepatic *bile ducts* are tubes with a highly folded lining.

The *epithelium* is composed of pale, tall columnar cells.

The relatively thick wall is mostly fibro-elastic tissue.

Mucous glands occur in the wall.

Smooth-muscle is deficient or lacking.

It occurs dependably only in the lower levels of the common duct.

Even here it does not constitute a complete longitudinal coat.

3. Functional correlations.

All tubes of the duct system, inside the liver or outside it, transport bile.

In addition, the extrahepatic ducts add mucus to the biliary fluid.

Chapter XXI

The Respiratory System

This apparatus conducts air and provides for gaseous interchanges in the lungs.
It consists of two portions, specialized for different purposes.
   One is a set of *conducting passages*, whose function is piping air to and from the lungs.
      These are: *nose; naso-pharynx; larynx; trachea; bronchi;* and *bronchioles.*
   The other is the *respiratory seat* where intimate interchanges occur between air and blood.
      This comprises: *respiratory bronchioles; alveolar ducts; atria;* and *alveolar sacs.*

I. THE NASAL CAVITY

The *nose* is a hollow organ covered with skin, provided with muscles, supported by cartilage and
         bone, and lined with a mucous membrane.
   A *nasal septum* partitions it into two passages.
Each *nasal cavity* consists of a *vestibule*, and of *respiratory* and *olfactory regions*.

1. Vestibule.

   This dilated region is a sort of anteroom, supported by cartilages on its medial side.
   Its lining is continuous with the skin, but changes character as it advances inward.
      The stratified, squamous *epithelium* loses keratinization and layering.
   Coarse *hairs* are numerous near the external orifice.
   Sebaceous and *sweat glands* occur also.

2. Respiratory region.

   In man this territory includes nearly all the septum and lateral walls.
      The lateral wall of each nasal cavity bears three *nasal conchae*.
      These shelf-like elevations greatly increase the area of the mucosal lining.
   The *epithelium* is pseudostratified and ciliated, with numerous *goblet cells*.
      The exact composition varies in regions either sheltered or exposed to passing air.
         Even small areas of stratified epithelium may occur over the projecting conchae.
      Goblet cells sometimes concentrate locally in small glandular pits.
      The *basement membrane* varies regionally from thin to very thick.
   The fibrous *lamina propria* becomes infiltrated with lymphocytes.
      Eosinophils, plasma cells and macrophages may also be represented.
      There are mixed *sero-mucous glands*, especially in the more exposed regions.
   A type of cavernous *erectile tissue* occurs in the deeper levels of the lamina propria.
      This is a vascular plexus; it is composed of large, thin-walled, modified veins.
      Such a system of vessels ordinarily serves to warm the passing air.
      But in response to irritation it can distend with blood and produce turgidity.
         However, its structure is unlike genital erectile tissue in two respects.
            The plexus is supplied by small veins, not by arterioles.
            The muscle is in the walls of vessels, not in septa between cavernous spaces.
   A definite *submucosa* is lacking, although the deep, cavernous lamina propria is unusual.
      The deepest level of the lamina propria fuses with the subjacent periosteum.

3. Olfactory region.

This specialized portion of the wall occurs on the superior concha and adjacent septum.
 The epithelium contains slender cells that continue brainward as *nerve fibers*.
 Specialized *serous glands* occur in the lamina propria.
Further details will be found in the account dealing with sense organs (p. 296).

4. Diagnostic features.

The *respiratory mucosa* is surfaced with pseudostratified, ciliated epithelium.
 Goblet cells are fairly abundant in it.
 Mixed, *sero-mucous glands* and prominent, broad *veins* occur in the lamina propria.
 The deepest level of the lamina merges with the periosteum of underlying bone.
The *olfactory mucosa* has characteristics summarized on p. 296.

5. Functional correlations.

The entire tract, from the nostrils into the lungs, is a two-way thoroughfare for air.
 These parts also warm, humidify and filter the air in transit.
The epithelial lining is overlaid with a film of secreted mucus.
 Mucus serves to entrap particulate matter, such as dust and bacteria.
In the nasal cavity the cilia beat backward in the direction of the naso-pharynx.
 This continuous action propels the mucus onward and cleans the epithelial sheet.
The nasal glands furnish about one pint of fluid daily.
 These secretions inactivate bacteria rapidly.

II. THE PARANASAL SINUSES

The *sinuses* are sacculations that extend from the nasal cavities into nearby bones.
 They include the *frontal*, *sphenoidal*, *maxillary* and *ethmoidal sinuses*.
The *mucosa* resembles that of the respiratory region, but is thin and less specialized.
 The *epithelium* is lower and contains fewer goblet cells.
 A *basement membrane* is, for the most part, not visible with the light microscope.
 Glands are fewer and smaller, and venous *erectile plexuses* do not occur.
Cilia propel the mucous coating toward the narrow openings of the sinuses.
 Here it joins the moving mucus of the nasal cavities.

III. THE NASO-PHARYNX

The *naso-pharynx* is lined regionally with either pseudostratified or stratified epithelium.
 Its structure is described on p. 211.

IV. THE LARYNX

The *larynx* is a short, firm tube that is supported by *cartilages* and *muscles*.
 It also contains the *vocal folds*, commonly called *vocal cords*.
The larynx is interposed between the naso-pharynx and trachea.
 Prominent at its inlet is the flap-like *epiglottis*.

1. Mucosa

The lining *epithelium* is not uniform in type throughout.
 Surfaces subject to wear and tear are covered with *stratified squamous epithelium*.
 These are the vocal folds, ary-epiglottic folds and most of the epiglottis.
 A few *taste buds* occur on the epiglottis and nearby surfaces.
 Below the level of the vocal folds, the epithelium is *pseudostratified*.
 It contains *goblet cells* and bears *cilia*.

The cilia, as in all the lower respiratory passages, stroke toward the pharynx.

A *basement membrane* is present, but it is thin.

At the junction of the two types, ciliated stratified columnar epithelium may occur.

The *lamina propria* is rich in elastic fibers.

It contains small, mixed *sero-mucous glands*, except in the vocal folds.

A diffuse lymphocytic infiltration and a few *solitary nodules* occur.

There is no clearly defined *submucosa*.

Yet the glands and richest elastic tissue occupy a deep, special level.

The *vocal folds* are two apposed folds of the mucous membrane.

Each encloses an elastic band that constitutes a *vocal ligament*.

The exposed surface is covered with stratified squamous epithelium.

Bordering and paralleling each fold laterally is a *vocal muscle*.

2. Cartilaginous wall.

The supporting wall contains *cartilaginous plates*, united by ligaments.

The cartilages maintain the larynx as a constantly open tube.

The larger plates are composed of *hyaline cartilage*.

Included are the thyroid, cricoid, and arytenoids (in large part).

These begin to calcify early (the thyroid of males, at puberty).

Other (mostly smaller) cartilages are composed of *elastic cartilage*.

Included are the cuneiform, corniculate, arytenoids (tips) and epiglottic.

3. Laryngeal muscles.

Some neighboring muscles attach to the cartilages; these are *extrinsic muscles*.

Other muscles interconnect the cartilages themselves; these are *intrinsic muscles*.

4. Diagnostic features.

The larynx is mostly lined with ciliated *pseudostratified epithelium*.

The vocal folds and epiglottis are covered with *stratified squamous epithelium*.

The *lamina propria* contains small, mixed, *sero-mucous glands*.

Sectioned *cartilages* (mostly hyaline) are encountered in the peripheral wall.

Attached to them are *skeletal muscles*.

The highly elastic *epiglottis* and *vocal folds* are distinctive features.

One or both will be included in a representative section.

5. Functional correlations.

The *extrinsic muscles* elevate and depress the larynx as a whole; they aid in *swallowing*.

Some *intrinsic muscles* of the larynx are concerned with changing the *pitch* of sound.

The size of the opening between the vocal folds is varied for the passing air.

Also the tension on the vocal folds is increased and diminished.

Other muscles bend down the epiglottis and close the inlet during swallowing.

Unimpeded breathing is aided by the cartilages which keep the larynx open.

V. THE TRACHEA AND CHIEF BRONCHI

The *trachea* is a relatively thin-walled semirigid tube, about 4.5 inches long and 1 inch wide.

Near the lungs it bifurcates into two chief *bronchi*, similar to the trachea in structure.

The mucosa-lined tube is supported and held open by prominent *cartilages*.

1. Mucosa.

The lining *epithelium* is pseudostratified; all superficial cells bear microvilli.

All of the cells are specialized into ciliated cells or scarcer goblet cells.

The epithelium rests upon a very thick, compound *basement membrane*.

Its primary layer (basal lamina) is reinforced by thick reticular and elastic layers.

The *lamina propria* is a relatively thin, fibrous layer.

There is no muscularis mucosae, but a substitute stratum occupies the same level.
Here elastic fibers form a longitudinally directed *elastic layer*.
Accumulations of lymphocytes occur in the *reticular tissue* of the lamina propria.

2. Submucosa.

A deeper, gland-containing stratum can be designated a *submucosa*.
Many small, *sero-mucous glands* characterize this layer.
They are most frequent at the level of the interspaces between successive cartilages.
Fat cells may be represented, as well.

3. Adventitia.

This tunic contains cartilages, interconnected by fibrous membranes.
There are 16 to 20 *tracheal cartilages*, and about half as many in each chief bronchus.
Each is shaped like a C or Y; they nearly encircle the trachea, but open posteriorly.
This open interval, facing the esophagus, is filled-in by two components.
One is a membrane of fibro-elastic tissue.
The other is the *trachealis muscle*, composed of mostly circular smooth-muscle fibers.
It is the sole representative of a muscular coat.
Submucosal glands often penetrate into the muscle and even extend outside it.
Cartilages show degenerative changes in old age, and many partially calcify.

4. Diagnostic features.

The lining *epithelium* is pseudostratified, bearing cilia and goblet cells.
The *basement membrane* is the thickest in the body.
Mixed *sero-mucous glands* occur in the submucosa.
The *adventitia* tends to show a thick, horseshoe-shaped cartilage 'ring.'
Some transverse sections, however, may contain more than one cartilage-unit.
This is owing to the oblique direction or irregular shape of some cartilages.
Sections cut between rings usually lack cartilage.
Longitudinal sections display a series of oval, cartilaginous masses.
Muscle is lacking, except for some *smooth muscle* between the ends of cartilages.

5. Functional correlations.

The walls of the trachea and bronchi are held open mechanically by the cartilages.
This prevention of collapse makes breathing easier.
Such rings also provide these tubes with considerable flexibility and extensibility.
Membranous regions of the tube, facing the esophagus, yield to its expansions.
This includes the membranes between rings, and muscle between cartilage ends.
The larger air passages, in general, subserve several practical functions.
They conduct and condition the air on its way to the respiratory alveoli.
They also protect the lungs by trapping dust and bacteria in mucus.
Cilia sweep such particles upward whence they are lost by coughing.
Local friction, as by chronic coughs, can produce stratified squamous epithelium.

VI. THE LUNG

The *lungs* occupy paired pleural cavities in the chest; these are lined with a serous membrane.
Each lung lies free within its cavity, except for a stalk carrying an air tube and vessels.
These organs develop like a gland, and maintain a similar structural plan.
Their fundamental component is a system of branching *air tubes*, ending in compound *sacs*.

A. STRUCTURAL PLAN:

Each lung subdivides into nearly separate *lobes*, and these into indistinct *lobules*.
The larger lobules are bounded by *interlobular septa*.
The lung is attached at the *hilus*, where a chief bronchus and vessels enter.

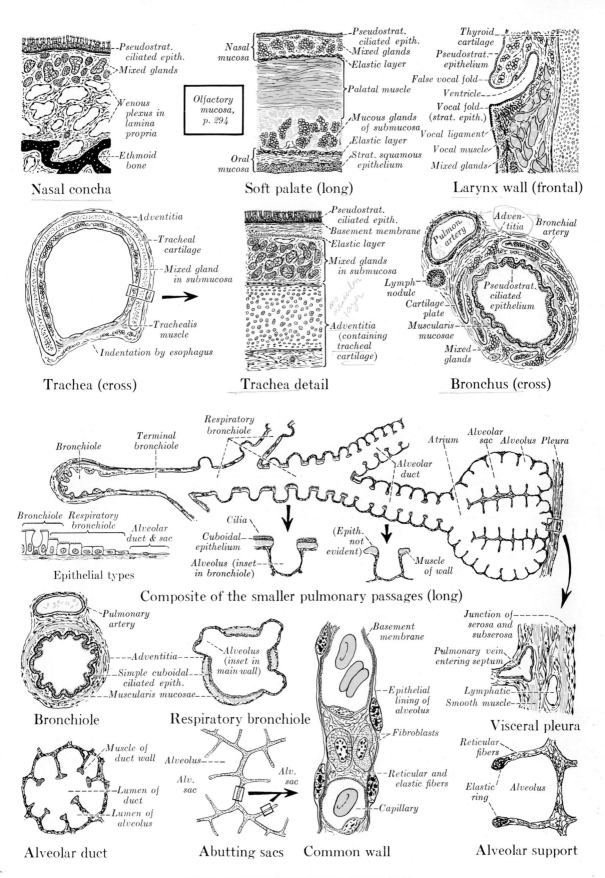

Nasal concha

- Pseudostrat. ciliated epith.
- Mixed glands
- Venous plexus in lamina propria
- Ethmoid bone

Olfactory mucosa, p. 294

Soft palate (long)

Nasal mucosa
- Pseudostrat. ciliated epith.
- Mixed glands
- Elastic layer
- Palatal muscle
- Mucous glands of submucosa
- Elastic layer
Oral mucosa
- Strat. squamous epithelium

Larynx wall (frontal)

- Thyroid cartilage
- Pseudostrat. epithelium
- False vocal fold
- Ventricle
- Vocal fold (strat. epith.)
- Vocal ligament
- Vocal muscle
- Mixed glands

Trachea (cross)

- Adventitia
- Tracheal cartilage
- Mixed gland in submucosa
- Trachealis muscle
- Indentation by esophagus

Trachea detail

- Pseudostrat. ciliated epith.
- Basement membrane
- Elastic layer
- Mixed glands in submucosa
- Adventitia (containing tracheal cartilage)

Bronchus (cross)

- Pulmon. artery
- Adventitia
- Bronchial artery
- Lymph nodule
- Cartilage plate
- Muscularis mucosae
- Mixed glands
- Pseudostrat. ciliated epithelium

Composite of the smaller pulmonary passages (long)

- Bronchiole
- Terminal bronchiole
- Respiratory bronchiole
- Atrium
- Alveolar sac
- Alveolus
- Pleura
- Alveolar duct
- Cilia
- Cuboidal epithelium
- Alveolus (inset in bronchiole)
- (Epith. not evident)
- Muscle of wall

Epithelial types
- Bronchiole
- Respiratory bronchiole
- Alveolar duct & sac

Bronchiole

- Pulmonary artery
- Adventitia
- Simple cuboidal ciliated epith.
- Muscularis mucosae

Respiratory bronchiole

- Alveolus (inset in main wall)

Common wall

- Basement membrane
- Epithelial lining of alveolus
- Fibroblasts
- Reticular and elastic fibers
- Capillary

Visceral pleura

- Junction of serosa and subserosa
- Pulmonary vein entering septum
- Lymphatic
- Smooth muscle

Alveolar duct

- Muscle of duct wall
- Lumen of duct
- Lumen of alveolus

Abutting sacs

- Alveolus
- Alv. sac
- Alv. sac

Alveolar support

- Reticular fibers
- Elastic ring
- Alveolus

THE RESPIRATORY ORGANS

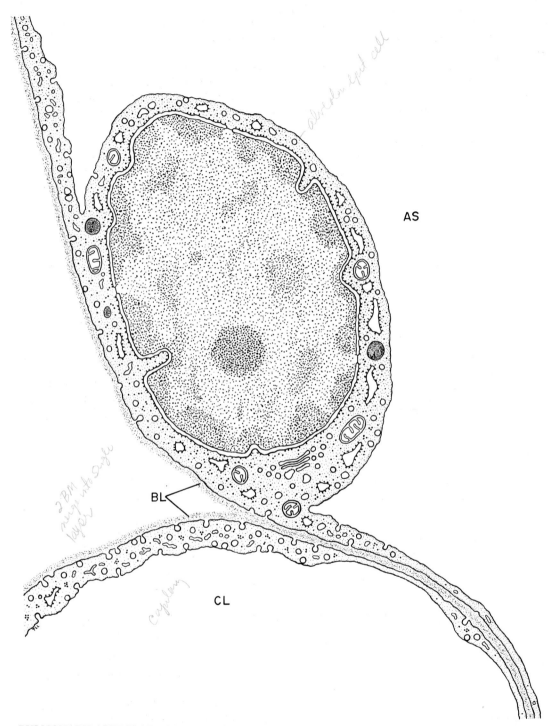

AS

BL

CL

PULMONARY ALVEOLAR EPITHELIUM.   This cell is so thin that only the region of the nucleus bulges into the alveolar lumen (AS). The perinuclear cytoplasm contains sparse organelles. Where the alveolar cell abuts against a capillary (CL) the two basal laminae (BL) merge into a single layer. Both the alveolar cell and the endothelial cell show pinocytotic vesicles in relation to the plasma membranes at both surfaces, and similar detached vesicles occur in the interior cytoplasm.

Here the two portions of the pleura become continuous.

The *parietal pleura* lines the thoracic wall.

The *visceral pleura* is reflected so as to enclose the lung.

The pleurae are typical serous membranes, moistened by fluid.

The system of branching air tubes is divided into conducting and respiratory divisions.

The *conducting tubes* include branches of the *bronchi* and all ordinary *bronchioles*.

They correspond to the excretory ducts of a gland, and function as air conduits.

The *respiratory tubes* consist of *respiratory bronchioles, alveolar ducts, atria* and, terminally, *alveolar sacs;* all contain at least some air cells, or *alveoli*.

They correspond to the smaller ducts and alveoli of a gland.

Each participates, by its alveoli, in the exchanges of pulmonary functioning.

The smaller subdivisions of this system are closely crowded and somewhat displaced.

Hence sections of a collapsed lung give a poor picture of the true spatial relations.

Accompanying the air passages are fibrous tissue, smooth muscle, vessels and nerves.

B. LOBULATION:

The right lung is divided into three major *lobes*, the left lung into two lobes.

Internally there can be recognized small, rather poorly defined *lobules*.

It is commonly considered that an ordinary bronchiole and all branching passages beyond it constitute a unit that is a *pulmonary lobule*.

This unit also has been called a *secondary lobule*.

Lobules abutting on the lung-surface are pyramids whose bases measure $1/2$ to 1 inch.

Such bases can be seen marked off on the surface of the lung.

They show well in a fetus or when outlined by pigment deposited in the septa.

The sides of such a lobule are bounded by incomplete *interlobular septa*.

Lobules located deeper within the interior assume irregular, angular shapes.

Some recognize a much smaller unit within the secondary lobule as the *primary lobule*.

It consists of a respiratory bronchiole and all the terminal subdivisions beyond it.

Several of these primary lobules associate to constitute a secondary lobule.

C. DETAILED STRUCTURE:

1. Framework.

Each lobed lung is intimately invested with a fibro-elastic membrane.

This is the fibrous layer of the *visceral pleura*; it also contains smooth muscle.

Extending inward are *interlobular septa* that enclose secondary lobules fairly well.

At the apex of a lobule they join the connective tissue that surrounds bronchi.

The lobules of the lung are permeated with *reticular networks* and *elastic networks*.

These support the bronchioles, smaller air tubes and alveolar sacs.

2. Conducting tubes.

The air tubes within the lung diminish progressively in size and complexity.

Different names are given to successive segments with changing features.

A. BRONCHUS.

The *epithelium* gradually reduces in thickness and layering.

The larger bronchi within the lungs have *pseudostratified epithelium*.

Cilia and goblet cells occur, as in the chief bronchi and trachea.

In the smallest bronchi the epithelium becomes *simple columnar*.

Cilia are still abundant, and goblet cells are numerous.

A *muscularis mucosae* encircles the thin *lamina propria* as interlacing spirals.

It gradually replaces the elastic layer of the trachea and chief bronchi.

Its contraction causes the mucosa to appear folded.

Nevertheless, some elastic fibers are retained even in the smallest tubes.

The *submucosa* contains mixed, *sero-mucous glands*.

These glands also project into the spaces between the cartilages.

They decrease in number and size as the bronchi grow smaller.

Solitary *lymph nodules,* when present, lie here (*i.e.,* outside the m. mucosae).

The *adventitia* contains separate *cartilaginous plates* instead of C-shaped rings.
> They overlap in the larger bronchi, but are scarce in the smaller divisions.
> Some *lymph nodes* may occur in the adventitia of the largest bronchi.

B. BRONCHIOLE.

The largest bronchioles are about 1 mm. in diameter; the smallest, 0.5 mm.
> The latter (*terminal bronchioles*) number some 50 in each secondary lobule.

The *epithelium* reduces gradually to a low columnar type, still ciliated.
> Goblet cells become infrequent and disappear in the smaller tubes.

The *muscularis mucosae* is relatively heavier than at higher or lower levels.
> It forms a spiraling network of fibers that dominates the *lamina propria*.
> Many elastic fibers intermingle with the smooth muscle, as in bronchi.

An *adventitia* remains; but cartilage, glands and lymph nodules no longer occur.
> In this loss of firm support, the mucosa is thrown into longitudinal folds.

In bronchioles and all smaller ducts patency is not maintained by cartilages.
> The elastic framework of lung tissue pulls on all sides of these tubes.

3. Respiratory tubes.

A. RESPIRATORY BRONCHIOLE.

This conduit is a short branching tubule, 0.5. mm. or less in diameter.
> About two arise from each terminal bronchiole; each subdivides once or twice.
> Structurally it is transitional between a conducting and respiratory tube.

The *epithelium* ranges from a low columnar type to a low cuboidal layer.
> Goblet cells do not occur, but cilia are still present in the larger tubes.
>> This insures that mucus will not collect and plug the lumen where it cannot
>> be moved upward by ciliary action.

The thin *supporting wall* consists primarily of collagenous fibers.
> It retains a spiral network of smooth-muscle and elastic fibers.

Alveoli appear as little outpouchings that interrupt the main wall at intervals.
> They project beyond the ordinary wall as thinner, box-like insets (*cf.* p. 249).
> Alveoli increase in number progressively at lower levels of the bronchiole.

B. ALVEOLAR DUCT.

Each respiratory bronchiole gives rise to several branching *alveolar ducts*.
> They are relatively long, thin-walled tubes, studded with alveoli.

The main wall of the duct resembles a sieve, with large, closely set holes.
> Its lining epithelium is reduced to flattened, inconspicuous cells.
> Outside are spirals of smooth muscle and some connective tissue.

The duct is thickly beset with single alveoli outpouched from the main wall.
> Also clusters of alveoli (*alveolar sacs*) open into its lumen.

Alveoli are the most abundant and conspicuous feature of the alveolar duct.

C. ATRIUM.

Each makes an antechamber between an alveolar duct and several air sacs.
From 3 to 6 atria branch off from the end of each alveolar duct.
Some do not assign a special name to these 'atria.'
> They regard them merely as terminal branches of alveolar ducts.

4. Alveolar sacs and alveoli.

A. GENERAL FEATURES.

From 2 to 5 single or compound *alveolar sacs* open off each atrium.
Each sac is composed of a variable number of thin-walled, minor compartments.
These cubicles are primary *alveoli*, all opening into the main lumen of the sac.
In the normal adult each ranges from 100 to 300 μ in diameter.
The total number of alveoli is estimated at 700,000,000.
> The surface area, when normally distended, may equal 75,000 square yards.

An individual alveolus, or air cell, is like a six-sided box with its top open.
> Thus the interior of an alveolar sac has an open, honeycombed appearance.

Both the sacs and their component alveoli are packed as snugly as possible.
Identical relations exist in any membrane-septum that separates two cavities.
That is, a side wall separating two alveoli of the same sac is identical with the common floor serving abutting alveoli of different sacs.
It will be noted that such a septum is always a common partition.
It is like a common wall that separates adjoining rooms in a house.
Some adjacent alveolar sacs communicate by *alveolar pores*, 10 to 15 μ wide.
These apertures perforate the floor common to two alveoli.
They can provide a pathway for air if a tiny bronchiole becomes blocked.
Also they can prevent local overdistention by exudate, etc.

B. ALVEOLAR DETAILS.

An inconspicuous *alveolar epithelium* lines the interior of an alveolus.
It is too thin (0.05 μ minimum) to be resolved convincingly by light microscopy.
The epithelium bears a lipoprotein film, known as a *surfactant.*
It reduces surface tension and aids alveolar recoil during expiration.
Interspersed in the epithelium are *great alveolar cells,* bearing microvilli.
These rounded, pale cells contain layered bodies (the source of surfactant?)
A very thin *basal lamina* underlies the highly squamous alveolar epithelium.
It merges with a similar lamina of a capillary wherever the two abut.
Such direct union gives a thickness, lumen to lumen, of as little as 0.3 μ.
So thin a 'barrier' facilitates gaseous interchanges between air and blood.
In these places only three layers constitute the air-blood barrier.
These are alveolar epithelium, fused basal laminae and capillary endothelium.
In areas between capillaries the alveolar lamina adjoins septal tissue directly.
The unperforated *capillaries* form a very closely spaced, two-dimensional network.
This constitutes by far the bulkiest component of the septum.
Its total area in a lung has been estimated at 150 square yards.
Their *basal laminae* unite with that of alveolar epithelium wherever they abut.
The supporting tissue of an alveolar side-wall or floor is a meshwork of fibers.
Most abundant are reticular fibers, but there are elastic fibers also.
Elastic fibers encircle the mouth of each alveolar sac and alveolus.
Within the sac and its alveoli smooth muscle fibers are entirely lacking.
Regions of a septum, not occupied by capillaries and fibers, contain cells.
These are fibroblasts, macrophages and some wandering leucocytes.

5. *Pleura.*

The pleura forms a lining to the wall of each thoracic cavity (parietal pleura).
At the hilus of each lung it reflects over the lobes (visceral pleura).
Both divisions are normally in contact, surface to surface.
Only a thin film of secreted pleural fluid intervenes between the two.
Both are *serous membranes* (p. 160), essentially alike in structure.
The exposed surface of a pleural membrane is *mesothelium.*
Directly underlying is a dense layer of collagenous and elastic fibers.
At deep levels there are larger veins and lymphatic vessels.
This deep tissue becomes continuous with interlobular septa.
Nerves, sensory endings and scattered plates of smooth muscle occur also.

6. *Vessels and nerves.*

A. BLOOD VESSELS.

There are two sets: one is for respiration; the other nourishes the air tubes.
The pulmonary arteries and veins carry blood that participates in respiration.
The *pulmonary artery* follows branching air ducts, conveying impure blood.
It lies on, or is attached to, the wall of the bronchus and bronchiole.
It ends in capillary networks wherever pulmonary alveoli exist.
Pulmonary veins collect purified blood from alveoli, and from the pleura.

For a considerable distance they run in the septa between lobules.
> Here they pursue solitary courses, and this is a distinctive feature.
They ultimately join the bronchi and are attached to their walls.
> A vein is situated opposite to the similarly attached pulmonary artery.
Bronchial arteries nourish the air tubes and accompanying pulmonary arteries.
They are much smaller than the pulmonary arteries and veins.
They differ by coursing within the walls of the air tubes and arteries.
Such vessels do not extend peripherally beyond the respiratory bronchioles.
> Here anastomoses are made with capillaries from the pulmonary arteries.
Branches of the arteries supply also the interlobular septa and pleura.
> This blood is returned by the pulmonary veins.
True *bronchial veins* are said to occur only at the hilus of the lung.

B. LYMPHATICS.

A profuse superficial *pleural network* receives lymph from interlobular septa.
> Valves prevent backflow, and draining trunks conduct the lymph to the hilus.
A *deep set* of lymphatics accompanies the air tubes and pulmonary artery.
> It begins with the alveolar ducts and drains toward the hilus of the lung.

C. NERVES.

The *vagus nerve* and *sympathetic system* supply the air tubes and blood vessels.
> There are constrictor (vagal) and dilator (sympathetic) fibers to the tubes.
Some sensory endings are described in relation to muscle and epithelium.

D. BIRTH CHANGES:

The fetal lung has a compact, glandular appearance, unlike the fully expanded organ.
> Even at birth, alveoli are small and the lung does not fill its pleural cavity well.
With breathing, the air passages dilate greatly and the whole lung expands.
> Such a lung will float in water, whereas the lung of a still-born sinks.
Within two months after birth some alterations occur in the small ducts.
> Terminal bronchioles bud off alveoli and become respiratory bronchioles.
> Respiratory bronchioles acquire more alveoli and become alveolar ducts.

E. REGENERATIVE ABILITY:

Loss of the mucosa in the trachea and bronchi is repaired by cell migration and mitosis.
> The new epithelium differentiates ciliated cells and gland cells.
After tissue destruction in the lung, by surgery or disease, healing is by scar tissue.
> There is no evidence of a capacity of pulmonary tissue to regenerate as such.

F. DIAGNOSTIC FEATURES:

Bronchi within the lungs show several cartilage-plates in the adventitia.
> These decrease in size in the smaller divisions and become scarcer.
> The mucosa differs from that of the trachea in two particulars.
>> It is folded and possesses a muscularis mucosae.
> Hence separate cartilage-plates and a muscularis mucosae securely identify these tubes.
>> The presence of adjacent lung tissue can be expected.
Ordinary *bronchioles* possess a simple columnar, ciliated epithelium.
> Cartilage and glands are lacking; goblet cells are sparse or absent.
> The muscularis mucosae is well developed in relation to the size of the tube.
> Alveoli, with a chick-netting appearance, always surround the bronchiole.
Respiratory bronchioles differ from the terminal bronchioles in an important respect.
> They have thin alveoli that protrude here and there through gaps in the main wall.
>> Sections that miss these alveoli can be mistaken for the smallest bronchioles.
> Also the epithelium shortens even to a low cuboidal type.
Alveolar ducts differ from respiratory bronchioles by an increased number of alveoli.
> These alveolar interruptions in the wall make a continuous series.
> Smooth muscle is reduced to tiny, local knobs in what remains of the main wall.
>> Such a knob, surmounting a septal wall between two alveoli, resembles a drumstick.

No epithelial lining is easily recognizable in this tube or its alveoli.

A longitudinal section can be likened to rows of doorless rooms opening off a hallway.

Alveolar sacs consist of box-like alveoli arranged about a main, central lumen.

The walls between alveoli show no easily determinable structural details.

A differential characteristic over alveolar ducts is the absence of muscular knobs.

Sections cutting across the central lumen of an alveolar sac (or alveolar duct) resemble a circle of doorless rooms opening off a central rotunda.

Tangential sections that miss the central lumen cut through several alveoli.

These show as a thin network about polygonal spaces, like chick netting.

G. FUNCTIONAL CORRELATIONS:

The primary purpose of the lungs is to serve as the seat of *respiratory exchanges*.

This is accomplished through the breathing of air.

Yet quiet breathing draws on only 5 per cent of the lungs' capability.

The smooth pleural surfaces are kept moist with a serous fluid.

This fluid-film enables the lungs to glide without friction during breathing.

During *inspiration* the conducting system of air tubes increases in length and diameter.

As the chest expands, the lungs also increase in size and draw in air.

This is the consequence of negative pressure developing in the pleural cavities.

The lung, in expanding, stretches elastic tissues everywhere within the organ.

If the pleural cavity is opened, pressures equalize and the lung collapses.

This shrinkage is the result of elastic recoil.

Such retraction is the condition seen in ordinary sections of the uninflated lung.

During *inspiration*, the respiratory division of the pulmonary tubes also expands.

Probably the volume increase is due to elongation and distention of alveolar ducts.

Seemingly the alveoli change volume but little, although they do change shape.

During *expiration*, it is the elastic tissue that provides for recoil in both the conducting and respiratory divisions; muscular force is used only in hard breathing.

There is a double spiral of muscle in bronchi, bronchioles and alveolar ducts.

This arrangement both contracts these tubes and shortens them.

The relatively heaviest concentration of muscle is in the bronchioles.

As might be expected, these tubes are subject to strongest asthmatic spasms.

The lungs act as intermediaries in respiratory *gaseous exchanges*.

These exchanges take place through a film of fluid, and a very thin layer of tissue.

The transfers probably are accomplished by processes involving physical diffusion.

Oxygen is given to the blood, and carbon dioxide is removed from it.

The lungs also have excretory functions.

Nearly a quart of water is eliminated daily from the lungs.

Volatile agents, taken into the body, are excreted by them; carbon dioxide is exhaled.

The *air-filtering* service of the respiratory system is a significant activity.

Inspired particulate matter adheres to the lining of respiratory tubes.

In the conducting tubes this foreign material is removed in a mass movement.

Here (and in respiratory bronchioles) cilia are present and beat upward.

They force mucus and its entrapped particles upward, whence it is expelled.

In so doing, mucus is also kept from accumulating and occluding the air ducts.

Alveolar ducts and alveolar sacs lack cilia to move and expel foreign particles.

Instead, *alveolar phagocytes* (or *dust cells*), of uncertain origin, become active.

They most probably are aroused monocytes, outwandered from alveolar septa.

Once free in the lumen, they engulf dust, smoke particles or bacteria.

Some cells deposit this material in the septa, lymphoid tissue and lymph nodes.

In this way the lungs of a city dweller, in particular, become blackened.

Other dust cells move upward to the respiratory bronchioles.

Thence cilia or coughing bring them to the pharynx.

In certain types of heart disease the phagocytes contain broken-down hemoglobin (hemosiderin) and are called 'heart-failure cells.'

Chapter XXII

The Urinary System

The *urinary system* consists of the *kidneys* and the urinary passages leading away from them. The latter include the *calyces, renal pelvis* and *ureter* that stand in relation to each kidney. Additional parts are the *urinary bladder* and its drainage duct, the *urethra.*

I. THE KIDNEY

The *kidney* is a compound tubular gland, adapted to filtering wastes from the blood. It is located in the lumbar region, just outside the dorsal peritoneum.

A. STRUCTURAL PLAN:

The *kidney* is a flattened, bean-shaped organ, about 4.5 inches long.
It is surrounded by a thin, fibrous *capsule*, which is weakly attached.
A concave indentation, the *hilus* and *renal sinus*, contains associated structures (p. 259).
The interior of the kidney is almost wholly *parenchyma.* very little TC
  Trabeculae or other gross supporting tissues are replaced by delicate *reticulum.*
The parenchyma consists of many long, tortuous secretory canals (*nephrons*).
  These become continuous with tree-like systems of *excretory ducts.*
  A nephron and its excretory duct, together, comprise a *uriniferous tubule.*
The parenchyma is plainly divisible into a cortex and a more centrally located medulla.
  The *cortex*, brownish in life, has an irregular inner border (next to the medulla).
    It overlies the bases of the pyramids and dips down between them.
      These latter, displaced portions of cortex invade the medullary territory.
      They constitute the *renal columns* (of Bertin).
    A magnifying lens shows that the cortex is not uniform in texture.
      It is subdivided into alternating radial tracts.
    The lighter tracts are radially striate and hence named the *pars radiata.*
      Since they are continuous with the striate medulla they became called 'medullary rays'; *cortical rays* is a more appropriate name.
    The darker tracts have a granular appearance when cut and viewed with a lens.
      This is because the convoluted tubules, composing them, are cut irregularly.
      Hence this part is called the *pars convoluta*; another name is *labyrinth.*
      Among the tubules, in fresh specimens, bright red points are seen.
        These are globular vascular tufts, or *glomeruli*, at the blind ends of tubules.
  The *medulla* is gray in fresh material.
    It usually consists of 10 to 15 *pyramids*, whose apices point toward the hilus.
      Two or three pyramids commonly fuse and end in one common *papilla.*
      Hence there are fewer papillae (6 to 15) than pyramids.
    The pyramids have a radially striate appearance as they diverge from papillae.
      This is because the tubules and vessels in them are straight.
    Its tip bears 10 to 25 pits where the main trunks of excretory ducts open.

B. LOBULATION:

A *lobe* consists of a pyramid, together with the cortex overlying it; there are up to 21 in all.

252

Their boundaries are prominent on the surface of a fetal kidney.

Such external lobation is permanent in reptiles, birds, oxen and bears.

They become blurred and fused in the adults of some mammals (including man).

Lobes are not outlined internally by trabeculae or other obvious landmarks.

The kidney of many mammals has a single pyramid, and hence but one lobe.

Example: rodents; cat; monkey.

A *lobule* is a smaller unit than the lobe.

It is a natural functional unit whose core is a ray. *(cortical ray / medullary ray)*

It consists of a cortical ray, plus all adjoining parts of the labyrinth whose secretory tubules drain into collecting tubules located in that ray.

Such lobules are staked off by interlobular blood vessels, coursing radially (p. 257). *(interlobular vessels)*

Like the functional 'portal lobule' of the liver, it is not a well outlined unit.

It is best demarcated when bounding vessels have been injected with colored fluid.

C. Detailed Structure:

1. Framework.

The thin and firm (but weakly attached) *capsule* consists mostly of collagenous fibers.

The *interstitial connective tissue* is extremely scanty, especially in the cortex.

It consists almost wholly of reticular tissue, inconspicuous with ordinary stains.

Some collagenous fibers do occur, but their distribution is limited.

They surround blood vessels, glomerular capsules and large papillary ducts.

Each uriniferous tubule is enclosed throughout its length by a *basement membrane*.

Reticular fibers support the amorphous basal lamina.

2. Uriniferous tubule.

The kidney is a compound tubular gland; the tubules are very long and closely packed.

A complete *uriniferous tubule* consists of two component parts.

These components have separate embryonic origins, but become linked secondarily.

The *secretory tubule,* or *nephron,* is unbranched and about 35 mm. long.

Some portions of it are straight, while other portions are highly convoluted.

There are about 1,300,000 tubules in each kidney.

Their combined length in each kidney totals some 38 miles.

Their total interior area in each kidney equals 25 to 30 square meters.

The *collecting tubule* belongs to a branched, tree-like system of excretory ducts.

Their main stems are named *papillary ducts;* 10 to 25 open on a papilla. *(Tub. collectores, de Bellini)*

These ducts are all straight; the length of a drainage course is about 21 mm.

All uriniferous tubules have the same general form, composition and relations.

Some minor differences depend on the position of a nephron in the cortex (p. 254).

Nevertheless, to know one tubule and its blood supply is to understand the kidney.

Since the tubules intermingle so intimately, simple inspection of sections does not identify surely all the portions that belong to any particular nephron.

Each nephron, however, is a compact mass, except for a long, looped portion.

Reconstruction and teasing methods have isolated complete nephrons successfully.

3. Subdivision of a tubule.

A total *uriniferous tubule* consists of a number of consecutive portions or segments.

These differ both structurally and functionally.

It is customary to designate these distinctive segments as 'tubules.'

Usage makes the term *proximal* indicate 'nearer the glomerulus.'

Similarly, *distal* indicates 'nearer the papilla.'

Beginning at the blind, proximal end these parts are, in order, as follows:

A. Secretory Portion.

Glomerular capsule (of Bowman).

Neck.

Proximal tubule.

Convoluted portion.

Straight portion.

This is the first (descending, thick) segment of Henle's loop.

Thin segment of Henle's loop (second segment of Henle's loop).

Distal tubule:

Straight portion.

This is the third (ascending, thick) segment of Henle's loop.

Convoluted portion.

B. EXCRETORY (OR DUCT) PORTION.

Arched collecting tubule (or junctional tubule).

Straight collecting tubule.

Papillary duct (of Bellini).

4. Nephron variations correlated with position.

The chief variation is in Henle's loop—its length, position and composition.

Nephrons located *high in the cortex* have short Henle's loops.

That is, the loop does not dip far into the medulla.

The thin segment does not extend down to the apex of the loop.

Nephrons located *near the medulla* have long Henle's loops.

That is, the loop dips far down into the pyramid.

Its medullary portion is up to three times longer than the highest, shortest loop.

The thin segment passes around the apex and part way up the ascending limb.

All intergrades between these two extreme types naturally occur.

Tubules with short-dipping loops are much more numerous (7:1, it is said).

5. Tubule characteristics.

The *epithelium* is specific for each segment of a secretory tubule (nephron).

By contrast, the epithelium of all excretory ducts is of one structural type.

The epithelium of the entire uriniferous tubule rests on a *basement membrane*.

This membrane is inconspicuous without special staining.

A. RENAL (OR MALPIGHIAN) CORPUSCLE.

This is a spheroidal body, about 0.2 mm. wide, located in the labyrinth.

It consists of a vascular *glomerulus*, nearly enveloped by a double-walled cup.

The thin cup is an indented epithelial sac, named the *glomerular capsule*.

In development the corpuscle arises when a group of capillaries becomes grown around by the expanded, blind end of the secretory tubule.

The two components of a renal corpuscle are separate but associated entities.

1. *Glomerulus.*

This is a *rete mirabile* (p. 129), interrupting an arteriole in its course.

It is lobulated and contains tangled vessels, resembling capillaries.

The *afferent arteriole* subdivides, each vessel branching and anastomosing.

But each loop-complex forms a separate lobule, largely distinct from others.

The combined length of the tortuous loops is about 1 inch.

Their total length in each kidney is some 16 miles; the total filtration surface of the capillaries is said to be more than 0.5 square yard.

The *efferent arteriole* is formed when the loops reunite as a single vessel.

Its lumen is smaller than that of the afferent since it carries less blood.

The points of entry and exit of the arterioles are close together.

This region is often called the *vascular pole* of the corpuscle.

The *endothelium* of the 'capillaries' is extremely thin (0.04 μ).

Only where nuclei occur can a little be seen with a light microscope.

Electron micrographs show many perforations, about 0.06 μ wide.

A minority thinks that some or all are closed by thin diaphragms.

The capillary loops are invested by a basal lamina 0.1 μ thick.

2. *Glomerular capsule.*

Another name for this double-walled, epithelial cup is *Bowman's capsule*.

It has a parietal and a visceral layer, separated by a narrow *capsular space*.
    The two components are continuous at the vascular pole.
        Here is the rim where the visceral layer reflects over the glomerulus.
    Both layers are squamous epithelium; only the parietal layer is easily seen.
    The *parietal layer* forms a smooth external capsule, spheroidal in shape.
        Cell boundaries and a thin basement membrane are demonstrable.
    The *visceral layer* takes an irregular course, dipping inward between the lobules.
        Its cells (*podocytes*) give off processes that branch into smaller processes.
        These *pedicels* alone rest on capillaries, their basal laminae merging.
        Pedicels interdigitate intricately with those of adjacent podocytes.
        The apparent gaps between them are closed by thin diaphragms.
    3. *Mesangium.*
        This designates the intercellular material that embeds the capillary loops.
        Its cells are presumably pericytes belonging to the connective-tissue group.
            These are suspended in an amorphous substance containing fine filaments.
B. NECK.
    The parietal layer continues into the *neck* of the nephron at the *urinary pole*.
    This pole of the corpuscle is almost directly opposite the vascular pole.
    The neck is a very short segment of rapid epithelial transition.
    The flat, capsular cells elevate to a cuboidal and then low columnar cell-type.
C. PROXIMAL TUBULE.
    This is a long (14 mm.) and broad (40 to 60 μ) segment of the nephron.
        It consists of a convoluted portion and a straight portion.
    The *convoluted portion* lies wholly in the labyrinth, near its renal corpuscle.
        It is remarkably contorted and hence is cut irregularly in sections.
    The *straight portion* leaves the labyrinth, enters a ray and passes down it.
        Within the ray it pursues first a wavy and then a straight course.
        It terminates in the boundary zone of the medulla.
    Both portions are similar in structure; differences are quantitative.
        Yet some chemical responses suggest regional specializations.
    The component *cells* of a tubule are low columnar (actually pyramidal) in shape.
        Freshly obtained cells appear opaque and granular.
            They disintegrate rapidly and are difficult to preserve faithfully.
    Cell limits usually are not plain, owing to the presence of fluted side-walls.
        These foldings interlock complexly with those of neighboring cells.
    The *nuclei* are large, pale and spheroidal.
        Only 3 to 4 nuclei show in a transverse section at any level.
    The *cytoplasm* stains deeply with acid dyes.
        The basal half, when well fixed, tends to show vertical striations.
            Such represent mitochondria held in the bays of the folded walls.
        The free surface bears a prominent *brush border* of microvilli, 1.0 μ long.
            It may appear homogeneous if the fixation is poor, or may even be lost.
            In the latter instance the cell appears shorter, with a ragged top.
    The appearance of a cell varies with its state of rest or activity.
        Active cells become shorter; their lumen, wider; their brush border, taller.
D. LOOP (OF HENLE).
    This is a hairpin-shaped, recurring portion of the nephron.
    Each limb lies partly in the cortex and partly in the medulla.
    Three different segments of the nephron comprise the total loop.
        1. *Descending, thick segment* (straight portion of proximal tubule).
        2. *Thin segment.*
        3. *Ascending, thick segment* (straight portion of distal tubule).
    The *apex of the loop* varies in composition, correlated with its location.
        If the loop dips deep into the medulla, a long thin segment makes the loop.
        If the loop lies high in the medulla, the ascending thick segment is involved.

E. THIN SEGMENT OF LOOP.

In the boundary zone of the medulla there is a sudden transition from the straight tubule to a slender segment 2 to 10 mm. long and only 15 μ wide.

This *thin segment* runs a direct, radial course in the medulla.

If it extends past the apex of Henle's loop, it makes a sharp hairpin bend.

It may be short, or long and recurved, as explained in topic 4 on p. 254.

(It resembles a capillary somewhat, but is larger, thicker walled and its nuclei, 3 to 5 in transverse sections, are relatively closer spaced.)

The interlocking *cells* are squamous, with a pale-staining cytoplasm.

The somewhat flattened nuclei cause local bulgings into the lumen.

An obvious *brush border* is lacking from this level onward in the nephron.

Nevertheless, sparse stubby microvilli project into the lumen.

F. DISTAL TUBULE.

This tubule is about 14 mm. long and 20 to 50 μ in diameter.

It consists of an ascending, thick portion and a convoluted portion.

The *straight portion* (9 mm.) comprises the ascending, thick segment of Henle's loop.

There is an abrupt transition from the thin limb into cuboidal epithelium.

The component cells stain more deeply acidophilic than those of the thin limb.

They resemble those of the distal convoluted portion (see below).

Yet some chemical responses suggest regional specializations.

Entering a ray the thick segment ascends, and then passes into the labyrinth.

It ends between the two arterioles of its own glomerulus.

The region in contact with the afferent arteriole is specialized.

This *macula densa* is an elliptical cluster of taller, crowded cells.

Nuclei are close together; the Golgi complex is beneath the nucleus.

It constitutes one-half of the juxtaglomerular apparatus (p. 257).

The *convoluted portion* (5 mm.) differs from the proximal convoluted portion.

It is shorter, somewhat narrower and much less tortuous.

Most of its convolutions occur near its own Bowman's capsule.

Several characteristics distinguish the distal from the proximal portion.

The *epithelium* is lower (cuboidal) and the lumen is larger.

Cells are smaller and their boundaries more distinct.

Hence 5 to 8 nuclei show in a transverse section, instead of 3 to 4.

The *cytoplasm* stains less intensely with acid dyes.

Small, scattered microvilli are present, but no true brush border.

Extensive infoldings of the plasma membrane and vertical mitochondria produce the appearance of vertical striations.

G. ARCHED COLLECTING TUBULE.

This short, junctional segment connects the nephron with an excretory duct.

Its short course (difficult to find in sections) passes from a labyrinth to a ray.

From 7 to 10 arched tubules join a single, straight collecting tubule.

Hence there are far fewer collecting tubules than nephrons in the kidney.

H. STRAIGHT COLLECTING TUBULE.

In rays and the outer zone of the medulla, these tubules run straight courses.

Here each is an independent duct, not joining others.

In the inner zone of the medulla they unite with similar ducts.

Successive unions produce large straight tubes, the *papillary ducts* (of Bellini).

From 10 to 25 papillary ducts converge and open separately on a papilla.

The total length of a drainage course averages about 21 mm.

The diameters of all ducts in the tree-like system range from 40 to 200 μ.

Transverse sections show an even, nearly circular external outline.

The *epithelium* is very different from that of secretory tubules in the nephron.

The cells are cuboidal to tall columnar in shape, and regularly arranged.

Cell boundaries are distinct, and the tops tend to bulge into the lumen.

Nuclei are dark-staining and located at one level, toward the base.

The *cytoplasm* is pale and clear, never staining deeply.

In arched tubules and proximally in collecting tubules there are some dark cells.

These resemble the cells of the terminal portion of the distal tubule.

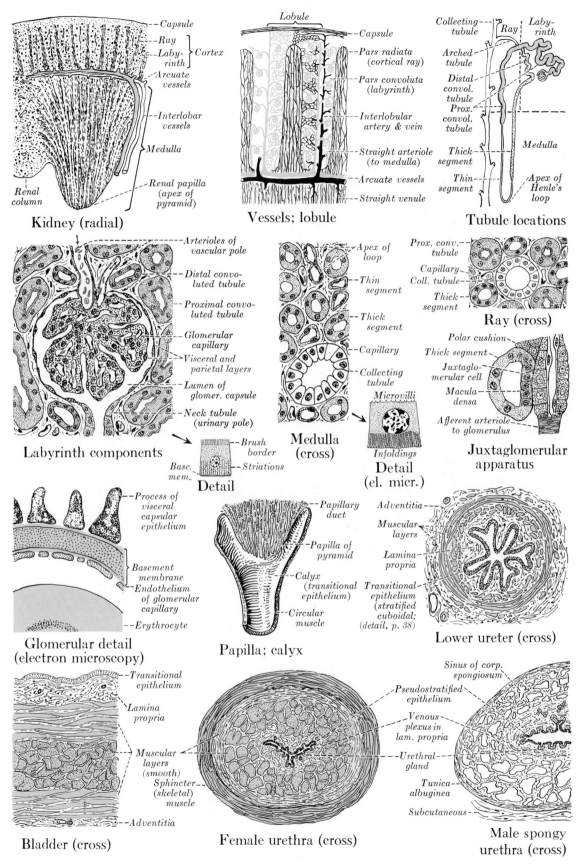

Kidney (radial)

Capsule
Ray
Labyrinth } Cortex
Arcuate vessels
Interlobar vessels
Medulla
Renal papilla (apex of pyramid)
Renal column

Vessels; lobule

Lobule
Capsule
Pars radiata (cortical ray)
Pars convoluta (labyrinth)
Interlobular artery & vein
Straight arteriole (to medulla)
Arcuate vessels
Straight venule

Tubule locations

Collecting tubule
Ray
Labyrinth
Arched tubule
Distal convol. tubule
Prox. convol. tubule
Thick segment
Thin segment
Medulla
Apex of Henle's loop

Labyrinth components

Arterioles of vascular pole
Distal convoluted tubule
Proximal convoluted tubule
Glomerular capillary
Visceral and parietal layers
Lumen of glomer. capsule
Neck tubule (urinary pole)

Detail

Brush border
Striations
Basc. mem.

Medulla (cross)

Apex of loop
Thin segment
Thick segment
Capillary
Collecting tubule
Microvilli

Detail (el. micr.)

Infoldings

Ray (cross)

Prox. conv. tubule
Capillary
Coll. tubule
Thick segment

Juxtaglomerular apparatus

Polar cushion
Thick segment
Juxtaglomerular cell
Macula densa
Afferent arteriole to glomerulus

Glomerular detail (electron microscopy)

Process of visceral capsular epithelium
Basement membrane
Endothelium of glomerular capillary
Erythrocyte

Papilla; calyx

Papillary duct
Papilla of pyramid
Calyx (transitional epithelium)
Circular muscle

Lower ureter (cross)

Adventitia
Muscular layers
Lamina propria
Transitional epithelium (stratified cuboidal; (detail, p. 38)

Bladder (cross)

Transitional epithelium
Lamina propria
Muscular layers (smooth)
Sphincter (skeletal) muscle
Adventitia

Female urethra (cross)

Male spongy urethra (cross)

Sinus of corp. spongiosum
Pseudostratified epithelium
Venous plexus in lam. propria
Urethral gland
Tunica albuginea
Subcutaneous

THE URINARY ORGANS

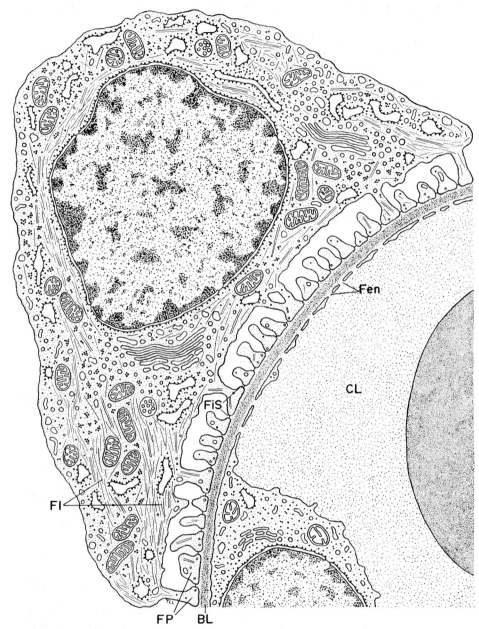

Fen

CL

FiS

Fl

FP   BL

GLOMERULAR CAPSULE DETAIL.   At the right is part of a glomerular capillary whose thin endothelium has multiple fenestrations (Fen); its lumen (CL) contains an erythrocyte. At the left is an epithelial cell of the visceral layer of the glomerular (Bowman's) capsule. Such a podocyte projects many foot-like processes (FP), called pedicels. A narrow gap, or filtration slit (FiS) separates neighboring pedicels, but each gap seems to be bridged by a thin membrane. The cytoplasm contains rough endoplasmic reticulum, free ribosomes, Golgi complexes, mitochondria, vesicles, microtubules and filaments (Fi). A thick basal lamina (BL) is intermediate between the expanded ends of pedicels and endothelium. It is the basal lamina and pedicel slit-membranes that form a filtration barrier between blood plasma and the cavity of the glomerular capsule.

6. Locations of tubule segments.

All uriniferous tubules have their component segments distributed similarly.
The locations of these segments are constant and in definite, recognizable regions.
There are three chief topographical regions in the kidney, each easily identified.
These are: (1) cortical labyrinth; (2) cortical ray; (3) medulla.
In each region, three different tubular segments can be recognized easily.
These prominent and important parts are marked by asterisks in the list.

A. CORTICAL LABYRINTH.
*Glomerular capsule (of Bowman).
Neck.
*Proximal tubule (convoluted portion).
Ascending, thick segment of Henle's loop (terminal portion).
*Distal tubule (convoluted portion).
Arched collecting tubule.

B. CORTICAL RAY.
*Proximal tubule (straight portion); descending, thick segment of Henle's loop.
*Ascending, thick segment of Henle's loop (main portion).
*Collecting tubule.

C. MEDULLA.
Proximal tubule (straight portion); descending, thick segment of Henle's loop.
(Limited to boundary zone, adjacent to cortex.)
*Thin segment of Henle's loop.
*Ascending, thick segment of Henle's loop (proximal portion).
*Collecting tubule; papillary duct.

7. Blood vessels.

The blood supply is rich; one-fifth of all blood traverses the kidneys each minute.
The various vessels, with special names, are successive portions of vascular trees.

A. ARTERIES.
Interlobar arteries branch off the renal artery and pass up between pyramids.
Each becomes an *arcuate artery* as it bends horizontally to form a short arch.
These lie in the plane of junction of cortex and medulla.
Each gives off vertical branches, named *interlobular arteries.*
An *interlobular artery* ascends radially in the axis of each labyrinth.
These vessels serve to stake off the edges of functional renal lobules.
Some terminal branches supply the capsule, and the cortex just beneath.
Most of the interlobular twigs become *glomerular arterioles* (afferent; efferent).
Afferent and efferent vessels are connected by several 'capillary loops.'
The tunica media of the *afferent arteriole*, near its entrance, is modified.
Its substitute cells are large, pale-staining and lack myofibrils.
These epithelioid cells contain granules subject to variation in number.
This myo-epithelial cuff is one-half of the *juxtaglomerular apparatus.*
It is closely associated with the macula densa of the distal tubule (p. 256).
The *efferent arteriole* has a smaller lumen than the afferent arteriole.
This inequality serves to promote filtration pressure in the glomerulus.
Arteriolae rectae arise from glomerular efferents, located near the medulla.
They dip into the medulla and vascularize it.
Renal arteries tend to be 'end arteries,' the sole supply of regions served.
If occluded, such an affected region suffers acutely from lack of blood.

B. CAPILLARIES.
Capillary plexuses surround the tubules of both the cortex and medulla.
Their supply is from the efferent arterioles of glomeruli.
Their endothelium is perforated with pores, as in the glomerulus (p. 254).
All blood to the glandular tissue has first passed through glomeruli.
Probably each set of convoluted tubules receives the blood that just previously
passed through its own glomerulus and left by the efferent arteriole.

In the cortical rays the blood comes from the nearest glomerular efferents.
The pyramids are supplied by the arteriolae rectae.

C. VEINS.

Stellate veins lie beneath the capsule and drain into interlobular veins.
Interlobular veins course medullaward in company with interlobular arteries.
They receive blood from the capillary bed of the cortex in general.
Arcuate veins parallel the course of corresponding arteries.
They receive the interlobular veins.
Venulae rectae drain the medulla and join the arcuate veins directly.
Hence these vessels have relations quite different from arteriolae rectae.
Interlobar veins course alongside the pyramids and make their exits.

8. Lymphatics.

There are networks in the capsule that join those of adjacent organs.
Another set is related to the uriniferous tubules and associated blood vessels.
These lymphatics accompany the vessels and leave the kidney at the hilus.

9. Nerves.

Both sensory and motor fibers accompany the blood vessels and innervate them.
Fibers to the tubules have also been described by some workers.

D. REGENERATIVE ABILITY:

Renal epithelium, especially that of the proximal tubule, can repair injuries.
After bichloride poisoning, multinucleate masses of cytoplasm appear in this tubule.
Within 10 more days, normal structure and function may be restored.
Regeneration is restricted to the replacement of cells dying by disease or aging.
Parts of nephrons can be replaced by new cells, but no new nephrons are formed.
Total nephron loss is compensated for effectively by the hypertrophy of other tubules.
Cells enlarge and become highly efficient in increasing functional activity.
Experimentally, removal of 80 per cent of the kidneys is compatible with survival.

E. DIAGNOSTIC FEATURES:

The kidney is the only compound gland highly deficient in connective tissue.
The *renal corpuscle* is a specific diagnostic feature, easily recognized.
Regions of a kidney, cut in any *radial plane*, show cortex and medulla.
The *cortex* contains alternate, parallel regions that differ in appearance.
The convoluted portion has renal corpuscles and irregularly cut tubules.
The rays consist of parallel tubules, cut lengthwise.
The *medulla* contains parallel tubules throughout its extent.
These show a fan-shaped spreading from the papilla of a pyramid to its base.
All the tubules are cut nearly lengthwise.
Regions cut *transversely* (*i.e.*, tangential to kidney curvature) have two appearances.
They show either cortex or medulla, depending on the level of section.
The *cortex* contains two different kinds of lesser regions.
A convoluted area is a continuous field of renal corpuscles and irregular tubules.
The rays are groups of tubules, cut transversely, surrounded by a convoluted field.
The *medulla* contains tubules, all cut transversely; collecting tubules are prominent.
Because of the curvature a total section may show regional differences.
Centrally the plane is transverse; peripherally it is somewhat radial.
The labyrinth, rays and medulla contain three main components each.
The three in such a territory are diagnosed by epithelial characteristics.

F. FUNCTIONAL CORRELATIONS:

The kidney does not secrete like other glands, but serves more as a filter.
This helps to maintain the composition, pH, and osmotic pressure of blood.

A chief function is to eliminate body wastes and foreign matter from the blood.
(A notable exception is carbon dioxide, which is eliminated mostly from the lungs.)
Also blood-volume is kept constant and its constituents maintain normal values.
Regional differences in nephron structure reflect differences in function.

1. Capsule function.

The *renal corpuscle* is a filtration apparatus that rests at intervals.
Blood pressure in glomerular capillaries provides the required filtration-energy.
The path of the blood-plasma filtrate is: capillary lumen→capillary pores→basal
lamina→pedicel-gap membrane→lumen of glomerular capsule.
The basal lamina and pedicel membrane are the two barriers to large molecules.
Capsular urine is essentially identical with plasma, less its large proteins and fats.
The method of filtration is held to be a passive physical process, overcoming resistance.
About 200 liters of fluid pass daily into the Bowman's capsules (140 ml./min.).
This is about 10 per cent of the amount of blood that flows through the kidneys.
The final concentrate of about one liter is greatly altered in composition.

2. Tubule functions.

The *proximal tubule* is characterized by vital cell activity (not simple diffusion).
Resorption removes glucose and amino acids, and most of the water and inorganic ions.
Urea and other useless catabolic products remain in the urine mostly or wholly.
Secretion introduces certain organic acids and organic bases into the urine.
The urine, reaching the thin segment of the loop, remains isosmotic to blood.
In *Henle's loop* passive diffusion produces different effects in the two limbs.
In the thin descending limb water is removed and sodium added.
This results in the urine becoming hypertonic.
In the thick, ascending limb sodium is lost; the urine becomes hypotonic.
In the *distal convoluted tubule* active transport again takes place.
More sodium is lost; it is replaced with potassium, hydrogen and ammonia.
This is the primary site of acidification.
Some water is passively lost in the presence of the antidiuretic hormone.
The urine, however, remains hypotonic to blood plasma.
The *collecting tubules* determine the final high concentration of urine.
Water is passively removed because the epithelium becomes permeable.
It does so in the presence of the antidiuretic hormone.
An activity of the *juxtaglomerular apparatus* is becoming established.
Its relation to *renin*, a secretion inducing vasoconstriction, is demonstrable.

II. THE RENAL PELVIS, URETER AND URINARY BLADDER

A. STRUCTURAL PLAN:

The *hilus* of the kidney is a slit-like orifice, opening into an expanded *renal sinus*.
The sinus is a capacious flattened cavity, filled with various things.
Chief of importance is the *renal pelvis*, or expanded ureter, and its branches.
Other components are vessels, nerves, fat and connective tissue.
The pelvis subdivides into 2 or 3 *major calyces*, and these into 7 to 14 *minor calyces*.
A minor calyx is a tube, infolded to form a double-walled cup.
The inner wall fits over the projecting tip (papilla) of a pyramid.
Its epithelium is continuous with that of the numerous papillary ducts.
The *ureters* are paired tubes, about 12 inches long, that course behind the peritoneum.
They connect the renal pelvis with the *urinary bladder,* also retroperitoneal.
All these parts are conventionally constructed, hollow organs.
They have much the same basic structure and can be treated as a unit.
Quantitatively their walls increase in thickness from above downward.
Along with the urethra, they serve as excretory passages to the exterior.

B. DETAILED STRUCTURE:

1. Mucosa.

The lining *epithelium* is stratified—the so-called transitional type.

In the calyx its cells make 2 to 3 layers; in the ureter, 4 to 5; in the bladder, 6 to 8.

The exact appearance and thickness vary with stretching, due to organ-distention.

In an empty bladder the cells range from rounded to club-shape.

Under distention the cells become thin and seem to reduce to 2 or 3 layers.

Actually the cells stretch and thin, and also may 'slip by'.

In general, *glands* are lacking except in the vicinity of the urethral orifice.

Here occur some small ingrowths, resembling urethral glands (see beyond).

There is a delicate *basement membrane*, not seen with the light microscope.

Because of this, capillaries may seem to indent the lower epithelial surface.

The *lamina propria* consists of thin fibers, mostly collagenous.

Prominent papillae do not indent the epithelium, as in highly stratified types.

Hence the junction between epithelium and lamina propria is quite even.

Nevertheless, thin folds, bearing capillaries, may indent the epithelium.

Diffuse lymphoid tissue and occasional *solitary nodules* sometimes occur.

2. Submucosa.

A clearly demarcated *submucosal layer*, like that of various organs, does not exist.

For this reason many refuse to recognize the presence of a submucosa.

Yet the deeper layers are looser, more elastic and could be so considered.

This laxity permits longitudinal *folding* of the lamina propria of the ureter-bladder.

In the *ureter* about five major and minor folds are characteristic.

This gives a regular, stellate pattern to the transversely cut lumen.

In the relaxed *bladder* the mucosa is thrown into thick, irregular folds.

3. Muscularis.

The *muscular tunic* contains 2 to 3 loosely arranged and rather ill-defined layers.

The smooth muscle occurs in discrete *bundles*, separated by connective tissue.

The inner layer is arranged longitudinally; the layer next outside, circularly.

In addition, the lower third of the *ureter* and all of the *bladder* have a third, outermost coat whose muscle is arranged longitudinally.

In the *pelvis* and *calyces* the muscle is thin and largely circular.

About each papilla there is a sort of sphincter.

In the *bladder* the muscular coat is robust and the bundles interlace.

The three layers are not sharply separable as such; the middle layer is thickest.

At the urethral orifice the circular muscle is densely arranged in thin bundles.

This constitutes the *internal sphincter* of the bladder.

4. Adventitia.

The fibrous, external tunic blends with the surrounding connective tissue.

In the *renal pelvis* it becomes continuous with the capsule of the kidney.

The *ureter* lies outside the peritoneum.

The superior surface only of the *bladder* is covered with peritoneum.

Hence the outer tunic becomes a *serosa* in this restricted region.

5. Vessels and nerves.

Blood vessels run in the adventitia; they supply the muscularis, form a plexus in the submucosa and another plexus beneath the epithelium.

Lymphatics also gather into plexuses in the submucosa and muscularis.

In the bladder they are said to occur in the muscularis only.

Nerves form a plexus, with ganglia, in the adventitia.

Motor nerves supply the muscularis.

Sensory nerves extend through the mucosa and into the epithelium.

C. Regenerative Ability:

Gaps in the epithelial lining heal readily from the edges of the wound.
Injury-defects in the muscle are replaced by scar tissue.

D. Diagnostic Features:

So-called *transitional epithelium* is a specific feature of the pelvis, ureter and bladder.
Glands are lacking, except for a few at the bladder outlet.
The *muscular layers* consist of bundles, rather than closely knit sheets.
The innermost layer is longitudinal smooth muscle.
Next there is a circular layer of smooth muscle.
An outermost, longitudinal layer occurs in the lower ureter and bladder.
The *ureter* is a small tube with a rather symmetrical, stellate lumen.
The radial arms of the lumen usually branch at their ends.
The *bladder* is a large organ, and only sections from sample blocks are seen.
It has a thick wall, heavy muscularis and an irregularly folded mucosa.
Sections usually are cut from randomly oriented blocks of bladder-wall.
This makes the direction of the muscle coats seem variable.

E. Functional Correlations:

Urine comes from the papillary ducts at the rate of 15 drops a minute.
The *calyces* are said to show milking movements, allegedly to aid the passage of urine.
Similarly, the ureter exhibits rhythmically peristaltic movements, downward.
The *ureters* pierce the wall of the bladder obliquely, pursuing an intramural course.
Their lumina in these regions tend to be closed by pressure of the bladder contents.
This prevents backflow of urine.
Also a flanking fold of the bladder mucosa acts as a guarding valve.
Epithelium and longitudinal muscle constitute the only wall of the intramural ureter.
Contraction of this muscle opens the lumen of the ureter for downward flow.
The *bladder* is a reservoir for temporary urinary storage; its normal capacity is one pint. 250 cm
There is little evidence of absorption (except for bloating of the superficial cells).
A stratified epithelium serves as a barrier against the hypertonic urine.
This prevents further exchanges between the blood and urine.
The plastic and elastic transitional epithelium is well adapted to changing demands.

III. THE URETHRA

A. Female Urethra:

This terminal segment of the urinary tract is a short duct, about 1.5 inches long.
It extends from the bladder to its outlet into the vestibule.

1. Mucosa.

The *epithelium* near the bladder is transitional stratified.
Next comes a longer segment with considerable stratified squamous.
Some areas in it are pseudostratified; others are stratified columnar. ← H†m 77 ?
Finally, near the outlet, there is stratified squamous epithelium.
Occasional nests of mucous cells occur within the epithelium.
Also there are some small diverticula containing mucous cells.
These *urethral glands* are more numerous in the male urethra (see beyond).
The epithelium rests upon an inconspicuous *basement membrane*.
The *lamina propria* lacks papillae, but is folded longitudinally.
This gives the lumen an irregular, crescentic shape.

2. Submucosa.

A deeper stratum, rich in elastic fibers and veins, could be considered a *submucosa*.
Many, however, interpret this layer as belonging to the lamina propria.

The veins constitute a plexus of prominent, thin-walled channels.

They represent a sort of spongy, *semi-erectile tissue*.

3. Muscularis.

There is a rather thick coat of *smooth muscle*.

The inner layer is arranged longitudinally.

There is considerable intermingling with the venous plexuses of the submucosa.

The outer layer is arranged circularly.

At the neck of the bladder it condenses, forming an *involuntary sphincter*.

Bundles of circular *skeletal fibers* occur outside the smooth fibers.

This voluntary muscle is the *constrictor urethrae*.

It is deficient on the posterior surface (facing the vagina).

At the lower end of the urethra it forms a *voluntary sphincter*.

4. Adventitia.

This coat is indefinite because of fusions with surrounding structures.

Dorsally there is merging with the fibrous coat of the vagina.

Elsewhere the muscular coat and neighboring constrictor urethrae muscles adjoin.

B. MALE URETHRA:

This tube is 8 inches long; only its stem is homologous to the female urethra.

This is because the segment below the urethral crest serves also as a genital duct.

Here it corresponds to the urogenital sinus (permanent vestibule of females).

It has three regional segments, with different neighboring relations.

The *prostatic urethra*, next to the bladder, is only 1.5 inches long.

It bears the elevated urethral crest on its posterior wall.

The prostatic utricle and paired ejaculatory ducts open onto this crest.

The *prostate gland* surrounds and discharges into this segment of the urethra.

The *membranous urethra*, between the prostate and penis, is 0.5 inch long.

It is surrounded by muscles and other components of the urogenital diaphragm.

The *cavernous urethra* (or *spongy urethra*) extends for 6 inches through the penis.

1. Mucosa.

The *epithelium* varies regionally; also the distribution shows individual variations.

Near the bladder it is transitional in type.

Most of the remainder is variably pseudostratified or stratified columnar.

Near the meatus it becomes stratified squamous.

Intra-epithelial *glands* (*i.e.*, nests of mucous cells) are common.

The epithelium rests on a thin *basement membrane*.

The *lamina propria* resembles that of the female urethra, already described.

Branching mucous tubules extend into the lamina propria, and even deeper.

They are *urethral glands* (of Littré), best developed in the cavernous urethra.

Their ducts contain intra-epithelial nests or pockets of mucous cells.

They open into local recesses of the lumen, produced by epithelial pocketings.

2. Submucosa.

A well defined *submucosa* is not distinguishable as such.

As in the female, there is a deeper layer containing many veins.

The entire cavernous urethra is ensheathed by true *erectile tissue* (corpus spongiosum).

It is customarily considered as a part of the penis proper.

That is, it is not a specialized submucosa of the urethra.

3. Muscularis.

A *muscular tunic* occurs chiefly in the prostatic and membranous segments.

The inner layer of smooth muscle is arranged longitudinally.

The outer layer of smooth muscle is arranged circularly.

It is best developed at the neck of the bladder, forming a *sphincter* there.

Except proximally, the cavernous segment lacks typical smooth-muscle layers.
(Instead, longitudinal muscle is distributed in the true erectile tissue.)

4. Adventitia.

There is no typical *adventitial tunic*.
The prostatic urethra is surrounded by the tissue of the prostate gland.
The membranous urethra is encircled by a sphincter of skeletal muscle belonging to
the deep transverse perineal muscle.
The cavernous urethra is surrounded by erectile tissue and a dense outer sheath.
Neither is considered as belonging to the urethra itself.

C. Vessels and Nerves:

The general pattern is similar to that described on p. 260.

D. Diagnostic Features:

The *epithelium* changes from level to level, and is variable at some levels.
Represented are transitional, pseudostratified, stratified columnar and squamous.
Diverticula with mucous cells (urethral glands) are characteristic features.
The *lamina propria* is notable for its prominent venous spaces.
The *muscle arrangement* is: inner layer, longitudinal; outer layer, circular.
(The male prostatic and cavernous urethrae lack muscle layers, as such.)
The *female urethra* throughout has a heavier musculature than the male.
It can be confused only with the male membranous urethra (see below).
The male *prostatic urethra* is surrounded by that gland, and hence is distinctive.
The projecting urethral crest gives the lumen a crescentic shape.
The male *membranous urethra* resembles the female urethra closely.
However, its lumen tends to be stellate, not crescentic as in the female.
Both abut peripherally on adjacent skeletal muscle.
The male *cavernous urethra* is surrounded by cavernous erectile tissue.
This segment of the urethra is included within the penis as a component of that organ.

E. Functional Correlations:

The *female urethra* is exclusively a urinary drainage duct from the bladder.
Only the stem of the *male urethra* is similarly an exclusive urinary duct.
The remainder (membranous; cavernous), therefore, is a joint urinary and genital canal.
It is a permanent retention of the embryonic urogenital sinus.
The secretion of the urethral glands is lubricative only.

Chapter XXIII

The Male Reproductive System

The male reproductive organs include the following parts:

The *testes*, or male sex glands.

The *ducts* of the testes, and the *auxiliary glands* associated with them.

The *penis*, or copulative organ.

I. THE TESTIS

The *testis* is functionally a double gland.

Its exocrine product is chiefly the sex cells; hence it is a *cytogenic gland.*

An internal secretion is elaborated by certain cells; hence it is also an *endocrine gland.*

A. STRUCTURAL PLAN:

The *testis* is an ovoid gland, about 1.8 inches long.

It is surrounded by a thick capsule, the *tunica albuginea.*

Along the posterior border the capsule projects inward, like a ridge.

This thickened, inturned crest is named the *mediastinum testis.*

Thin, fibrous partitions (*septula*) radiate from the mediastinum to the capsule proper.

The compartments, thus formed, are wedge-shaped lobules (*lobuli testis*).

Within the lobules are located the contorted *seminiferous tubules.*

These lie in a bed of loose connective tissue, containing groups of *interstitial cells.*

B. DETAILED STRUCTURE:

1. Framework.

The *tunica albuginea* is a thick, tough capsule that encases the testis.

It is composed of dense fibro-elastic tissue, and appears white in life.

The innermost layer is the *tunica vasculosa;* it is looser and more vascular.

Along the posterior margin of the testis is the thickened *mediastinum testis.*

It corresponds to a hilus region; ducts, vessels and nerves connect here.

The *septula testis* are thin fibrous partitions, incomplete and branching.

These radiate from the crest-like mediastinum to the inner surface of the capsule.

They divide the testis into about 250 compartments, or *testis lobules.*

Each lobule is a pyramidal mass, with its apex toward the mediastinum.

Since the septula are incomplete partitions, the lobules communicate in places.

(Within the lobules are seminiferous tubules, embedded in a fibrous stroma.)

Each seminiferous tubule is surrounded by a layered *sheath* of fibrous tissue.

This is a local condensation of the general connective tissue within a lobule.

The connective-tissue *stroma* occupies the angular spaces between tubules.

This material is a soft loose tissue, containing fine collagenous fibers.

It also contains vessels, nerves and several types of cells.

Most interesting are the specific *interstitial cells*, or 'cells of Leydig.'

These are large ovoid cells, usually occurring in groups.

Their rounded chromatic nucleus contains one or two prominent nucleoli.

The acidophilic cytoplasm is rich in inclusions, such as lipid, pigment, etc.

Many cells also contain peculiar rod-shaped *crystalloids* (of Reinke).
These are albuminous bodies, characteristic of the human testis.
There are smooth endoplasmic reticulum and mitochondria with tubular cristae.
Both are characteristic of steroid-producing endocrine glands.
Less differentiated spindle-shaped cells are viewed as replacing stages.

2. Seminiferous tubules.

Each lobule of the testis contains 1 to 4 highly contorted *seminiferous tubules.*
A tubule is 30 to 80 cm. long and about 0.2 mm. wide.
Their combined length in some 500 tubules of a human testis is about 275 yards.
A tubule rarely shows blind side-branches or a blind ending.
Instead, simple or branched tubules join with other tubules into arched loops.
They may even unite, by lateral branches, with tubules of adjoining lobules.
At the apex of a lobule each *contorted tubule* loses its convolutions and becomes a *straight tubule.*
A contorted, seminiferous tubule is lined with a specialized, stratified epithelium.
This is known as the *germinal* or *seminiferous epithelium.*
Most of its cells are sex cells; some others are auxiliary, supporting elements.
The epithelium rests upon a *basement membrane* whose thickness varies with age.
This tubular membrane is surrounded by a layered *sheath* of fibrous tissue.
Centrally the epithelium borders upon an axial lumen.
Not until the prepuberal time do the 'tubules' acquire a definite, central canal.
Some atrophic tubules begin to appear in the third decade of life.

A. SUSTENTACULAR CELLS.
These elements (also called *Sertoli cells*) are supporting and nutritive cells.
Relatively few in number, they are spaced at fairly regular intervals.
Their shape is tall and pillar-like.
The base rests on the basement membrane of the tubule.
The free end extends in a radial direction and reaches the lumen.
The sex cells are crowded between the Sertoli cells and indent them.
As a result, their sides bear branching, wing-like processes.
The cell outline is so irregular and indistinct that it cannot be fully traced.
The *nucleus* is located some distance above the base of the cell.
It is ovoid, pale and radially oriented; its surface is often grooved.
The nucleolus is prominent and of a peculiar, compound type.
There are a chief mass and two accessory masses.
The *cytoplasm* has a reticular appearance in fixed preparations.
It contains fibrils, lipoid droplets and tapering crystalloid bodies.
Spermatids attach to Sertoli cells during their transformation period.
Apparently these supporting elements also serve as nurse cells at this time.
They successfully withstand various influences that destroy the sex cells.

B. SEX CELLS.
The *germ cells* (or sex cells) make up a stratified layer 4 to 8 cells deep.
The cells differentiate progressively, from periphery to lumen, in the tubule.
Proliferation (never amitotic) pushes cells toward the lumen.
Those nearest the lumen transform into spermatozoa.
They detach and become carried away as free cells.
This sequence of events is known as *spermatogenesis;* in man it requires 64 days.
Six major stages in this process are recognized and named.
A cross-section of a tubule at any level shows several of these different stages.
But the particular combination of stages changes at different levels.
This is because the stem-cells proliferate singly and not in groups.

1. *Spermatogonia.*
These cells (12 μ in diameter) lie upon the *basement membrane.*
They are the only sex cells present until the time of puberty.

Human spermatogonia contain 23 pairs of chromosomes (*i.e.,* a double set).

When cells divide, some daughter cells remain as stem-cells.

Others proliferate and differentiate into primary spermatocytes.

2. *Primary spermatocytes.*

These represent spermatogonial cells that are undergoing growth.

They become the largest germ cells seen (18 μ) and have prominent nuclei.

They lie just lumenward of the spermatogonia.

Division of the primary spermatocytes is by a modified mitosis, named *meiosis.*

In this process the nuclei and cytoplasm divide twice; the chromosomes once.

Its characteristic feature is the reduction of the double set of chromosomes, present in the young primary spermatocyte, to a single set of 23.

Before dividing, the individual chromosomes of each pair come into contact.

Each member consists of two spiral filaments, named *chromatids.*

Such a group of four chromatids (in two chromosomes) is a *tetrad.*

On dividing, the individual chromosomes of each tetrad separate bodily.

That is, each member (two chromatids) passes into different daughter cells.

As a result of this reduction, the chromosome-number is halved (46 to 23).

Yet the single set contains one of each kind originally present.

(An exception occurs in the unequal sex-determining pair, p. 267.)

3. *Secondary spermatocytes.*

These are daughter cells of the primary spermatocytes.

They are about two-thirds the size of the primaries and lie nearer the lumen.

Almost as soon as they are formed, they divide and produce *spermatids.*

Hence few of them are seen in a section of a tubule.

This cell division is essentially like that of an ordinary mitosis.

The two chromatids of each chromosome separate and move apart.

Each passes into one daughter cell or the other.

Now only a single set of 23 chromosomes characterizes each cell.

4. *Spermatids.*

These daughter cells of the secondary spermatocytes cease dividing.

They are about 9 μ in diameter and lie close to the lumen.

Spermatids occur as a cluster of eight cells, connected by cytoplasmic bridges.

This is because the final spermatogonial division was incomplete.

5. *Spermiogenesis.*

Next, the spermatids separate and attach to Sertoli cells.

They undergo a drastic transformation into highly atypical cells.

These have a *head, neck, body* and long *tail.*

The nucleus condenses greatly and forms most of the sperm head.

The Golgi apparatus elaborates an *acrosome* at the apex of the head.

A surrounding acrosomal vesicle undergoes collapse.

It spreads over the upper two-thirds of the head as the *head cap.*

The *proximal centriole* locates in the neck, just beneath the head.

The *distal centriole* takes position just tailward of the proximal one.

From it an *axial filament* grows out and becomes the core of the tail.

It is a flagellum, with the same set of filaments as in cilia.

That is, one central pair is surrounded by nine other pairs.

The *distal centriole* disappears, but a mass near it takes form.

This ring, or *annulus,* moves down to the lower end of the sperm's body.

The general cytoplasm supplies a thin investment over the head.

It also extends as a *sheath* along the neck, body and tail.

In the tail it forms a set of coarse fibers about the axial filament.

Mitochondria group about the body as a spiral *mitochondrial sheath.*

The excess of cytoplasm is sloughed off as an unused remnant.

6. *Spermatozoa.*

Mature sperms detach, yet are not commonly seen free in the lumen.

This is because they are carried into the ducts as fast as formed.

Human spermatozoa have a total length of about 60 μ.

The *head* (5 μ) is pear-shaped and flattened.

The short *neck* and longer *body* (5 μ) interconnect the head and tail.

The *tail* (50 μ) is long, extremely slender and vibratile.

3. *Vessels and nerves.*

Blood vessels enter the testis at the mediastinum.

Some supply the tunica vasculosa (the inner layer of the tunica albuginea).

Others follow the septula inward, and form networks about the tubules.

Lymphatics drain the interstitial tissue.

Nerves follow the blood vessels, but endings within the tubules seem doubtful.

C. REGENERATIVE ABILITY:

The testes are incompetent to repair wounds other than by producing scar tissue.

The interstitial cells, nevertheless, can proliferate when the occasion requires.

Sex cells are highly susceptible when subjected to certain environmental conditions.

For example, slightly elevated temperature causes widespread decline and destruction.

Yet recovery can follow a severe decline if normal temperature is restored.

D. DIAGNOSTIC FEATURES:

There are *epithelial tubules*, surrounded by distinct connective-tissue sheaths and embedded in a more or less cellular *stroma*.

The irregularly sectioned tubules take a multiplicity of shapes (C, J, S, etc.).

The *epithelium*, 4 to 8 cells deep, is a specialized stratified cuboidal type.

Actually, the cells are rounded to polyhedral in shape.

Some, next to the lumen, may show transformation stages into spermatozoa.

Prepuberal 'tubules' are mostly solid; sustentacular (Sertoli) cells dominate the field.

Senile tubules vary, but typically show atrophy and a reduction or loss of sex cells.

Yet some aged individuals may have quite normal appearing testes.

E. FUNCTIONAL CORRELATIONS:

The *exocrine function* of the testis is to produce male sex cells.

For this reason it is a type of cytogenic gland.

Spermatogenesis and the differentiation into spermatozoa depend on several factors.

A *hormone (FSH)* of the hypophysis is a stimulating, necessary agent.

Vitamins (especially E) are also indispensable.

A suitable *temperature* is critical; such is furnished by the scrotum.

This has to be slightly lower (1.5 to 2.5° C.) than that in the abdominal cavity.

In man, *spermatogenesis* is a continuous process, all stages not showing at the same level.

In some individuals it may continue even into extreme old age.

Local tubules, especially after age 35, show signs of atrophy.

Furthermore, in illness there may be temporary regressive changes.

Spermatozoa are adapted to swimming and penetration of the relatively huge egg.

The nucleus has been condensed to the limit imposed by close chromosome packing.

Cytoplasm has been reduced to the minimum consistent with flagellate swimming.

The locomotor apparatus is 92 per cent of the total length of the cell.

The effective and important contributions to a new individual are thus limited to chromosomes and, seemingly, the centriole.

The *sex-determining role* of spermatozoa is correlated with two types that are produced.

Half of the secondary spermatocytes acquire a female-determining chromosome (X).

An equal number acquire a smaller male-determining chromosome (Y).

One or the other then continues into each spermatid and spermatozoön.

This is the only chromosome-pair whose members are wholly unlike.

The chief *endocrine secretion* of the testis is a steroid hormone, *testosterone*.

The weight of evidence favors the interstitial cells as the source of this hormone.

Testosterone controls secondary sex characters, the sex impulse and the proper maintenance of the genital ducts and accessory glands.

Its production depends on stimulation by the LH (or ICSH) hormone of the hypophysis.

Castration before puberty results in the nondevelopment of secondary sex characters.

Castration after puberty results in some retrograde changes (*eunuchism*).

II. THE SCROTUM

The *scrotum* is a divided pouch of the integument, each compartment containing a testis.

It was invaded by the testes, which migrated from an original abdominal position.

1. Structure.

The *scrotum* is specialized integument, somewhat modified from ordinary skin.

The *epidermis* is changeable in thickness, as the scrotum is lax or contracted.

It is also more pigmented than that of the body in general.

The *dermis* contains sparse hair follicles and large sebaceous and sweat glands.

The *subcutaneous* has a thick layer of smooth muscle that comprises the *dartos tunic*.

It also is notable for the absence of fat cells.

The twin cavities of the scrotum were produced by the invasion of two peritoneal sacs.

These serosal extensions pushed into the subcutaneous tissue in late fetal life.

They then detached from the general peritoneum and became closed sacs.

Such a serosal sac is named the *tunica vaginalis*.

Its *parietal layer* makes a lining to the scrotal wall and its dividing septum.

Its *visceral layer* is reflected over three-fourths of the testis and epididymis.

The surface mesothelium corresponds to the germinal epithelium of an embryo.

Both layers become continuous along the posterior, attached border of the testis.

2. Diagnostic features.

The scrotum, penis and areola mammae have integument of the same specialized type.

Differences in pigmentation, glands and muscle content are largely quantitative only.

3. Functional correlations.

Each vaginal sac contains enough serous fluid to afford its walls frictionless play.

The tissue anchoring the testis still allows it considerable freedom of movement.

The muscle-content of the scrotal wall responds to temperature conditions.

The scrotum contracts when cold and relaxes when warm.

This makes the testes hug the body closely or become pendulous, respectively.

The scrotum acts as a thermoregulator, which is an adaptation, since sex cells are susceptible to injury by a temperature equaling that of the interior body.

The muscular dartos tunic is responsible for the *dartos reflex*.

This is a writhing movement of the general scrotal wall when it is stroked locally.

III. THE MALE GENITAL DUCTS

The *male ducts* differ structurally at seven levels along their course.

For this reason they have been given different regional names.

A. TUBULI RECTI:

At the apex of a lobule each seminiferous tubule becomes a single, short *straight tubule*.

The diameter of the duct narrows to about 25 μ.

Only the sustentacular (Sertoli) cells remain, arranged as a simple epithelium.

The component cells are columnar or cuboidal elements with fatty inclusions.

B. RETE TESTIS:

The straight ducts open into a network of canals within the mediastinum.
> These are irregular, anastomosing channels of variable breadth.

Their lining is a *simple epithelium*, cuboidal to columnar in shape.
> Some cells bear a single flagellum.
> There is a delicate *basement membrane*, but no specific lamina propria.
> That is, the epithelium lines clefts in the fibrous stroma of the mediastinum.

C. DUCTULI EFFERENTES:

About 10 to 15 *efferent ductules* emerge from the upper part of the rete testis.
> Each forms a spirally wound *lobule of the epididymis*, conical in shape.
> Each ductule is about 3 inches long, when straightened, and 0.2 to 0.4 mm. in diameter.
> The several lobules comprise most of a mass named the *head of the epididymis*.

The individual tubules are embedded in connective tissue, and are surrounded by a very thin layer of smooth-muscle fibers, circularly arranged.

The *epithelium* is mostly simple columnar, but it varies in a characteristic pattern.
> Externally the tubule has a fairly smooth contour.
> Internally it is indented by closely spaced pits.
> > This is owing to the presence of much shorter cells in these local areas.

> Tall cells make a lining for the general lumen.
> > Some of these are ciliated; others bear microvilli.
> > The finely granular cytoplasm is acidophilic.
> > > It contains fat droplets and pigment granules.

> The shorter cells form cup-like pits; these are *intra-epithelial glands*.
> > The cytoplasm is clear, pale and contains pigment granules.
> > Some of these cells may bear cilia also.

The *cilia* of both cell-types beat toward the epididymis and move spermatozoa along.
> These are the only motile cilia in the entire duct system.

Both the nonciliated tall- and short cells are said to be *secretory*.
> Blebs of secretion sometimes adhere to their free surfaces.
> In addition, there are a few rounded, basal cells that do not reach the lumen.

The epithelium rests upon a distinct *basement membrane*.

The winding tubules, at their ends, change gradually into the epithelium of the epididymis and join individually with that duct.

D. DUCTUS EPIDIDYMIDIS:

A compact mass, the *epididymis*, stretches along the posterior side of the testis.

A single, coiled duct courses throughout the extent of this mass.
> It is the *duct of the epididymis*, often called by the last of these names alone.

In the upper part (head) of the epididymis the duct receives the efferent ductules.
> In the middle and lower regions ('body' and 'tail') only the coiled duct is present.

The total duct is highly tortuous, nearly 20 ft. long and about 0.4 mm. wide.

The duct has a smooth cylindrical outline, inside and out.
> The *epithelium* is thicker than in the efferent ductules, and is uniform in thickness.
> The duct is surrounded by a definite *basement membrane* and a thin layer of circular *smooth muscle;* it lies embedded in a fibrous stroma.

The *epithelium* is pseudostratified; it contains basal cells and tall columnar cells.
> The rounded basal cells contain fatty droplets.
> The tall cells contain secretion droplets, granules, vacuoles and pigment.
> > At the apex there is a pencil of nonmotile (often clumped) cytoplasmic processes.
> > Although long named *stereocilia,* they are extremely long (30 μ) microvilli.

E. DUCTUS DEFERENS:

The duct of the epididymis enlarges into the *deferent duct*, which soon straightens.
> It traverses the inguinal canal and courses behind the peritoneum toward the urethra.

This is a typically organized tubular organ, about 18 inches long and 2 to 3 mm. wide.
The wall is relatively very thick and the lumen relatively narrow.
In the scrotum and inguinal canal the ductus deferens courses within the *spermatic cord*.
It is easily palpable through the scrotum and the soft cord.
Other contents of the spermatic cord are the following:
Testicular artery and the pampiniform system of veins.
Lymph vessels and nerves of the testis and epididymis.
Fascias and the striated *cremaster muscle* enclose the spermatic cord.
The muscle is responsible for the *cremasteric reflex* when the thigh is stroked.
Leaving the cord, the duct courses behind the pelvic peritoneum toward the urethra.
It ends in a short dilated segment, near the prostate, known as the *ampulla*.

1. Mucosa.

The *epithelium* is pseudostratified; many of the tall cells bear *stereocilia*.
It is essentially like the epithelium of the duct of the epididymis.
There is a delicate *basement membrane* and a thin *lamina propria*.
The latter contains many elastic fibers.
The mucosa is thrown into 4 to 6 longitudinal folds.
In transverse section the lumen is, therefore, stellate.

2. Submucosa.

There is no definite *submucosal layer* although the deeper level of the lamina propria
contains numerous blood vessels.

3. Muscularis.

The *muscular coat* is very heavy; on palpation it gives the duct a cord-like feel.
It is thickest in the pelvic part of its course.
The inner layer is a relatively thin sheet of longitudinal smooth muscle.
The middle, circular layer is strongly developed.
It is loosely arranged, and longitudinal bundles intermingle with it.
This layer is especially well represented in the pelvic course of the duct.
The outer longitudinal layer is also robust.

4. Adventitia.

The fibrous *external tunic* is typical, blending with adjoining tissues.

F. Ampulla of Ductus Deferens:

Terminally the duct dilates into an irregular spindle-shaped tube, the *ampulla*.
Here the lumen is larger and the mucosa much more folded.
Thin *mucosal folds* branch and anastomose, thereby producing pocket-like *recesses*.
From these recesses, occasional outpocketings invade the muscularis.
The appearance resembles somewhat the arrangement in the seminal vesicle (p. 272).
The simple columnar *epithelium* gives indications of secretion.
The *muscularis* shows much interlacing of circular and longitudinal bundles.
It is the external longitudinal layer that retains its identity best.

G. Ejaculatory Duct:

This is the short (0.8 inch), slender, terminal segment of each male genital duct.
It appears as if it were formed by the union of the ampulla and seminal vesicle.
The duct pierces the prostate gland and opens into the urethra on the urethral crest.
The *mucosa* is highly folded, much like that of the ampulla.
The simple columnar to pseudostratified *epithelium* is apparently secretory.
Some mucosal outpocketings occur, like those from the recesses of the ampulla.
Except at the upper end, the *supporting wall* consists of fibrous tissue alone.
In the terminal portion cavernous vascular spaces occur, as in the urethra.

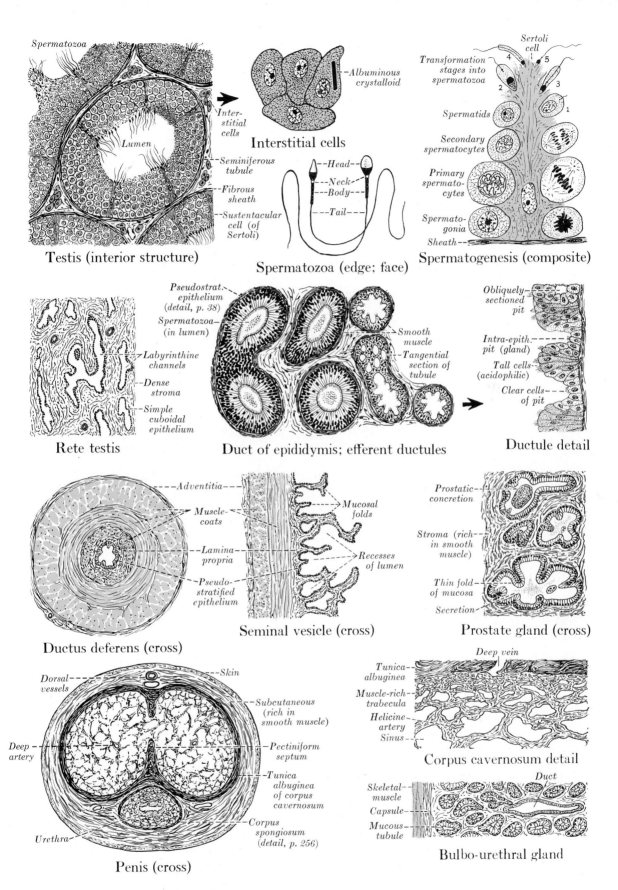

Spermatozoa

–Albuminous crystalloid

Inter-stitial cells

Interstitial cells

–Head–
–Neck–
–Body–
–Tail–

Inter-stitial cells
Lumen
–Seminiferous tubule
–Fibrous sheath
–Sustentacular cell (of Sertoli)

Testis (interior structure)

Spermatozoa (edge; face)

Sertoli cell
Transformation stages into spermatozoa
Spermatids
Secondary spermatocytes
Primary spermato-cytes
Spermato-gonia
Sheath–

Spermatogenesis (composite)

Pseudostrat. epithelium (detail, p. 38)
Spermatozoa (in lumen)

–Smooth muscle
–Tangential section of tubule

–Labyrinthine channels
–Dense stroma
–Simple cuboidal epithelium

Obliquely-sectioned pit
Intra-epith.-pit (gland)
Tall cells-(acidophilic)
Clear cells-of pit

Rete testis

Duct of epididymis; efferent ductules

Ductule detail

–Adventitia–
–Muscle-coats
–Lamina propria
–Pseudo-stratified epithelium

→Mucosal folds
→Recesses of lumen

Prostatic-concretion
Stroma (rich in smooth muscle)
Thin fold-of mucosa
Secretion–

Ductus deferens (cross)

Seminal vesicle (cross)

Prostate gland (cross)

Dorsal--vessels
–Skin
–Subcutaneous (rich in smooth muscle)
–Pectiniform septum
Deep-artery
–Tunica albuginea of corpus cavernosum
Urethra–
–Corpus spongiosum (detail, p. 256)

Deep vein
Tunica-albuginea
Muscle-rich--trabecula
Helicine-artery
Sinus

Corpus cavernosum detail

Duct
Skeletal-muscle
Capsule–
Mucous-tubule

Penis (cross)

Bulbo-urethral gland

THE MALE REPRODUCTIVE ORGANS

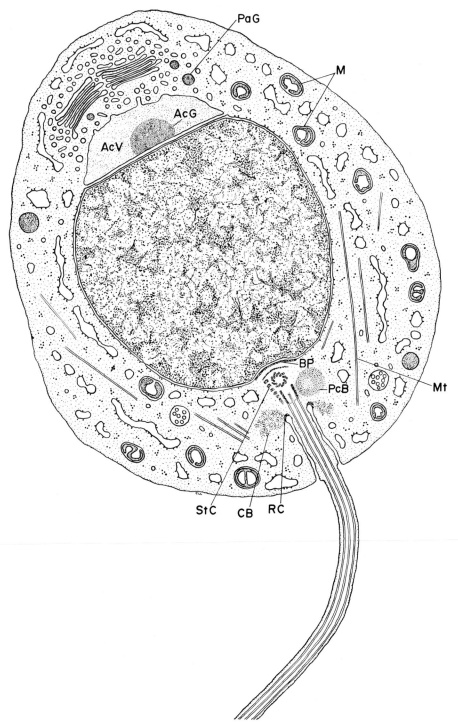

SPERMATID. The cytoplasm of a transforming spermatid shows various specializing organelles. Mitochondria (M) are atypical; microtubules (Mt) are prominent, as is the apically located Golgi complex. Associated with the Golgi are membrane-bounded proacrosomal granules (PaG) which coalesce and form a large, dense acrosomal granule (AcG). This granule is contained within a highly dilated acrosomal vesicle (AcV), applied to the apical pole of the nucleus. At the opposite pole of the nucleus is a centriole, cut lengthwise, that is giving rise to a long flagellum. Nearer the nucleus is another centriole, cut transversely, in close relation to a dense basal plate (BP) applied to the nuclear membrane. Flanking this centriole are striated columns (StC) and a paracentriolar body (PcB). A chromatoid body (CB), closely associated with a reflection of the plasma membrane (RC) will produce the ring, or annulus.

H. Vessels and Nerves:

These auxiliaries are distributed according to the general plan described on p. 260.

I. Diagnostic Features:

The rete testis, efferent ductules and epididymis are all embedded in a fibrous stroma.
  None has a conspicuous muscular layer.
The *rete testis* appears as a localized set of irregular-calibered, *communicating channels.*
  The channels are well spaced in a bed of dense fibrous tissue.
  Their *epithelium* varies from simple cuboidal to a columnar type.
The *efferent ductules* are tortuous tubules that become sectioned in various planes.
  They are characterized by a unique type of *epithelium*, containing intra-epithelial pits.
  Externally the cell bases produce a fairly even contour.
  Internally the contour is uneven, showing in sections as a scalloped lumen.
    These *crests* and *troughs* are produced by alternate groups of tall and short cells.
      Some cells are ciliated; others show secretory blebs.
The *epididymis* is a fatter, winding duct, sectioned many times and in various planes.
  Its epithelium is not variable; its external and internal contour are both even.
    Transverse sections show as regular, *washer-shaped bands.*
  The *epithelium* consists of tall, falsely ciliated cells and rounded basal cells.
    The half of the epithelial cells bordering the lumen is free of nuclei.
  Spermatozoa, stored in the lumen, can be expected in normal postpuberal ducts.
The *ductus deferens* has a wall that is very thick in comparison to lumen size.
  The *epithelium* resembles that of the epididymis.
    However, it is folded so as to produce a stellate lumen (in transverse section).
  The muscular coat is exceptionally thick, showing three layers.
    The inner and outer layers are longitudinal; the middle layer, circular.
The *ampulla* of the ductus deferens has complicated, thin mucosal folds.
  The epithelium is simple columnar.
  Its relatively thinner muscularis shows a markedly irregular arrangement.
    Longitudinal and circular bundles intermingle.
The *ejaculatory duct* has a mucosa resembling that of the ampulla.
  The tube lacks a muscular coat and is supported by fibrous tissue alone.
  Most of it courses within prostatic tissue.

J. Functional Correlations:

This system of ducts *transports* and *stores* spermatozoa.
Nonmotile spermatozoa pass through the *straight tubules* and *rete testis.*
  Fluid, secreted by the testis, washes them along; cilia are lacking.
  They traverse these passages quickly, so are rarely seen in sections.
The cilia of the *efferent ductules* are functional.
  Presumably they aid muscular action in moving spermatozoa to the epididymis.
The *epididymis* is a long storage duct, through which spermatozoa pass slowly.
  Progress is passive; the journey may take as long as six weeks.
  Here, also, spermatozoa ripen and acquire optimal fertilizability.
    At the same time, they become capable of motility, but remain immobile.
  The thick, viscid secretion supplies nutritive substance to be used by spermatozoa.
The *ductus deferens*, its ampulla and the ejaculatory duct are primarily for transport.
Powerful contractions of the epididymis, ductus deferens and urethra forcibly expel spermatozoa under the stimulus of climactic sexual excitement.
Efferent ductules, epididymis, ampulla and ejaculatory ducts give evidence of secretion.
  Their functional maintenance depends on stimulation by the testicular hormone.
The rete, efferent ductules and duct of the epididymis (proximally) absorb transport fluid.

IV. THE AUXILIARY GENITAL GLANDS

These organs are the paired *seminal vesicles,* and the *prostate* and *bulbo-urethral glands.*

A. SEMINAL VESICLE:

Each *vesicle* is a diverticulum off the adjacent ductus deferens, just below the ampulla.
It is a convoluted *glandular sac,* about 2 inches long and 0.7 inch wide.
If straightened, it would be a tube more than twice this length.
The lumen is irregular and highly recessed throughout; there are some side bays.
This organ does not develop fully until stimulated hormonally at puberty.
Some mammals (insectivores; carnivores; etc.) lack seminal vesicles.

1. Mucosa.

The *lining membrane* is remarkably folded into an intricate system of elevations.
High primary *folds* branch into secondary and tertiary folds.
The thin folds project far into the lumen and frequently merge with others.
As a result, the internal surface appears honeycombed.
The *recesses* are of different sizes, and all communicate with the lumen.
There are no true glandular alveoli, but only these alcoves between folds.
The capacious main lumen regularly contains stored *secretion.*
It is a yellowish, gelatinous, sticky, mucoid and weakly alkaline fluid.
It contains rounded, acidophilic masses; fixation coagulates the fluid.

A. EPITHELIUM.
The *epithelium* may be simple columnar; but it is usually pseudostratified.
Besides low columnar cells, there are rounded basal elements.
Cell height varies with secretion-storage, age and other influences.
The cells contain *secretory granules* and yellow, lipoidal *pigment.*
The pigment first appears after puberty; it colors the fresh mucosa.
Some cells show blebs of secretion on their free surface.

B. LAMINA PROPRIA.
This *lamina* is a thin layer of richly elastic connective tissue.
Thin extensions from it serve as supports for the epithelial folds.
The *basement membrane* is not easily recognizable; a *submucosa* is lacking.

2. Muscularis.

The *muscular coat* is relatively less heavy than that of the ductus deferens.
Internally, there are circular and oblique bundles of smooth muscle.
These bundles interlace considerably.
Externally there is a longitudinal layer of smooth muscle.

3. Adventitia.

The *external tunic* is thin and composed mostly of elastic fibers.
It blends with the surrounding connective tissue.
Many blood vessels and some autonomic ganglia occupy this layer.

4. Vessels and nerves.

The distribution follows the plan described on p. 260.

5. Diagnostic features.

The *seminal vesicle* is an elongate, saccular organ, folded upon itself.
A typical section through it appears to contain several separate compartments.
The *mucosa* forms high, thin folds that branch and anastomose.
Small, open recesses and obliquely sectioned, seemingly enclosed cavities are seen.
T- and L-shaped folds are common; between such large folds occur smaller ones.
Looping arches often bound cavities and enclose minor folds.

These are obliquely sectioned recesses.

The *epithelium* is mostly pseudostratified, but may be simple in some regions.

The capacious *lumen* of the adult constantly contains *secretion.*

It commonly appears as a deeply staining, acidophilic, net-like coagulum.

It may contain small acidophilic masses, but fixation often destroys them.

Some spermatozoa are usually seen in the lumen of specimens taken after death.

A well-developed *muscular coat* surrounds the organ.

Yet, relatively, this is far less imposing than in the ampulla of the ductus deferens.

6. Functional correlations.

The *epithelium* of the seminal vesicles (and prostate) depends on hormonal support.

It is the male hormone, *testosterone*, that exerts this direct influence.

Castration before puberty results in underdevelopment and secretory failure.

Castration after puberty is followed by involution and loss of secretory power.

Administration of testis extract promptly restores the cells to function.

The seminal vesicle functions primarily as a gland with a voluminous lumen (4 ml.).

It secretes and stores the viscid part (20%) of seminal fluid, rich in fructose (30%).

Folding of the mucosa increases the secretory surface and aids distention.

Storage of spermatozoa is seemingly incidental and inconstant.

They probably enter incidentally, as the result of backflow.

This may occur during sexual excitement without ejaculation, or after death.

In some mammals spermatozoa are never found in these organs.

B. Prostate Gland:

This gland, about 1.5 inches in diameter, surrounds the urethra as it leaves the bladder.

It is really an aggregate of 30 to 50 tubulo-saccular glands, grouped in 5 *lobes*.

These empty into the prostatic urethra by 15 to 30 ducts.

The glands are not fully developed until puberty, and then under hormone influence.

1. Capsule and stroma.

The whole gland is surrounded by a fibro-elastic *capsule*.

Its inner zone, in particular, is rich in smooth muscle.

A dense, very abundant *stroma* embeds the alveoli in a compact mass.

The stroma constitutes an ensheathing system that joins the capsule.

It constitutes one-fourth of the volume of the total organ.

The fibro-elastic stroma contains a rich intermixture of *smooth-muscle* strands.

There is no easily demonstrable *basement membrane.*

2. Parenchyma.

The elongate *tubules,* with saccular recesses, vary greatly in size and shape.

They are irregular, varicose and branching; some become cystic.

The saccules and their ducts have lumina dilated with secretion.

The *epithelium* is remarkably folded into large and small folds.

These festoons are supported by thin extensions of the fibro-muscular septa.

The *epithelial cells* are cuboidal to columnar in shape.

They contain *secretion granules* and yellowish, *lipoidal droplets*.

Some cells show cytoplasmic protrusions that seemingly detach, apocrine style.

In some places, basal cells occur also.

The *ducts* have an irregular lumen, the smaller ones resembling secretory tubules.

Terminal excretory ducts, near the urethra, have pseudostratified epithelium.

In them are patches of secretory cells.

3. Secretion.

Secretion is said to be continuous, but is especially active during coitus.

The *prostatic secretion* is thin, milky and faintly acid; its odor is distinctive.

It is rich in citric acid and acid phosphatase; it contains lipid.

The secretory product makes up most of the bulk (75%) of the seminal fluid.
Yet removal of the gland does not necessarily incur reproductive incapacity.
Fixation coagulates the fluid into an acidophilic, granular mass.
The secretion frequently contains ovoid *prostatic concretions* (corpora amylacea).
Many of these acidophilic secretion-condensations are lamellated.
Their size is extremely variable, but the average diameter is 0.25 mm.
They consist of protein and carbohydrates.
Concretions first appear in adults and become increasingly abundant with aging.
Large concretions (up to 2 mm.) are often retained, and may calcify into *calculi.*

4. Vessels and nerves.

Blood vessels, lymphatics, nerves, ganglia and sensory corpuscles are abundant.
They are found in the capsule and stroma, and are numerous alongside the organ.

5. Diagnostic features.

There are many long, wide-lumened, irregular tubules — not closely spaced.
These are embedded in a dense, abundant, fibro-muscular *stroma.*
The stroma has a rich content of *smooth muscle* that shows well when stained.
The *columnar epithelium* forms many thin folds within alveoli.
Each is supported by a notably thin plate of stromal tissue.
Tangential sections of such folds often appear as isolated tissue-islands.
The *secretion* makes an acidophilic, granular mass in fixed preparations.
It may contain acidophilic *concretions*, usually lamellated.

6. Functional correlations.

The gland contributes an important component to the seminal fluid (p. 275).
Dependence on hormonal support parallels the behavior of the seminal vesicle (p. 273).

C. Bulbo-Urethral Gland:

These paired bodies, also called *Cowper's glands*, lie behind the membranous urethra.
Each is a compound tubulo-alveolar gland, the size of a pea.
It is a special, larger type of urethral gland (p. 262).

1. Capsule and stroma.

Each is surrounded by skeletal muscle and invested with a thin *capsule.*
Connective-tissue *septa* subdivide the organ into *lobules.*
These septa contain considerable skeletal muscle and some smooth-muscle fibers.
Within the lobules the *stroma* also may contain some smooth-muscle fibers locally.
Basement membranes surround the secretory tubules and ducts.

2. Parenchyma.

The *secretory end-pieces* of the gland are variable in size and form.
They may be tubular, alveolar or somewhat saccular.
These end-pieces either terminate blindly or connect by anastomoses.
The *epithelium* is variable in appearance.
Most alveoli consist of cuboidal to columnar, pale epithelium.
Some of them are dilated and lined with flattened epithelium.
The cytoplasm contains *mucigen droplets* and colloid spherules.
It also contains acidophilic, spindle-shaped inclusions.
The *nuclei* are flattened and basally located.
Other darker-staining alveoli, with rounded nuclei, are at rest functionally.
They somewhat resemble serous alveoli.

3. Secretion.

The *secretory product* is clear, viscid, glairy and stringy.
It is a mucoid substance, differing somewhat from true mucus.

Fixation precipitates the secretion into angular masses.
These stain brightly with acid dyes.

4. Ducts.

Within most lobules there are definite *ducts*, and these may be dilated locally.
In some regions the ducts are also secretory and appear as glandular tubules.
Also, the *main excretory ducts* contain patches of mucous cells, and even alveoli.
These ducts are 3 to 4 cm. long and open into the cavernous urethra.
They are surrounded by thin rings of smooth muscle.
Their epithelium is simple, but becomes stratified columnar near the outlet.

5. Diagnostic features.

The bulbo-urethral gland is a lobulated mucous gland, surrounded by skeletal muscle.
A minority of the alveoli may resemble a group of serous cells.
Some regions may lack intralobular ducts, recognizable as such.
Elsewhere the intralobular ducts are large and often dilated.
The main excretory ducts are equipped with some circular muscle.
They often contain mucous areas of epithelium, or even mucous diverticula.
The secretion shows angular masses, staining brightly with eosin.

6. Functional correlations.

The gland supplies a small amount of mucus under erotic stimulation (see beyond).
The spindle-shaped inclusions are said to dissolve in the mucus after discharge.

D. REGENERATIVE ABILITY:

Repair, leading to the replacement of specific cells, is limited in these glands.
Yet hypertrophy and hyperplasia occur with aging.
These responses also occur in response to hormonal stimulation.

E. SEMINAL FLUID AND EJACULATION:

1. Semen.

Seminal fluid (semen) consists of spermatozoa suspended in a thick, composite fluid.
The auxiliary genital glands furnish most of the fluid-bulk by far.
A slight amount is supplied by the system of genital ducts.
Semen is a whitish, opaque, gelatinous fluid, with a characteristic odor.
The ejaculate (about 3 ml.) contains some 250,000,000 spermatozoa.
Liberated spermatozoa are motile; they swim about 1.5 mm. per minute.

2. Ejaculation.

The forcible discharge of seminal fluid is the chief feature of the *orgasm*.
Its events are said to occur in a definite sequential series.
The *bulbo-urethral glands* discharge their product during erection.
Mucus, accumulated in the ducts and sacs, is expelled.
Perhaps additional discharge occurs during the orgasm.
The expelled mucus serves to lubricate the urethra.
The *prostate* is supposed to discharge first during actual ejaculation.
Its nearly alkaline fluid reduces the acidity of the urine-bathed urethra.
(Spermatozoa are highly susceptible to an acid environment.)
It also dilutes the thicker constituents of semen and augments sperm motility.
The *spermatozoa* are next forced down the seminal ducts.
Some of the supply, stored and ripening in the epididymis, is forced out.
This is accomplished by contractions of the muscle in that duct.
Passage through the ductus deferens is speeded by its massive muscle.
Lastly the *seminal vesicle* adds its thick secretion to the composite mass.
The spermatozoa are said to be pushed along by it, thus clearing the urethra.
Its content of fructose is a source of metabolic energy to spermatozoa.

These several components enter the urethra and mix with the mucus already there.
Semen is forced to the outside by the *bulbo-cavernosus muscle*.
It acts by compressing the bulb of the urethra.

V. THE PENIS

The *penis* serves both as a urinary outlet and as a copulatory organ.

A. STRUCTURAL PLAN:

The *penis* contains three cylinders of erectile tissue and the cavernous (or spongy) urethra.
One of the cylinders is the unpaired *corpus spongiosum*.
    It encloses the *cavernous* (or *spongy*) *urethra* and enlarges terminally into the *glans penis*.
Parallel and dorsal are two larger cylinders, the *corpora cavernosa*.
    However, they extend distad only to the region of the glans.
    They are united by a common median partition, the *pectiniform septum*.
Each corpus is enclosed by a fibrous sheath, the *tunica albuginea*.
    Internally each corpus (especially c. cavernosa) is a mass of unique erectile tissue.
All three cylinders are surrounded by muscular *subcutaneous tissue* and by thin *skin*.
    Terminally the skin reduplicates in a fold named the *prepuce*.
    It continues over the surface of the glans and then blends with the urethral outlet.

B. DETAILED STRUCTURE:

1. Skin.

The *skin* enveloping the penis is thin and soft, with tall papillae.
    It has only vellus-type hairs (except at base), and small sweat glands.
A thick *subcutaneous layer* attaches the skin to the erectile cylinders.
    This subcutaneous tissue is unusual in two regards.
        It has no fat, but contains considerable *smooth muscle*.
The *glans penis* is surrounded by the *prepuce*, a cylindrical fold of skin.
    The epithelium of the glans is united firmly to the fibrous tissue beneath.
        It becomes continuous with urethral epithelium at the urinary orifice.
    On the glans and the facing prepuce, the skin is moist like a mucous membrane.
        Sebaceous glands, usually described, are probably inconstant and rare.
        The odoriferous *smegma* consists mostly of cheesy, epithelial debris.

2. Corpora cavernosa.

These begin as *crura* and run side-by-side, dorsally, to tapered endings at the glans.
Each cylinder is enclosed by a robust fibrous sheath, the *tunica albuginea*.
    It has an inner circular and outer longitudinal layer of collagenous fibers.
    The common median wall, between the two corpora, is the *pectiniform septum*.
        Distally it has slit-like openings through which the blood sinuses communicate.
Trabeculae, continuous with the fibrous sheath, form a dense, internal framework.
    They carry blood vessels and intervene between the labyrinthine sinuses.
    Their structure is fibro-muscular, surfaced with endothelium.
The erectile *cavernae,* or *blood sinuses* are a prominent system of spaces (see beyond).

3. Corpus spongiosum.

This cylinder occupies a groove on the under-surface of the corpora cavernosa.
It is traversed axially by the *cavernous urethra,* already described (p. 262).
Terminally the corpus spongiosum expands into the conical, hood-like *glans penis*.
    This consists of dense connective tissue and plexuses of veins.
The external sheath (*tunica albuginea*) is thin and contains many elastic fibers.
    Hence it resists expansion feebly during erection.
    Its inner layer contains smooth-muscle fibers, circularly arranged.
Trabeculae are thinner and more elastic than those of the corpora cavernosa penis.

They also contain less smooth muscle.

The *cavernae*, or *sinuses*, grade into the smaller venous spaces about the urethra.

The glans contains a dense venous plexus; there is no tunica albuginea.

4. Erectile tissue.

This is a labyrinth of *blood sinuses,* better developed in the corpora cavernosa.

They are supplied by capillaries and special arterioles, and drained by venules.

In the corpora cavernosa the central sinuses are larger than peripheral ones.

In the corpus spongiosum the sinuses are nearly uniform in size.

The sinuses of the *flaccid penis* remain collapsed through tonic muscular compression.

Hence they then appear as mere clefts, lacking a significant blood-content.

During *erection* the sinuses become large cavities, engorged with blood.

The *trabeculae* of erectile tissue are the common partitions between adjacent sinuses.

They consist of *collagenous fibers, elastic networks* and strands of *smooth muscle.*

Their free surfaces are covered with the *endothelial lining* of the sinuses.

This endothelium is continuous with that of the communicating vessels.

These vessels both supply (arterioles; capillaries) and drain (venules).

5. Blood supply.

During the *flaccid state*, the *dorsal artery* of the penis provides circulating blood.

It supplies the tunica albuginea and larger trabeculae.

Here the arterial twigs break down into capillaries.

Their small amount of blood enters the sinuses and drains into the venules.

During *erection*, a *deep artery*, traversing each corpus cavernosum, is paramount.

These arteries give off trabecular branches that are called *helicine arteries.*

They are spiraling arterioles, many of which open directly into the sinuses.

The convolutions provide 'slack' to be taken up during erection.

The media is thick and the intima bears a longitudinal ridge of muscle.

Muscular tone causes these projecting ridges to plug the lumen.

Only when the muscle relaxes does blood pass through and flood the sinuses.

A *bulbar artery* supplies the corpus spongiosum.

Venules occur plentifully on the inner surface of the tunica albuginea of each corpus.

They drain the adjacent venous sinuses and join into somewhat larger vessels.

These radicles pierce the albuginea and unite as the *deep dorsal vein.*

The large central sinuses of the corpora cavernosa penis connect with special veins.

These have funnel-shaped valves that allow blood to leave only slowly.

6. Lymphatics and nerves.

A superficial *lymphatic plexus* occurs in the skin.

A deep network in the erectile tissue is also described.

Sensory nerve fibers terminate in a variety of sensory end-organs, many encapsulated.

Some (including genital corpuscles) are in skin and others in the urethra.

Motor nerve fibers supply the smooth muscle of blood vessels and trabeculae.

Still others supply the skeletal fibers of the bulbo-cavernosus muscle.

Reflexes are involved in the control of flaccidity, erection and ejaculation.

Sympathetic impulses constrict arterioles, thus maintaining tonic flaccidity.

They also are important in provoking the mechanism of ejaculation.

Parasympathetic impulses relax arterioles, and this leads to erection.

C. REGENERATIVE ABILITY:

Skin regenerates as elsewhere, except for its deep muscular layer which is indolent.

The *corpora cavernosa* and *corpus spongiosum* heal defects by filling-in of scar tissue.

D. DIAGNOSTIC FEATURES:

The *penis* is covered with skin; it contains the urethra and cavernous bodies.

The thin *skin* has only very fine hairs, except at the base of the organ.

The abundant *subcutaneous layer* is without fat, but contains smooth muscle.

The urethra is surrounded by a prominent cylinder of spongy *erectile tissue*.
Overlying this *corpus spongiosum* are the even larger, paired *corpora cavernosa*.
  They are enclosed by a thick, fibrous sheath and separated by a median septum.
  The interior consists of *erectile sinuses,* separated by fibro-muscular trabeculae.
The *glans* is surfaced with moist skin; highly vascular fibrous tissue envelops the urethra.
  Transverse sections vary in appearance, according to the level cut through.
    The prepuce may surround the glans, or do so incompletely.
    The glans may overlap the tapered ends of the corpora cavernosa.

E. Functional Correlations:

The urinary function of the *penis* is a feature that was acquired secondarily.
This is because the penis arose primarily as a *copulative organ* and seat of erotic excitation.
  Its evolution among mammals has paralleled that of the vagina and uterus.
  In some mammals a *penile bone* is a component in addition to erectile tissue.
  By contrast, the requisite rigidity in most mammals depends wholly on erectile tissue.
    Hence functional correlations pertain chiefly to the mechanism of erection.
In the *flaccid penis,* some blood passes from trabecular capillaries into the 'empty' sinuses.
  It is drained by the plexus of venules in the tunica albuginea.
During erection arterioles are the active agents; sinuses and venules are passive.
Effective *erection* is almost wholly a function of the *corpora cavernosa*.
  It begins with the relaxation of muscular tone in arteries and trabeculae.
  Blood is then able to force its way through the straightening helicine arterioles.
  The cavernous sinuses begin to fill, the large central ones first.
    This compresses the periphery, where venules underlie the firm tunica albuginea.
    The result is that venous drainage is severely hampered.
  By these means the sinuses are filled and put under pressure.
    Turgidity results because the fibrous tunica albuginea resists distention.
In the *corpus spongiosum*, rigidity is less marked.
  This is partly because the central and peripheral sinuses are about the same size.
    As a result, blood is not so well retained, and this tissue is less turgid.
  In addition, the tunica albuginea is thinner and more elastic.
    This permits distention and hence prevents the compression of peripheral veins.
  The glans contains only convoluted venules, and never attains significant rigidity.
At the termination of sexual excitement flaccidity is regained through *detumescence*.
  The arteries soon recover their muscular tone as the nervous control is regained.
    As a result, the blood supply to the sinuses is shut off.
  Flaccidity is resumed slowly because of the compression of peripheral venules.
    It is said that the central sinuses drain first through their valved veins.
      This results in a reduction in pressure peripherally where veins have been squeezed.
        The ordinary route of peripheral venous drainage is then restored.
  The residual blood content of the sinuses is pressed out by the muscular trabeculae.

Chapter XXIV

The Female Reproductive System

The female reproductive system includes the *ovaries* and a set of tubular organs.
 The latter are the *uterine tubes, uterus, vagina* and *external genitalia*.
  These organs have other functions than serving merely as a system of ducts.
The female organs are in a fully developed, functional condition for about 30 years.

not on tenario

I. THE OVARY

An *ovary* lies on each side of the uterus on the lateral wall of the pelvic cavity.

A. STRUCTURAL PLAN:

The *ovary* is an ovoid exocrine (cytogenic) and endocrine gland about 1.5 inches long.
 It is surfaced with a specialized layer of reflected peritoneum *(germinal epithelium)*.
One margin receives a mesentery (the *mesovarium*), which attaches to the *broad ligament*.
 This attached, ovarian border is the *hilus* where blood vessels enter.
The ovary consists of a cortex and medulla, not sharply delimited.
  The *cortex* is a compact layer, interrupted at the hilus.
   It contains *eggs*, in *follicles* of various sizes and degrees of development.
   It also contains discharged, transformed follicles *(corpora lutea)*, their degenerating
     remains *(corpora albicantia)* and *atretic follicles*.
  The *medulla* is a vascular and fibrous core, looser than the cortex.
   It reaches the 'surface' only at the hilus where it merges with the mesovarium.

B. DETAILED STRUCTURE:

1. Medulla.

The interior of the ovary, or *medulla* is a core of rather loose fibro-elastic tissue.
Abundant *blood vessels* enter at the hilus, and then take spiral courses inward.
The *stroma* contains scattered strands of smooth muscle (especially at the hilus).
Enlarging ovarian follicles encroach upon the medulla each month.

2. Cortex.

The *cortical zone* consists of a dense *stroma* that contains *follicles* with eggs.
 In a functional ovary many follicles are quiescent, or practically so.
  Others are undergoing progressive or regressive development.
The exact condition, however, depends upon the age of the ovary.
 Before *puberty* the ovary shows, with few exceptions, only *primitive follicles*.
 Sexual maturity is characterized by the presence of *growing* (and *ripe*) *follicles*.
  Also their end-products *(corpora lutea* and *albicantia; atretic follicles)* occur.
 In the later reproductive years the ova progressively decrease in number.
  After the menopause they disappear completely.
 The *senile cortex* becomes a narrowed zone of ordinary fibrous tissue.
All the descriptions that follow refer to the mature, functional ovary.

A. GERMINAL EPITHELIUM.

This surface layer is a specialized portion of the *peritoneal epithelium*.

Its cuboidal to columnar cells rest upon a thin *basement membrane.*

The epithelium detaches easily and is commonly lost from sections.

The name 'germinal,' inferring a source of eggs, is inappropriate.

(Primitive sex cells migrate from the yolk sac and colonize the ovary.)

B. STROMA.

The connective-tissue *stroma* is peculiar; it is much like an embryonic type.

It is compact, rich in cells and relatively poor in fibers.

The *cells* are spindle-shaped with elongate nuclei, somewhat like smooth muscle.

They have more potentialities than ordinary fibroblasts possess.

The *fibers* are thin, reticular threads that form a meshwork between the cells.

They are fine elements, like thin collagenous fibers but argyrophilic.

The *tunica albuginea* is a zone directly beneath the germinal epithelium.

It is less cellular, less vascular and more compact than the general stroma.

About the follicles the stroma specializes into distinctive envelopes *(thecae).*

They are characteristic of growing follicles and will be described with them.

C. OVA.

All the egg cells are large, spherical elements.

The most immature ova (technically *oögonia*) are about 20 μ in diameter.

When full grown, they are six times this size; volume increase is 200 times.

Such stages of progressive growth, bear the name *primary oöcytes.*

The *nucleus* is large and vesicular; the nucleolus, prominent and dark-staining.

The *cytoplasm* is opaque and granular, especially centrally.

The larger granules are particles of lipid substance.

A typically delicate *plasma membrane* borders the cytoplasm.

D. PRIMARY FOLLICLES.

A primitive ovum, before growth begins, is enclosed by a single layer of cells.

These flat elements, products of the germinal epithelium, are *follicle cells.*

Such a *primary follicle* measures 30 to 40 μ in diameter.

The greatest number of follicles occurs in the fetal ovary (400,000).

Destruction enters early and continues until none is left after some 50 years.

After puberty, however, some surviving follicles do grow each month.

E. GROWING, SOLID FOLLICLES.

In the initial stage of advance both ovum and follicle increase in size.

The growing egg is technically a *primary oöcyte;* it reaches its maximum size.

The *follicle cells* become first cuboidal, and then columnar.

Proliferation next produces a stratified, cellular ensheathment of the oöcyte.

Lipid granules appear and the thick *zona pellucida* organizes.

The zona is a refractile, glycoprotein membrane that envelops the oöcyte.

It is usually considered to be a product of the follicle cells.

Cells bordering the zona send long branching processes through it.

These mingle with short, thin *microvilli* from the oöcyte.

Nutritive substances are thought to reach the oöcyte by this route.

This phase of growth is a self-contained, ovarian function.

F. GROWING VESICULAR FOLLICLES.

These hollow sacs (also called *Graafian follicles*) occur in mammals alone.

Follicles about 0.2 mm. in diameter begin to collect pools of fluid.

This follicular fluid *(liquor folliculi)* is apparently secreted by the follicle cells.

It comes to occupy a single cavity, the *antrum*, within the follicular layer.

The fluid crowds the oöcyte and its neighboring follicle cells, to one side.

This eccentric, cellular mound constitutes the *cumulus oöphorus.*

A peripheral shell of cuboidal follicle cells then surrounds the antrum.

It is several layers deep and is named the *stratum granulosum.*

Meanwhile adjacent stroma has organized into a double-layered capsule, the *theca.*

The *theca interna* is largely vascular and cellular in composition.

Between it and the stratum granulosum is a basement or *glassy membrane.*
The *theca externa* is a denser and more fibrous layer.
Follicles of 0.5 mm. begin to expand toward the ovarian surface.
A *mature follicle* is probably completed 10 to 14 days after growth begins.
Although large (1 cm.), it bulges but little beyond the ovarian surface.
It occupies the full breadth of the cortex and indents the medulla.
The production of vesicular follicles is induced by a hypophyseal hormone (FSH).

3. Maturation and ovulation.

The full-grown 'egg' is actually still a *primary oöcyte,* and technically immature.
Before it is liberated from the follicle, an unequal cell division occurs.
The daughter cells are a *secondary oöcyte* and the tiny, first *polar body.*
The chromosome assortment in each is reduced to a single set of 23 chromosomes.
This reduction is the result of meiosis, as in spermatogenesis (p. 266).
At about this time the large follicle, covered with thinned cortex, ruptures.
This is *ovulation;* it is, in part, the result of a weakened wall and cortex.
The follicular fluid oozes out, carrying the loosened or free oöcyte with it.
Some follicle cells adhere to the ovum and comprise the *corona radiata.*
Ovulation occurs at about 28-day intervals, and roughly in alternate ovaries.
The time is about midway between two menstrual onsets.
Usually only one secondary oöcyte is set free in each cycle.
The free oöcyte probably remains fertilizable for something less than one day.
If fertilized by a spermatozoön, the oöcyte undergoes a second maturation division.
This results in a *mature ovum (oötid)* and a tiny, *second polar body.*
Each still retains a complete single set of chromosomes (*cf* p. 266).
Thus, only one daughter cell of a primary oöcyte becomes functional.
This is a sacrifice in number, to insure adequate size to one functional egg.
If not fertilized, the oöcyte fragments and is phagocytosed or absorbed.

4. Corpus luteum.

The collapsed follicle becomes prominently folded and heals its rupture.
The cavity is filled with transuded serum and unexpelled follicular fluid.
There is sometimes a little bleeding within the cavity of the follicle.
More often, significant bleeding follows later vascularization.
The follicular wall transforms into a temporary glandular body, the *corpus luteum.*
It is called a *corpus luteum of ovulation* if pregnancy does not follow.
It is called a *corpus luteum of pregnancy* if pregnancy ensues.
(Corpus luteum spurium and c. l. verum are other terms used, respectively.)
There is no essential difference between the two, except size and length of life.
In pregnancy the glandular mass grows to a larger size and lasts longer.
The epithelial cells of the stratum granulosum begin a new kind of specialization.
They transform directly into a cell-type different in structure and function.
These cells enlarge greatly into spheroidal elements, but they rarely divide.
The transformed granulosa cells are called *granulosa lutein cells.*
Their abundant cytoplasm is clear; it increasingly acquires lipid droplets.
Lutein cells become arranged in cords and masses, separated by capillaries.
The theca interna also produces epithelioid elements called *theca lutein cells.*
These have less cytoplasm than granulosa cells and are easily distinguishable.
They aggregate peripherally, especially where the wall is indented by folding.
They are smaller, stain more intensely and have smaller, darker nuclei.
Capillary sprouts and spindle-shaped cells of the theca interna invade the main mass.
Some fibroblasts organize a delicate *reticulum* throughout the corpus luteum.
Other fibroblasts reach the internal surface of the luteal wall and spread along it.
Here they form a fibro-gelatinous lining about the central cavity.
They also organize the central coagulum and absorb it.
The *corpus luteum of ovulation* attains its highest development at the ninth day.

At this same time the involution of this ordinary corpus luteum begins.
The former rich and intimate vascularization of the granulosa mass declines.
Granulosa lutein cells undergo fatty degeneration; lipochrome pigment increases.
 The corpus luteum now first assumes a bright yellow color.
Theca lutein cells also become less conspicuous and gradually disappear.
Regression is well advanced after two weeks, but continues for several months.
 Hence several stages, from different cycles, are always found in an ovary.
 There is gradual reduction to a hyaline scar named the *corpus albicans*.
The *corpus luteum of pregnancy* is large because its cells continue to grow.
 In the second month it attains a diameter of 2 to 3 cm., but is relatively pale.
 Involution begins promptly, but reduction proceeds slowly and variably.
 After pregnancy the final decline and replacement proceed at a rapid rate.
 Yet the resulting corpus albicans is large and quite persistent.

5. Atresia of follicles.

The process of *atresia* is a characteristic feature in immature and mature ovaries.
 This process is one of degeneration (involution) of ovarian follicles.
 It occurs abundantly between fetal life and puberty.
 It also continues, less actively, throughout the functional sexual years.
 The duration of the active sexual span in woman is 30 years or more.
 Only about 400 follicles reach full maturity during this time.
 Yet follicles are seen constantly at various stages of growth.
 All unsuccessful follicles are destined to involute and disappear.
 The depletion is nearly complete at the time of the menopause.
 Within 3 to 4 years thereafter all residual follicles have succumbed.
Atresia may attack follicles when they are young, growing or practically mature.
 The *ovum* is primarily attacked, but the causative factors are unknown.
 The ensuing process is a reaction that brings about the absorption of dead material.
Atresia in *primary follicles* involves first a degeneration of the *ovum*.
 This is followed by similar changes in the *follicular cells*.
 The empty space, at the end of the process, is then filled-in with stromal tissue.
Atresia in *growing* and *vesicular follicles* introduces more complicated changes.
 The first degenerative signs tend to appear in the *ovum*, as in primary follicles.
 After this the follicular epithelium (granulosa) undergoes fatty degeneration.
Cells of the *theca interna* develop much like those in a corpus luteum.
 They become epithelioid cells, arranged in vascularized, radial cords.
 The appearance of a well advanced stage is much like a corpus luteum.
 But there is (or was) a degenerating ovum in the interior of the follicle.
The *zona pellucida* swells, stains deeply and may persist by itself for a long time.
The *glassy membrane* may likewise thicken, fold, hyalinize and persist.
 Eventually connective tissue penetrates it and replaces interior residues.
The final fate of such a follicle is fibrosis and shrinkage.
 The scar-tissue mass looks like a corpus albicans, but is smaller.

6. Interstitial cells.

Groups of epithelioid cells sometimes show in the ovarian stroma of mammals.
 The cytoplasm of such spheroidal cells contains fine lipoidal droplets.
 They are best seen in rodents, where they constitute the '*interstitial gland.*'
In the adult, human ovary they are either absent or very poorly represented.
All such cells derive from the internal theca of follicles undergoing atresia.
 Accordingly, they are most abundant when atresia is commonest.
 In the human this is the first year of life.
These elements are lingering products of atresia, dispersed by growth processes.
 They are not comparable to the interstitial cells of the testis.

7. Vessels and nerves.

Blood vessels from the hilus spiral through the medulla and invade the cortex.

Capillary networks are abundant in the theca interna of follicles.

Lymph capillaries begin in the theca externa of follicles and unite into larger vessels.

Such collecting vessels enter the medulla and leave at the hilus.

Nerve fibers follow the blood vessels and supply their muscular coat.

Other fibers form plexuses about the follicular epithelium.

Some sensory fibers and lamellar (Pacinian) corpuscles occur in the stroma.

C. REGENERATIVE ABILITY:

Ovaries are notoriously incompetent in effecting repair beyond healing by scar tissue.

D. DIAGNOSTIC FEATURES:

The ovary has a cortex and a thicker medulla, different structurally.

The *medulla* is fibrous and contains prominent blood vessels.

The *cortex* is bounded by a cuboidal *epithelium.*

This layer, however, is commonly lacking in sections from preserved ovaries.

The cortical *stroma* is highly cellular and deficient in obvious fibers.

Its spindle-shaped cells resemble somewhat swirling groups of smooth muscle.

Follicles, before puberty, are mostly primordial, with a single epithelial layer.

Between puberty and the menopause, *growing follicles* of all sizes can be expected.

Also a *corpus luteum* (at some stage) and *corpora albicantia* are commonly seen.

The cell columns of the c. luteum resemble slightly those of suprarenal cortex.

Atretic follicles are encountered in almost every section.

After the menopause, follicles disappear and the ovary shrinks.

The thinned cortex is replaced by fibrous tissue.

E. FUNCTIONAL CORRELATIONS:

As an *exocrine gland* the ovary produces eggs; it is a *cytogenic gland.*

The production of such a large cell, with much cytoplasm, is an adaptive specialization.

It must furnish the actual building material for the body of a new individual.

Endocrine synthesis produces two important hormones.

Estrogen is elaborated by cells of the theca interna.

This occurs during the growth of vesicular follicles and also of the corpus luteum.

At puberty estrogen is responsible for the growth of the genital tract and breasts.

It also brings out the secondary sexual characters and the sex drive.

After menstruation it directs the proliferative repair of the uterine mucosa.

During pregnancy it dominates the growth of the uterus and mammary glands.

Progesterone is produced by the corpus luteum (granulosa lutein cells).

It brings the estrogen-primed uterine mucosa to a condition fit for pregnancy.

During pregnancy it preserves the uterine mucosa and embryo.

It probably aids in producing growth of the mammary gland.

The ovary, itself, is activated and governed by hypophyseal *gonadotropic hormones* (p. 179).

II. THE UTERINE TUBE

The egg-conducting *uterine tube* is also called the *oviduct* and the *Fallopian tube.*

It extends from the ovary to the uterus in a fold of peritoneum.

This mesentery (*mesosalpinx*) attaches to the broad ligament.

The tube is 4 to 5 inches long, and is unique in not uniting directly with its gland.

The uterine tube shows four regional divisions:

The *infundibulum* flares and opens trumpet-fashion; it bears fringed folds (*fimbriae*).

The *ampulla* is a dilated region, comprising two-thirds of the length of the tube.

The *isthmus*, slender and narrowed, connects with the uterus.

A continuation of the canal through the uterine wall is called the *intramural portion*.
The wall of the uterine tube thickens progressively toward the uterus.
Conversely, the lumen diminishes remarkably in this direction (from 8 to 1 mm.).

1. Mucosa.

The *epithelium* is mostly simple columnar, but sometimes has basal cells.
Some cells are *ciliated*, the direction of their stroke being downward.
Other groups of cells contain granules and secrete a *mucoid substance*.
However, no true glands are present in the uterine tube.
So-called *peg cells* are presumably depleted secretory cells.
Slight changes in height occur, and a cyclic loss and renewal of cilia.
A *basement membrane* occurs, but is inconspicuous with the light microscope.
The *lamina propria* is highly cellular; collagenous fibers are thin and sparse.
The cells are spindle-shaped or angular, separated by thin fibers.
The whole mucosal lining is thrown into characteristic longitudinal *folds*.
Next to the uterus the folds are few (3 to 4), low and simple.
Toward the ovarian end the thin folds are many, high and intricate.
The primary folds branch and interconnect, lengthwise.
They also give rise to subordinate folds in a most complicated manner.
This system of folds subdivides the *lumen* into a labyrinth of narrow clefts.
At the rim of the flaring tube, close to the ovary, the mucosal lining of the tube and
the peritoneal mesothelium of the serosa become continuous.

2. Submucosa.

The lamina propria extends without change all the way to the muscular coat.
Hence there is no recognizable *submucosa*.

3. Muscularis.

This tunic of smooth muscle becomes progressively thicker toward the uterus.
The *inner layer*, circularly arranged, is well developed.
The *outer layer* is thin and loosely distributed in longitudinal bundles.
It does not make a closed layer, but is best developed near the uterus.
There is no distinct boundary between the two muscle coats.

4. Serosa.

The uterine tube is loosely invested with a *serosal fold* of reflected peritoneum.
This is continuous into that portion of the broad ligament called the *mesosalpinx*.
The muscle-bundles of the longitudinal coat are embedded in this relatively thick layer.

5. Vessels and nerves.

The distribution follows the plan described on p. 260.

6. Diagnostic features.

The *uterine tube* is a specialized egg duct, with characteristic features.
The *epithelium* is simple columnar.
Cilia occur on some cells, but routine sections often fail to show them.
The *lamina propria* is characterized by its highly cellular composition.
(The uterus is the only hollow organ sharing this type of tissue.)
A *circular muscle layer* is complete and clearly seen.
The outer, *longitudinal layer* is arranged in scattered bundles.
Only close to the uterus does it approximate a closed layer.
The *serosa* is loosely applied; its deeper levels contain the longitudinal muscle.
Wide quantitative variations are seen at different levels of the duct.
Toward the *ovarian end*, the tube is much larger.
Its muscularis is thin and the lumen wide.
The mucosa is remarkably folded into a complex series of thin plates.

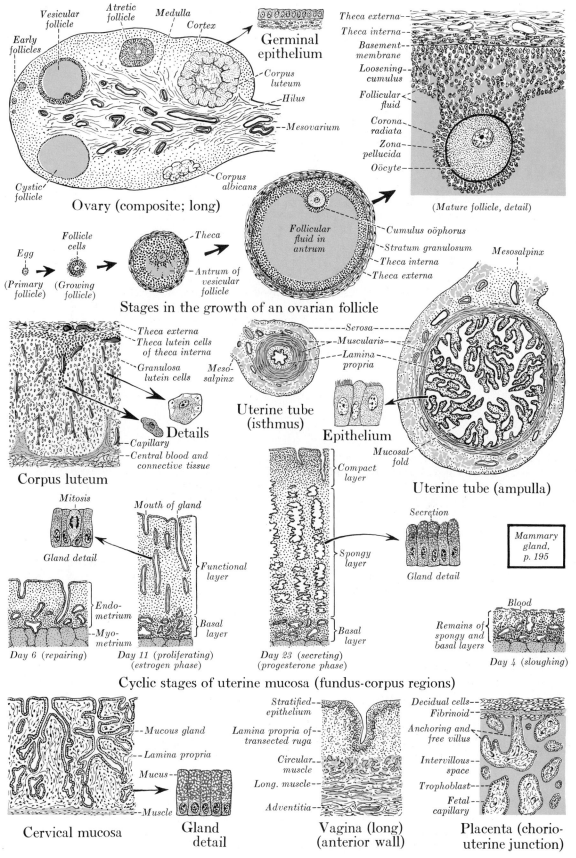

Vesicular follicle · Atretic follicle · Medulla · Cortex

Early follicles

Germinal epithelium

Corpus luteum

Hilus

Mesovarium

Cystic follicle

Corpus albicans

Ovary (composite; long)

Theca externa
Theca interna
Basement membrane
Loosening cumulus
Follicular fluid
Corona radiata
Zona pellucida
Oöcyte

(Mature follicle, detail)

Egg

(Primary follicle)

Follicle cells

(Growing follicle)

Theca

Antrum of vesicular follicle

Follicular fluid in antrum

Cumulus oöphorus
Stratum granulosum
Theca interna
Theca externa

Mesosalpinx

Stages in the growth of an ovarian follicle

Theca externa
Theca lutein cells of theca interna
Granulosa lutein cells

Meso-salpinx

Serosa
Muscularis
Lamina propria

Details

Capillary
Central blood and connective tissue

Corpus luteum

Uterine tube (isthmus)

Epithelium

Mucosal fold

Uterine tube (ampulla)

Mitosis

Mouth of gland

Compact layer

Secretion

Mammary gland, p. 195

Gland detail

Functional layer

Spongy layer

Gland detail

Endo-metrium
Myo-metrium

Basal layer

Basal layer

Blood

Remains of spongy and basal layers

Day 6 (repairing)

Day 11 (proliferating) (estrogen phase)

Day 23 (secreting) (progesterone phase)

Day 4 (sloughing)

Cyclic stages of uterine mucosa (fundus-corpus regions)

Mucous gland

Lamina propria

Mucus

Muscle

Cervical mucosa

Gland detail

Stratified epithelium
Lamina propria of transected ruga
Circular muscle
Long. muscle
Adventitia

Vagina (long) (anterior wall)

Decidual cells
Fibrinoid
Anchoring and free villus
Intervillous space
Trophoblast
Fetal capillary

Placenta (chorio-uterine junction)

THE FEMALE REPRODUCTIVE ORGANS

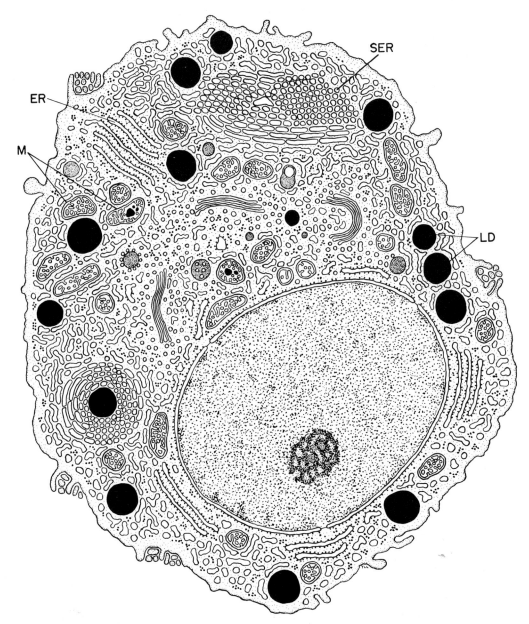

GRANULOSA LUTEIN CELL. This specialized follicular cell shows a prominent nucleolus within a pale, eccentric nucleus. Rough endoplasmic reticulum (ER) is sparse. The cytoplasm contains free ribosomes, but its chief component is the tubules of smooth endoplasmic reticulum (SER). Mitochondria (M) have vesicular to tubular cristae. Golgi complexes are multiple; nearby are multivesicular bodies and dense bodies. A few lipid droplets (LD) occur.

The lumen is thereby reduced to a labyrinth of narrow spaces.
Toward the *uterine end*, the tube is much smaller.
Its muscularis is thicker, and the lumen is greatly reduced.
The mucosal folds become fewer, lower and simpler.

7. *Functional correlations.*

The uterine tube receives the ovum and transports it to the uterus.
Reception may be accomplished by cilia, which wave the egg inward.
This is aided by the fimbriae, which become turgid and sweep over the ovary.
Downward *transportation* is probably the result of muscular activity.
The tube serves as a meeting place for the egg and sperm.
Tubal contractions, rather than swimming ability, force spermatozoa up the tube.
Fertilization occurs usually in the ampullary region.
The mucoid secretion is lubricative; it also nourishes eggs in transit.
The open, fimbriated end of the tube is always a potentially dangerous feature.
It provides an avenue for the passage of infection into the peritoneal cavity.

III. THE UTERUS

The *uterus* lies between the bladder and rectum; it occupies a midregion in the broad ligament.
It is a hollow, pear-shaped organ, about 3 inches long, with a thick muscular wall.
It receives the uterine tubes and opens into the vagina.
Regional divisions into *fundus, corpus* and *cervix* are recognized.
A transitional zone, between corpus and cervix, is designated the *isthmus.*
The cervix projects for a short distance into the vaginal cavity.
Structurally the fundus and corpus are alike; hence only two regions demand consideration.

A. STRUCTURAL PLAN:

The *uterus* is organized according to the general plan for hollow organs.
The several tunics are represented as in the oviduct, but they receive special names.
These are: *endometrium* (mucosa); *myometrium* (muscularis); *perimetrium* (serosa).
The endometrium is notable for its *cyclic changes*, ending in extensive destruction.
The entire wall participates in the changes and enlargement entailed by pregnancy.

B. DETAILED STRUCTURE:

1. *Endometrium.*

This layer, elsewhere called a *mucosa*, abuts directly against the muscular coat.
Its thickness and structure in the fundus-corpus vary cyclically month by month.
It is simplest to describe first the average condition, as at the middle of the cycle.
At this time the total thickness is about 2 to 3 mm.

A. SURFACE EPITHELIUM.
In the *fundus-corpus* it is a simple columnar layer, with groups of ciliated cells.
In the *cervix* the cells are taller and have basally located nuclei.
Some cells are ciliated, but most contain much mucus toward the free end.

B. GLANDS.
The *uterine glands* extend through the full thickness of the mucosa.
They are spaced apart by a distance about four times the breadth of a gland.
There are two regional types: in the fundus-corpus; and in the cervix.
1. *Fundus and corpus.*
This region embraces the upper two-thirds of the uterus.
The slightly tortuous *fundic-corporal glands* make a vertical palisade of tubules.
Usually called simple tubular, they may branch toward their basal ends.
The component *cells* (some ciliated) are like those on the surface.
They undergo periodic changes in a monthly secretory cycle (see beyond).
Their secretion is *mucoid,* gaining in *glycogen* as the changes advance.

2. *Cervix.*

    This region corresponds to the lower one-third of the uterus.

       Cervical glands consist of tall *mucous cells* and are highly branched.

         These glands sometimes become occluded and dilate with secretion.

           Such cysts are called *Nabothian follicles,* or ovules of Naboth.

       Cervical glands undergo only slight changes during the menstrual cycle.

         However, the secretion of mucus does vary somewhat during the cycle.

         In pregnancy the cervical glands both enlarge and proliferate.

c. Lamina Propria.

    The connective-tissue framework is composed of *reticular fibers.*

       A *basement membrane* is present, but quite inconspicuous.

    The *stromal cells* are very abundant, occupying the spaces of the fibrous mesh.

       They are small, angular cells with a large ovoid nucleus.

       Wandering lymphoid cells and other leucocytes also are to be seen.

    There is a superficial resemblance to lymphoid tissue in this cellular layer.

    In the *cervix* the stroma is firmer, more fibrous and less cellular.

       Longitudinal folds, the *plicae palmatae,* are produced.

2. Myometrium.

    The *muscularis* is a relatively massive coat of smooth muscle, 0.6 inch thick.

       It is arranged in bundles, separated by connective tissue.

       The muscle fibers are large, varying cyclically between 40 and 90 μ in length.

       In pregnancy the muscle fibers become relatively huge elements, 600 to 800 μ long.

         They also increase in number; new fibers differentiate (and old fibers divide?).

    There are three layers of muscle, somewhat blended due to interconnecting bundles.

       The *inner layer,* mostly longitudinal, is the so-called *stratum submucosum.*

       The *middle layer,* the thickest coat, is arranged obliquely circular.

         Many large vessels give it a spongy texture; it is the *stratum vasculare.*

       The thin *outer layer,* mostly longitudinal, is the *stratum supravasculare.*

    The muscle of the *cervix* is relatively deficient and is arranged in irregular bundles.

       Intermixed white and elastic fibers produce a firm consistency.

       An outer, more longitudinal layer of muscle continues into the vagina.

3. Perimetrium.

    This is a typical *serosa,* continued from the peritoneum of the broad ligament.

    It is lacking caudally on the anterior wall, where the bladder abuts.

4. Vessels and nerves.

    Blood vessels from the broad ligament penetrate to the middle layer of the myometrium.

       One set of *arterial extensions* supplies the basal part of the endometrium.

       Another set, specialized as *coiled arteries,* extends to higher levels.

         Here each branches into a terminal tuft of arterioles.

       Veins in the endometrium are thin-walled, forming a varicose meshwork.

         A plexus of larger vessels occurs in the vascular stratum of the myometrium.

    Lymphatics form plexuses in the mucous, muscular and serous coats.

       They are extremely abundant, yet are wholly absent in the superficial mucosa.

    Unmyelinated *nerve fibers* supply blood vessels and muscle bundles.

       Myelinated fibers enter the mucosa, but their endings are obscure.

C. Cyclic Changes:

    During the potential child-bearing years the endometrium undergoes periodic changes.

       The entire lining, except that of the cervix, is involved in this *menstrual cycle.*

       There is a building-up, followed by marked destruction and repair.

    Hence the appearance of the mucosa varies from day to day.

       A complete cycle consumes 21 to 35 days; the average is 28 days.

The first day of flow is numbered as day 1 of the cycle.

Five *stages* can be recognized in a continuous cycle of events.

These stages do not start and stop abruptly, but each passes insensibly into the next.

The times given for the following stages represent averages based on a 28-day cycle.

1. Resurfacing (day 5 or 6).

Even before all bleeding has ceased, *repair* begins to get under way.

Epithelial cells leave the surviving remnants of torn glands.

These remnants are located in the basal and deepest spongy layer of the membrane.

Cells glide over the denuded surface and epithelize it anew.

(Such spreading, without mitosis, characterizes early wound healing in general.)

2. Proliferative stage (days 7 to 14).

This phase is also called the *follicular stage*.

It extends and completes the postmenstrual repair; it is a period of growth.

It coincides with the growth of ovarian follicles and is induced by estrogen.

It is variable in duration, correlated with the length of the cycle.

The mucosa increases from 1 mm. (or less) in thickness to about 3 mm.

The *glands* proliferate, lengthen rapidly and finally become somewhat wavy.

Glycogen accumulates in the cells; only a thin mucoid secretion is given off.

Connective-tissue cells also multiply and rebuild the lamina propria.

They produce a new meshwork of *reticular fibers* as the restoration advances.

Coiled arteries are regrowing laggardly into the otherwise regenerated mucosa.

3. Secretory stage (days 15 to 27).

Other terms are the *progravid* or *luteal stage*; uterine competence is attained.

The time lapse between its start and the onset of bleeding tends to be 14 days.

This period is uniform in length, regardless of the length of the total cycle.

The glands gradually cease proliferating, but they become tortuous and swell.

Throughout a middle region, saccular ('baggy') outpocketings appear.

These are distended with a thicker *mucoid secretion*, rich in glycogen.

Such changes are induced by progesterone, secreted by the corpus luteum.

The *coiled arteries* spiral much more tightly and extend nearly to the surface.

By the end of this period, the endometrium is from 4 to 6 mm. thick.

This increase is due largely to the swelling of tissues and the accumulation of secretion and tissue fluid.

Three horizontal zones of the endometrium are given special names.

Nearest the surface is the *compact layer*, containing the straight necks of glands.

It is also characterized by enlarged stromal cells, of connective-tissue origin.

These are identical with the still larger *decidual cells* of pregnancy.

Deeper is the thick *spongy layer*, featured by the dilated portions of glands.

The compact and spongy layers together are often called the *functional layer*.

Deepest of all is the thin *basal layer*, containing the blind ends of glands.

It does not participate to any extent in the cyclic changes.

4. Ischemic stage (day 28).

One day or more before bleeding starts, the *coiled arteries* constrict intermittently.

The interruption of blood-flow continues for periods of several hours.

The functional layer becomes pale and shrinks.

It lacks blood, and loses glandular secretion and tissue fluid.

5. Menstrual stage (days 1 to 4 or 5).

The functional layer next undergoes necrosis and sloughs away.

Blood cells slip through the walls of intact capillaries.

At times the *coiled arterioles* relax locally and blood escapes from bursting vessels.

It also escapes from the injured capillaries whose blood supply has failed.

Pools of uncoagulated blood are thus formed in the lamina propria.
Patches of blood-soaked tissue separate off and are lost.
This exposes torn glands, arteries and veins.
Blood oozes (by reflux) from veins so opened.
The *discharge* contains blood, disintegrated epithelial and stromal cells, glandular
secretions, and sometimes tissue fragments; blood loss averages 35 ml.
The compactum and a variable amount of spongiosum are lost, leaving a raw surface.
The surviving stratum remains intact, although it has shrunk down considerably.
The straight arteries to the basal endometrium do not constrict during the cycle.
Hence the blood supply to this zone is adequate at all times.

6. Anovular cycle.

At times (especially in early adolescence) no follicle ovulates during a cycle.
In this instance neither corpus luteum nor progesterone are formed.
Menstrual break-down will then follow in an endometrium that has not advanced beyond
the proliferative stage.

D. PREGNANCY CHANGES:

1. Structural features.

An important organ, the *placenta*, features the period of pregnancy.
It is a composite organ produced partly by the uterus and partly by fetal tissue.
The *maternal component* is endometrium, continued even beyond the secretory stage.
The *fetal component* is supplied by the chorionic sac that encloses the embryo.
This is, of course, not fetal tissue proper, but rather auxiliary fetal tissue.
The maternal contribution, or *decidua basalis*, is not a complete endometrial thickness.
It lacks the superficial portion of the compact layer of the endometrium.
That is, it includes only the endometrium beneath the implanted chorionic sac.
A characteristic feature, in the first half of pregnancy, is the *decidual cells*.
These are enlarged, connective-tissue cells of uncertain significance.
The fetal contribution consists of a *chorionic plate* and its branching *villi*.
The *chorionic plate* is merely a portion of the chorionic sac about the embryo.
It is that local region of the membrane that lies deepest in the decidua.
Chorionic villi extend from the chorion, like branching trees.
Many end freely, but some fuse with the decidua as anchoring elements.
Both the chorionic plate and the villi have the same essential structure.
A *villus* contains a fibro-muscular core, embedding extensions of fetal blood vessels.
Its surface-covering is an epithelial tissue, named *trophoblast*.
In the first half of pregnancy two throphoblastic layers are recognizable.
The inner layer is composed of separate cuboidal cells, arranged one cell deep.
It is called the *cellular trophoblast* (cytotrophoblast).
The outer layer is without cell boundaries, and hence is *syncytial trophoblast*.
It shows a *brush border* and has its nuclei spaced fairly evenly in one row.
It arises by cells of the inner layer merging into a common mass.
In the last half of pregnancy the cellular trophoblast gradually disappears.
It finally ceases to proliferate, and its cells add to the syncytial layer.
The syncytial layer is mostly thin, but scattered clumps of nuclei occur in it.
These make local bulges called *syncytial knots*.
Where syncytium overlies capillaries, it is an especially thin layer.
Degenerative changes produce patches of *fibrinoid substance*.
In addition to the trophoblast, maternal blood is also involved.
The enlargement of myometrial *smooth-muscle fibers* during pregnancy is notable.
They increase in length 10 times, and also increase in number.
The *cervical glands* become larger and secrete mucus abundantly.
This forms a mucous plug that seals up the cervical canal.

2. Circulatory relations.

The fetal and maternal bloods follow wholly independent courses, without mixing.

(Occasionally small leaks of fetal blood do occur into the intervillous space.)

The *fetal vessels* comprise a closed circuit of small vessels and capillaries.

Uterine arterioles open by tiny nozzles into a labyrinthine *intervillous space.*

Veins drain the intermittently spurted blood away from this space.

The *intervillous space* was created at the expense of eroded decidual tissue.

It is carpeted everywhere with a continuous sheet of trophoblast.

That is, trophoblast covers the chorionic plate, villi and decidua basalis.

Like endothelium it does not provoke the clotting of blood.

The space and its lining are unique as a corridor for the passage of blood.

Hence all interchanges between the two circulations must cross a protoplasmic barrier.

E. REGENERATIVE ABILITY:

The *endometrium* is highly efficient in repairing injuries even when severe.

The course after delivery, curettage or other destruction is like postmenstrual repair.

F. DIAGNOSTIC FEATURES:

The *uterus* is a thick-walled organ with a distinctive mucosa (*endometrium*).

Its *epithelium* is simple columnar; some ciliated cells show if preservation is good.

The *glands* of the fundus and corpus are vertical tubules, not plainly branching.

They are not crowded, but are spaced well apart.

Their length, tortuosity and distention vary throughout the cycle.

The tubular *cervical glands* are obviously branched; they are mucus-secreting.

The gland cell (like the surface cell) is tall and pale, with a basal nucleus.

This type does not participate significantly in the cyclic changes.

The *lamina propria* is rich in cells and poor in fibers, like the uterine tube.

These cells enlarge in pregnancy into so-called *decidual cells.*

The *muscularis* is heavy and contains three layers, not sharply delimited.

Each layer shows interlacing bundles.

Sections through the *placenta* are featured by myriads of tissue-islands in a blood space.

These are sectioned *villi*, containing small vessels and bordered by epithelium.

The association of cuboidal cells and a syncytium is safely diagnostic of pregnancy.

In the last half of pregnancy, cuboidal cells lack; the syncytium collects in *knots.*

G. FUNCTIONAL CORRELATIONS:

The *uterus* is specialized toward receiving and rearing an egg within its mucosa.

It nourishes and protects the embryo, and expels it at the proper time.

In *childhood* the uterus is small, and its mucosa is thin.

Prepuberal growth is controlled by the increasing secretion of estrogen.

At *puberty* the uterus is brought into functional condition by an increase of progesterone.

After the *menopause* the uterus undergoes marked atrophy.

The same is true of the uterine tubes and vagina; estrogen-decline is responsible.

The significance of the *menstrual cycle* is that it anticipates each month the possibility of pregnancy and prepares a bed suitable for the fertilized ovum.

Postmenstrual, proliferative changes are directed by the follicular hormone (*estrogen*).

Postovulatory, secretory changes are governed by the luteal hormone (*progesterone*).

If pregnancy occurs, the egg implants during this favorable stage of upbuilding.

If *pregnancy fails*, the corpus luteum declines and its hormonal influence wanes.

The mucosa then is unstable; it breaks down, apparently from lack of hormonal support.

If *pregnancy supervenes*, the progravid changes continue under progesterone influence.

Hormone is supplied first by the persisting corpus luteum and later by the placenta.

The hormone-supported mucosa thereby becomes the *decidua* of pregnancy.

The stromal cells become the *decidual cells* of pregnancy.

Part of the decidua becomes the maternal portion of the placenta.

The placenta serves the fetus as a lung, food-intake apparatus and kidney.

Among its syntheses is a *chorionic gonadotropin* (by its cellular trophoblast).

The presence of this hormone in urine makes possible simple tests for pregnancy.

It also secretes *estrogen* and *progesterone* (probably syntheses by the syncytium).

The placenta acts as a *barrier* against particulate matter, such as micro-organisms.

Only chemical substances under a certain molecular size can pass through.

Hence fat and various blood proteins first break down into simpler products.

IV. THE VAGINA

The *vagina* is a fibro-muscular sheath, lined with a transversely folded mucosa.

Its upper end is continuous with the uterine cervix.

The lower end is bounded by the *hymen*, a transverse, annular fold of the mucosa.

It separates vagina from vestibule; stratified squamous epithelium covers both surfaces.

1. Mucosa.

This is continuous, by reflection, onto the outer wall of the protruding uterine cervix.

The thick *epithelium* is of the stratified squamous type.

It is unkeratinized and lacks glands; lubricative mucus comes from the cervix.

Transition into the simple epithelium of the cervical canal is abrupt.

The *lamina propria* is a thick feltwork of fine fibers, including an elastic network.

Lymphocytes and occasional *lymph nodules* occur.

Many lymphocytes invade the epithelium.

Papillae indent the epithelium; these are tall on the posterior wall.

Transverse ridges are responsible for the mucosal folds (*rugae*) of the vagina.

2. Submucosa.

A deeper, looser and more vascular layer exists, but is rather indefinite.

3. Muscularis.

Smooth muscle is arranged in interlacing bundles that occupy ill defined layers.

The *inner portion* is thin and contains more circular or spiral bundles.

The thicker, *outer portion* is preponderantly longitudinal; it continues onto the uterus.

At the lower end of the vagina there is a *sphincter* of skeletal muscle.

4. Adventitia.

A thin layer of dense, fibrous tissue merges into looser, adjoining connective tissue.

In front and behind, it blends with adventitia of the bladder and rectum, respectively.

It is rich in large blood vessels.

5. Vessels and nerves.

These follow the general plan described on p. 260.

6. Diagnostic features.

The vagina is lined with an unkeratinized, stratified squamous *epithelium*.

Papillae indent the epithelium; in the posterior wall they are tall.

The *lamina propria* is a thick, connective-tissue network.

A *muscularis mucosae* and glands are missing (differentiating it from the esophagus).

The *muscular coat* consists of smooth muscle, mostly longitudinal.

On its inner surface, a thin circular layer occurs.

The *adventitia* blends, in much of its extent, with that of other organs.

7. Functional correlations.

The vagina serves as a distensible *copulatory receptacle* and *birth canal*.

The epithelium contains a variable amount of glycogen.
   Its abundance is dependent on the periodic increase of *estrogen* prior to ovulation.
   Consequently, its fermentation to lactic acid in vaginal fluid is greatest then.
Midway of the cycle, keratohyalin granules accumulate in the more superficial layers.
   Superficial cells, then cast off, are faintly acidophilic and have small dark nuclei.
In some mammals the *estrous cycle* is accompanied by definite changes in the types and
         proportions of epithelial cells and leucocytes found free in the vaginal lumen.
   The exact stage can be determined by examining vaginal smears.
   In the human, less clearly marked cyclic changes occur at the time of ovulation.
      Yet smears will indicate the presence or absence of effective estrogen production.
      Also the follicular and luteal phases of the ovary can be distinguished.

V. THE EXTERNAL GENITALIA

The parts of the external genitalia are known collectively as the *vulva*.
   Its lateral boundaries are formed by the *greater lips*, within which are *lesser lips*.
The *vestibule* is a shallow cavity into which the urethra and vagina open.
   The *vestibular glands* also discharge into it, and the *clitoris* protrudes here.

1. Clitoris.

   The *clitoris* is a rudimentary and incomplete counterpart of the penis.
      It has two cavernous, *erectile bodies* and a rudimentary *glans* and *prepuce*.
      It lacks a urethra and corpus spongiosum.
   The whole organ is surrounded with thin, stratified squamous epithelium.
      It contains specialized sensory *nerve endings* of several types.

2. Vestibular glands.

   The *major vestibular glands* are also known as the glands of Bartholin.
      They are two bodies, located in the lateral walls of the vestibule.
         Each is about 0.5 inch long; its duct opens just outside the hymen.
      These glands correspond to the bulbo-urethral glands in the male (p. 274).
      They are *tubulo-alveolar glands*, structurally like those of the male.
         A lubricative *mucus* is discharged during sexual excitement.
   The *minor vestibular glands* are several small mucous glands located around the ure-
         thral opening and near the clitoris.
      They resemble the *urethral glands* (of Littré) of the urethra (p. 262).

3. Labia minora.

   These *lesser lips* form the lateral walls of the vestibule.
   Each is a long, high but relatively thin fold of mucous membrane.
      Tall connective-tissue *papillae* indent the stratified squamous epithelium.
      The basal layer of the epithelium contains *pigment granules*.
   Sebaceous glands occur on both surfaces of the fold.
      Neither hair follicles nor fat cells are found in the labia minora.

4. Labia majora.

   These *greater lips* are folds of skin that cover the labia minora.
      Within each fold there is a considerable amount of *fat*.
   The *inner surface* is soft, smooth and hairless.
      Its mucosa is much like that of the labia minora.
   The *outer surface* is covered with keratinized epidermis and bears coarse hairs.
   Both surfaces are supplied with sebaceous glands and sweat glands.

5. *Diagnostic features.*

The *clitoris* has two erectile columns, but lacks a urethra and surrounding spongiosum.
The *major vestibular glands* are essentially like the male bulbo-urethral glands (p. 274).
Each *labium minus* is a simple mucosal fold, clothed with stratified squamous epithelium.
   Sebaceous glands on both surfaces are a distinctive characteristic.
Each *labium majus* is a thicker fold, containing fat and having unlike surfaces.
   One surface is hairy skin; the other surface is soft mucous membrane.
      Both surfaces contain sebaceous glands and sweat glands.

6. *Functional correlations.*

The *vestibule* is a shallow urogenital sinus, corresponding to much of the male urethra.
The *clitoris* is an erectile organ and a receptor for erotic sensation.
The *labia minora* correspond to the undersurface of the penis, but remain ununited.
   They are lateral walls, bounding the vestibule.
The *labia majora* correspond to the halves of the scrotum, but remain ununited.
   They serve as guards to the lesser lips and shallow vestibule.

VI. THE MAMMARY GLAND

This organ is sometimes treated as a part of the female reproductive system.
Actually it is a specialized skin gland and belongs with the integumentary system (p. 200).

Chapter XXV

The Sense Organs

The distal process of a cranio-spinal ganglion cell conducts impulses centralward, like a dendron.
   Such a sensory nerve fiber loses its sheaths distally and ends as a *sensory receptor*.
   Each fiber branches near its end; the final naked twigs may bear berry-like tips.
Sensory receptors can be classified in different ways.
   One classification is based on the source of stimuli exciting the receptive endings.
      Exteroceptors are affected by stimuli external to the body itself.
         Example: touch; pressure; cutaneous pain and temperature; smell; sight; hearing.
      Proprioceptors are affected by stimuli arising within the body wall.
         Information is given concerning position and muscular tension.
         Example: excitation from muscles, tendons, joints and the ear.
      Interoceptors are affected by stimuli arising within the various visceral organs.
         Example: excitation from activities such as digestion, excretion and circulation.
   Another classification is based on the widespread or limited location of the receptors.
      General sensibility collects information from the body as a whole.
         Example: touch; pressure; pain; temperature; visceral sense; position; movement.
      Special sensibility is related to sense organs located in definite portions of the head.
         Example: smell; taste; sight; hearing; balance.

I. ORGANS OF GENERAL SENSIBILITY

These endings are rather simple structurally and are distributed widely throughout the body.
They can be classified on the basis of the *kind of tissue* in which the sensory fibers end.
Another grouping is based on whether or not the terminal fibers are *encapsulated*.
A combination of both types of criteria will be used in the descriptions that follow.

A. ENDINGS IN EPITHELIUM:
   1. Free endings.
      The innervated epithelium may be external (epidermis) or internal (mucosae).
      Nerve fibers, resolving into simple branches, terminate among the cells.
      Of special note are the *peritrichial endings* activated by movements of the hairs.
         The outer root sheath of a hair follicle is encircled by nerve fibers.
         Some fibers ascend in a palisade; endings are made on the glassy membrane.

   2. Terminal disks.
      Somewhat more specialized are the networks at the ends of certain nerve twigs.
      Each saucer-like plexus comes in contact with a single, modified epithelial cell.
      Such a receptive cell and its plexus are called a *tactile cell* and *-disk* (of Merkel).
         They occur in deep epidermis, in hair follicles and in the hard palate.

B. ENDINGS IN CONNECTIVE TISSUE:
   1. Free endings.
      A nerve fiber ends in bush-like *branchings*, in an interlacing *network*, or in a knot-like
         skein (*glomerulus*).
      Example: skin; serous and mucous membranes; periosteum; sclera.

2. Encapsulated endings.

This group is characterized by a *fibrous capsule* of varying thickness.

The capsule is continuous with the endoneurium of the nerve fiber.

A. GLOMERULI.

Branching nerve fibers form a tightly interlacing and anastomosing skein.

This spheroidal mass is enclosed by a thin, layered capsule.

Such corpuscles occur in the skin, mucous membranes, conjunctiva and heart.

Examples: *terminal cylinders* (of Ruffini); *end-bulbs* (of Krause); *genital corpuscles*.

B. TACTILE CORPUSCLES.

This receptor, ellipsoidal in shape, is also known as *Meissner's corpuscle*.

They occur in hairless skin, such as the palmar and plantar surfaces.

They are prominent in many of the papillae that indent the epidermis.

The largest corpuscles measure from 40 to 180 μ in length.

There is a fibrous capsule, and a core of flattened tactile cells.

The cells lie transversely, interspersed with horizontal fibrous shelves.

One or more nerve fibers enter and course upward, spiraling.

Branches end in net-like skeins in relation to the tactile cells.

C. LAMELLAR CORPUSCLES.

The commonest type is also known as a *Pacinian corpuscle* (or Vater-Pacinian).

Similar ones, but smaller and simpler, receive still other names.

They occur both in superficial and in deep locations in the body.

Lamellar corpuscles are macroscopic; the largest measure 2×4 mm.

Structurally this is the most complex type of encapsulated ending.

The *core* is a slender, protoplasmic cylinder, of semifluid consistency.

A single nerve fiber enters at one end and runs axially through it.

The fiber gives off lateral twigs and ends in a fibrillated knob.

The fibrous *capsule* is very thick and consists of many layers (up to 60).

These dense lamellae are arranged concentrically, like an onion.

C. ENDINGS IN MUSCLE AND TENDON:

1. Ordinary endings.

Some are simple *branchings*; others are *encapsulated endings*.

They lie between or on the fibers of muscle or tendon.

2. Neuromuscular spindles.

These are slender bundles that occur in a muscle, and mostly near its tendon.

They are oriented parallel to the long axis of the muscle.

A *spindle* is usually 2 to 4 mm. long and consists of 3 to 10 skeletal muscle fibers.

These fibers, in two sizes, are of the 'red' type (p. 103) and are notably thin.

The cluster of fibers is encapsulated with layered fibrous tissue.

Sensory nerve fibers enter, branch and spiral or spray about the muscle fibers.

They come into close apposition with the sarcolemma-sheaths.

Motor nerve fibers, terminating in typical *end-plates*, occur also.

3. Neurotendinous spindles.

Several groups of tendon fibers, near their junction with muscle, are involved.

The spindle-shaped bundle measures up to 3 mm. in length.

It is thinly encapsulated with connective tissue.

Nerve fibers enter, branch freely and end in clubbed enlargements on fibers.

D. REGENERATIVE ABILITY:

Free endings degenerate and regenerate as do peripheral nerve fibers in general (p. 121).

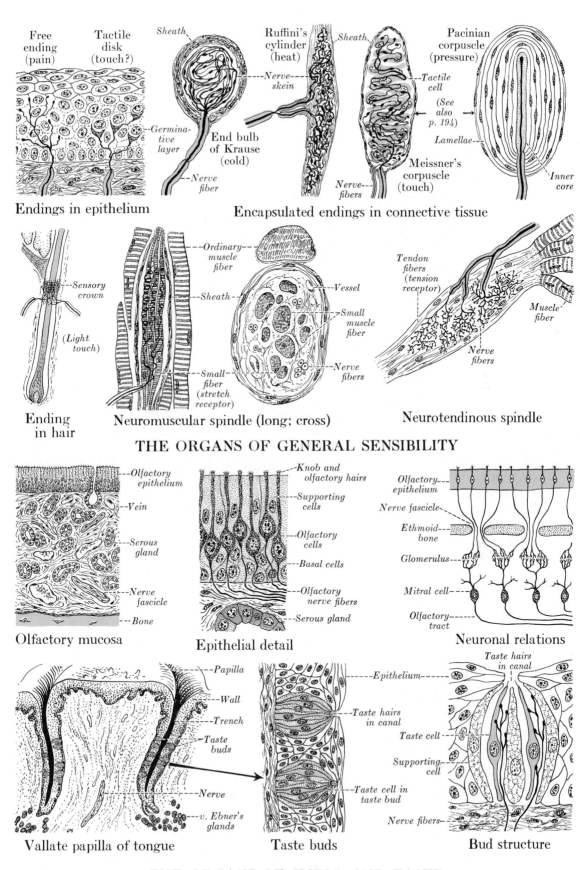

Free ending (pain) Tactile disk (touch?)

Sheath

Ruffini's cylinder (heat)

Sheath

Pacinian corpuscle (pressure)

Nerve-skein

Germina-tive layer

End bulb of Krause (cold)

Tactile cell

(See also p. 194)

Lamellae

Nerve fiber

Nerve-fibers

Meissner's corpuscle (touch)

Inner core

Endings in epithelium

Encapsulated endings in connective tissue

Sensory crown

Ordinary muscle fiber

Sheath

Vessel

Small muscle fiber

Tendon fibers (tension receptor)

Muscle fiber

(*Light touch*)

Small fiber (stretch receptor)

Nerve fibers

Nerve fibers

Ending in hair

Neuromuscular spindle (long; cross)

Neurotendinous spindle

THE ORGANS OF GENERAL SENSIBILITY

Olfactory epithelium

Vein

Serous gland

Nerve fascicle

Bone

Knob and olfactory hairs

Supporting cells

Olfactory cells

Basal cells

Olfactory nerve fibers

Serous gland

Olfactory epithelium

Nerve fascicle

Ethmoid bone

Glomerulus

Mitral cell

Olfactory tract

Olfactory mucosa

Epithelial detail

Neuronal relations

Papilla

Wall

Trench

Taste buds

Nerve

v. Ebner's glands

Epithelium

Taste hairs in canal

Taste cell in taste bud

Taste hairs in canal

Taste cell

Supporting cell

Nerve fibers

Vallate papilla of tongue

Taste buds

Bud structure

THE ORGANS OF SMELL AND TASTE

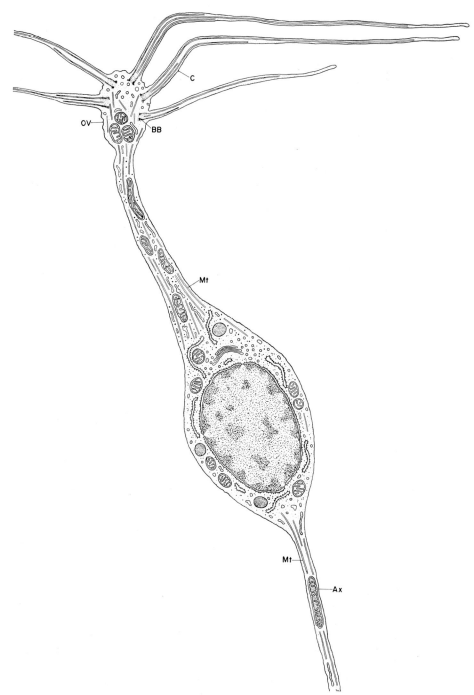

OLFACTORY CELL.   About the nucleus of this bipolar ganglion cell are ovoid mitochondria, some rough and smooth endoplasmic reticulum, a distally located Golgi complex, and a few lysosomes. In the distal process the mitochondria are elongate, some smooth endoplasmic reticulum occurs, and microtubules (Mt) are numerous. At its end the process dilates into a bulbous olfactory vesicle (OV) which projects above the general epithelial surface. From basal bodies (BB) long cilia (C) extend radially. In their more distal regions the characteristic tubular fibers are reduced in number. The proximal process becomes an axonal nerve fiber (Ax) that contains microtubules (Mt) and some elongated mitochondria. The fiber penetrates the basement membrane of the olfactory epithelium and joins others to constitute the olfactory nerve.

Information concerning encapsulated endings seems to be unknown, or at least unrecorded.
This lack includes data on their behavior after denervation and nerve regeneration.
Of interest would be data on their possible new formation in regenerated skin.

E. APPEARANCE IN SECTIONS.

Arborizations in epithelium and connective tissue are not seen after ordinary staining.
Special techniques (silver; methylene blue) demonstrate them satisfactorily.
Some of the *encapsulated endings* are readily recognizable.
Meissner's *tactile corpuscles* are identifiable in some dermal papillae of the skin.
Their location is limited to hairless surfaces (palm; sole; nipple; etc.).
Both the fibrous framework of the ellipsoidal corpuscle and the contained cells are ordinarily demonstrable.
Lamellar corpuscles are conspicuous near the junction of the dermis and subcutaneous.
Occasionally they are encountered in deep internal organs.
Example: pancreas; prostate; serous membranes.
The thick, concentric, onion-layered arrangement is unmistakable.
Glomeruli have a thin, layered capsule and a relatively voluminous, granular interior.
A *neuromuscular spindle* is seen but rarely, and then in a chance section.
Its encapsulation and contained, thin skeletal fibers are points of recognition.
Neurotendinous spindles are scarcely to be expected in ordinary sections.
Their site is not at locations where tissue samples are commonly taken.

F. FUNCTIONAL CORRELATIONS:

The stimulation of any receptor merely activates a conducted, nervous impulse.
Its translation into a conscious sensation occurs in a particular part of the brain.

1. Endings in epithelium.

Diffuse aborizations mediate the sensation of *pain*; (also touch, heat and cold?).
Peritrichial endings are *touch receptors* for hairy regions of the skin.
Terminal disks presumably mediate the sensation of *light touch*.

2. Endings in connective tissue.

Free endings, like those in epithelium, are concerned with *pain reception*, at least.
Functions usually assigned to certain encapsulated endings are as follows:
Krause's end-bulbs are *cold receptors*, for some regions at least.
Ruffini's terminal cylinders seemingly mediate the sensation of *warmth*.
Meissner's tactile corpuscles are point *touch receptors* for the hairless surfaces.
Pacinian lamellar corpuscles are thought to be concerned with *pressure sensibility*.

3. Endings in muscle and tendon.

These receptors furnish stimuli leading to adjustments in the *movements* and *positions* of the limbs and other parts of the body.
Neuromuscular spindles become *stretch receptors* when pulled upon.
They are stimulated when the muscle elongates passively during relaxation.
Neurotendinous spindles are *tension receptors*, responding to any pull.
This force may be due to active muscle contraction as well as to passive stretch.

II. THE SPECIAL SENSE ORGANS

1. THE OLFACTORY ORGAN

Combining the olfactory organ with the respiratory intake was introduced by lung fishes.
All higher vertebrates retained this feature, and some improved on it by evolving a palate.

A. STRUCTURAL PLAN:

The *olfactory region* of a nasal cavity includes the narrow roof and some adjacent mucosa.
The latter covers the superior concha and an equal extent on the nasal septum.
The area on each lateral and medial wall is about the size of a dime.
The olfactory organ is merely a highly specialized mucous membrane, brownish in color.
The receptive cells, within the epithelium, are bipolar ganglion cells.
They are the only ones to retain a primitive location in a surface epithelium.
Extensions of the olfactory cells become *nerve fibers* that pass to the brain.
The olfactory cell, with its fiber-process, is a neuron of the first order.
Other cells of the epithelium are insensitive *supporting elements*.

B. DETAILED STRUCTURE:

1. Olfactory epithelium.

The thick, yellowish *epithelium* is a pseudostratified type, without goblet cells.
The *olfactory cells* are spindle-shaped elements, with nearly spherical nuclei.
These nuclei occupy a middle- to somewhat deep zone in the epithelial layer.
The *distal part* of the cell is slender; it serves as a dendron.
It ends in a bulbous knob that bears 6 to 12 so-called *olfactory hairs*.
These long 'hairs' are poorly motile cilia that serve as sensory receptors.
The *proximal part* of the cell is drawn out into a thin axon-process.
This is the *olfactory nerve fiber* that makes connections within the brain.
It is an unmyelinated fiber that continues through the lamina propria.
Here it gains a neurolemma sheath.
Hence the total olfactory cell is a peculiarly located bipolar neuron.
The chief *supporting cells* are tall columnar elements, pigmented in the apical half.
Their *microvilli* give the appearance of a striated border.
The basal half of each cell is much narrower than the pigmented, apical half.
In addition there are conical *basal cells* that clasp clusters of nerve fibers.
Both nonsensory cell-types have an ovoid nucleus, characteristically located.
Their nuclei are nearer the cell top, or base, than those of olfactory cells.
Yet there is a prominent zone, free of all nuclei, near the free surface.

2. Lamina propria.

The *basement membrane* is too thin to be seen with the light microscope.
Superficially the lamina is delicately fibrous and contains many cellular elements.
Through it pass myriads of olfactory *nerve fibers* gathered in small bundles.
It contains the *olfactory glands* (of Bowman), which secrete continuously.
These are branched, tubulo-alveolar glands with a sero-mucous secretion.
Ducts convey the thin secretion to the surface of the mucous membrane.
More deeply the lamina is coarsely fibrous and fuses with the underlying periosteum.
In it occur about 20 prominent *fascicles* of nerve fibers.
These represent gatherings of the smaller bundles located at higher levels.
Each fascicle passes through an opening in the ethmoid bone to reach the brain.

C. REGENERATIVE ABILITY:

After destruction of olfactory mucosa, the ability to detect some odors may return.
This is probably owing to the survival of intact fragments of the original mucosa.
At least, the formation of new olfactory cells in the restored membrane is not known.

D. DIAGNOSTIC FEATURES:

The olfactory mucosa is surfaced with a thick *pseudostratified epithelium*, bearing cilia.
Nuclei are densely packed in a thick layer; goblet cells are lacking.
The lamina propria contains *serous glands*, and *nerve bundles* occur at a deep level.
This level lacks the venous plexuses, so prominent in the nasal respiratory region.
The mucous membrane lies upon bone.

E. FUNCTIONAL CORRELATIONS:

Olfactory stimulation is caused by gaseous, odoriferous substances in solution.
To this end the serous glands of the membrane bathe the surface with a watery fluid.
Continuous secretion serves also to freshen the fluid-film.
This prevents the retention of dissolved odors and lingering stimulation by them.
The actual receptive instruments are cilia (olfactory hairs) exposed at the surface in fluid.
No known differences in structure among olfactory cells are correlated with the discrimination of different kinds of odors.

II. THE GUSTATORY ORGAN

In fishes the organs of taste are widespread, occurring even on the gills, body and tail.
All higher vertebrates restrict them to the cavity of the mouth.

A. STRUCTURAL PLAN:

The *organ of taste* consists of numerous ovoid *taste buds,* about 70 μ tall.
They are most plentiful, in the adult, on the *vallate papillae* of the tongue.
Such a papilla bears about 200 taste buds on its sides.
The wall of the trench, opposite the papilla, bears about 50 buds.
These numbers are highly variable, and they decrease progressively with aging.
Taste buds are also plentiful midway in the folds that comprise the *foliate papillae.*
These papillae, however, are often regressive or rudimentary.
A few buds occur on the fungiform papillae, soft palate, pharynx and epiglottis.
In general, they are more numerous and widespread in the newborn than later.
A *taste bud* is a paler, ovoid specialization within a stratified squamous epithelium.
It contains *neuro-epithelial cells* and *supporting cells.*
It communicates with the free surface by a tiny *taste canal* opening by a *taste pore.*

B. DETAILED STRUCTURE:

A *taste bud* extends vertically from the basement membrane almost to the free surface of the stratified squamous epithelium.
The overlying layers of the general epithelium are pierced by a *taste canal.*
The shape of a bud is somewhat like a barrel, but is often narrower at the top.
Two cell types comprise a taste bud.
The *taste cells,* 4 to 20 in number, are slender, spindle-shaped neuro-epithelial elements.
The elongate nucleus occupies a middle position in these dark cells.
From the free end of the cell several long *microvilli* project into the taste canal.
(Mucoid fluid in the canal may coagulate into longer, misnamed *taste hairs.*)
The *supporting cells* are tall pale elements, with rounder light nuclei.
Most of these are at the periphery; they resemble thick barrel staves.
Some gustatory *nerve fibers* enter the bud, branch and make knobbed endings.
These endings touch the surface of the taste cells, and also the 'supporting cells.'
Other fibers end in twigs about the exterior of the taste bud.

C. REGENERATIVE ABILITY:

Taste buds are stable only when their innervation is intact.
Interference with the nerve supply leads to degeneration; removal is aided by phagocytes.
Immediate replacement is by ordinary epithelial cells, following local proliferation.
On reinnervation, after nerve regeneration, the buds differentiate anew.

D. DIAGNOSTIC FEATURES:

A paler, barrel-shaped *cluster of cells* lies vertically in a stratified squamous epithelium.
The commonest location in an adult is on the sides of a vallate papilla.
Smaller numbers occur in the wall surrounding the trench.

From the top of a bud a slender *canal* leads to the free surface of the epithelium.

Slanting sections may transect this canal variously, or fail to include it.

In preserved specimens, *'taste hairs'* may be seen within the canal.

E. FUNCTIONAL CORRELATIONS:

Various substances stimulate (the microvilli?) and educe the sensations of taste.

Such substances are effective only when in solution.

It is possible that the so-called supporting cells are inexactly named.

Primarily they may be replacing elements for the gustatory cells.

Taste cells are very short-lived, and transitional stages are demonstrable.

Moreover, the sensation of taste is not restricted to regions containing taste buds.

Actually, all the lingual mucosa innervated by gustatory nerves is responsive.

Sensitivity to the four taste modalities is different regionally in the tongue.

Even individual papillae may respond only to sweet, sour, salt or bitter.

Yet no recognizable differences occur in the structure of individual taste buds.

III. THE EYE

The visual organ consists primarily of the *eyeball* and *optic nerve.*

But it also includes various accessories (*extrinsic muscles; eyelids; tear apparatus*).

The several components of the visual organ are sheltered within the bony *orbit.*

A. STRUCTURAL PLAN:

The spheroidal *eyeball* consists of three *coats* that enclose certain *refractive media.*

The outer coat is the tough, fibrous *tunica fibrosa.*

Most of it is the opaque *sclera,* but anteriorly it becomes the transparent *cornea.*

The middle coat is the vascular and pigmented *tunica vasculosa* (or uvea).

Most of it is the relatively unspecialized *choroid.*

Near the front it becomes the muscular *ciliary body* and the *iris.*

The iris ends about a circular opening, the *pupil.*

The innermost coat is the *tunica interna,* or *retina.*

Its nerve fibers gather posteriorly and leave the eyeball as the *optic nerve.*

This coat becomes insensitive where it lines the ciliary body and iris.

A refractive *lens* lies just behind the pupil and iris.

It is held in position and is influenced to change shape by a *suspensory ligament.*

This *ciliary zonule* is a system of fibers that radiate to the muscular ciliary body.

The *vitreous body* is a jelly that occupies the large space behind the lens.

Watery *aqueous humor* occupies the space in front of the lens and vitreous body.

The *eyelids* are movable folds of skin that can cover fully the front of the eyeball.

The *lacrimal gland* secretes tears into the *conjunctival sac* (between eyelids and eyeball).

The *tears* are drained away by a *duct system* at the inner angle of the eye.

B. DETAILED STRUCTURE:

1. Fibrous tunic.

The outer coat consists of the *sclera* and the modified, transparent *cornea.*

A. SCLERA.

This firm, *external coat* ranges from 0.13 to 1.0 mm. in thickness.

It is expansive and is commonly known as the 'white' of the eye.

On it insert the tendons of the eye muscles.

In the region of the optic nerve the sclera thins into a sieve-like plate.

The outer scleral surface is a thin layer of loose, vascular *episcleral tissue.*

The middle region embraces the main scleral mass; it is the *substantia propria.*

It is composed mostly of densely woven collagenous fibers.

The inner surface is represented by the thin, pigmented *lamina fusca.*

It is transitional into the choroid (see the suprachoroid layer, beyond).

B. CORNEA.

The front, bulging portion of the eyeball is transparent and nonvascular.

Five layers can be distinguised in this *cornea,* from front to back.

1. The *corneal epithelium* is a thin, stratified squamous type.

   It contains only 5 to 6 layers of cells, and is moist and unkeratinized.

2. The *anterior limiting layer* (of Bowman) is a prominent, clear sheet.

   It is composed of collagenous fibrils arranged in an ultrafine feltwork.

3. The thick *substantia propria* contains about 60 collagenous lamellae.

   The fiber direction alternates in successive lamellae.

   Lamellae are permeated with polysaccharide that also embeds flat fibroblasts.

4. The *posterior limiting layer* (of Descemet) is thick and nearly structureless.

   It is somewhat elastic but probably consists of atypical collagen.

5. The *endothelium of the anterior chamber* is a low cuboidal epithelium.

   It is not a true endothelium, as named, since it is bathed by aqueous humor.

2. *Vascular tunic.*

This coat is primarily *vascular* and *pigmented,* yet one region contains muscle.

Ophthalmic blood vessels supply this tunic and the optic nerve separately.

It is bound intimately to the outer layer of the retina, but joins the sclera loosely.

Exceptions having firm union are at the cribriform plate and ciliary body.

It has two circular defects: one is the *pupil;* the other, about the optic nerve.

This middle coat comprises, from back to front, the *choroid, ciliary body* and *iris.*

A. CHOROID.

This coat extends forward two-thirds of the distance toward the pupil.

The soft, thin membrane is co-extensive with the light perceptive retina.

Four layers can be recognized, from outside inward, as follows:

1. The *suprachoroid layer* is a series of slanting plates that join the sclera.

   Each plate contains branched *pigment cells* and *elastic fibers.*

   Between the plates is a system of clefts, making the *perichoroid space.*

2. The *vascular layer* contains many vessels and stellate *pigment cells.*

3. A *chorio-capillary layer* forms a rather broad-bored network close to the retina.

   It supplies nutriment and oxygen to the subjacent retina.

4. The *basal lamina* (of Bruch) is a double-layered sheet.

   Its outer component contains fine elastic and collagenous fibers.

   An inner, homogeneous layer supports the pigment epithelium of the retina.

B. CILIARY BODY.

This division of the coat is a specialized circular band, forming a zone.

It is interposed between the expansive choroid and the iris.

It thickens progressively as it nears the iris, and here bears about 70 ridges.

Each ridge is a *ciliary process* that runs in a meridional plane.

The total set makes a wheel-like arrangement named the *ciliary crown.*

These processes anchor the fibers of the suspensory ligament of the lens.

Similar structural layers occur in the ciliary body as in the choroid.

But a unique and striking feature is the prominent *ciliary muscle.*

This mass of smooth muscle lies within the suprachoroid layer.

Its fibers run meridionally, radially and circularly.

Although a vascular layer exists, there is no specific capillary layer.

The *basal lamina* of the choroid continues into the ciliary body.

It serves as a basal support for the modified retina of this zone.

At least, the inner component does; the elastic component splits off.

The ciliary processes form *aqueous humor* and secrete it into the zonular space.

C. IRIS.

The *iris* is a washer-shaped marginal plate, bordering the pupillary opening.

At its attached border, it is continuous with the ciliary body.

Elsewhere it is suspended free in the aqueous space between cornea and lens.

Several layers can be distinguished, from front to back:

1. An indistinct, so-called *endothelium* covers the surface that faces the cornea.
   This is continuous with the more distinct lining of the cornea.
   It is lacking in some regions where crypt-like excavations occur.
2. An *anterior stromal layer* underlies the endothelium.
   It is nonvascular and contains few to many branched, pigmented cells.
   These *melanophores* determine the color (other than blue) of the iris.
   The thickness of the layer and its density of pigmentation are factors.
3. The *general stroma,* deeper in position, is a spongy fibro-elastic tissue.
   The fibers are fine, and most of the stromal cells are pigmented.
   Numerous blood vessels characterize this layer.

The posterior surface of the iris is clothed with a continuation of the retina.
   Its pigment layer specializes into *dilator-* and *sphincter muscles* (p. 302).

D. IRIS ANGLE.

The iris meets the sclero-corneal junction at an acute angle.
   This union subtends a space in front of the iris called the *iris angle.*
Here occurs a spongy meshwork belonging to the scleral and vascular coats.
   Its *spaces of the iris angle* (of Fontana) open off the anterior chamber.
Nearby is the more prominent, ring-shaped *scleral venous sinus.*
   This canal (of Schlemm) encircles the eyeball at the corneal margin.
   It drains by numerous branches into neighboring anterior ciliary veins.
The spaces of Fontana and canal of Schlemm do not communicate directly.
   Yet aqueous humor finds ready passage into the canal, and so out into veins.

3. Internal tunic (or retina).

This innermost ocular coat lines the tunica vasculosa throughout its extent.
The *retina* arose as a bulge of the brain wall that became a double-walled cup.
   The outer wall of the cup is the thin, insensitive *pigment layer.*
      This layer is commonly called the *pigment epithelium.*
   The inner wall is the *nervous layer* of the retina, or retina proper.
The nervous layer is an expansive membrane, most of which is photosensitive.
   (Blind portions are at the optic nerve, and on the ciliary body and iris.)
   It contains several delicate sublayers related to three sets of neurons.
   These neurons are linked together in neuron chains.
Three topographical regions of the internal tunic are recognized descriptively.
   These are, from back to front: an *optic-,* a *ciliary-* and an *iridical portion.*

A. PARS OPTICA.

This major expanse of the retina extends from the head of the optic nerve to the
      posterior border of the ciliary body.
   Here the truly nervous retina ends in a wavy line, the *ora serrata.*
Except for minor modified regions, the pars optica consists of 10 layers.
   All but the first belong to the nervous layer, or the retina proper.

1. *Pigment epithelium.*
   This single layer of *pigmented cells* is bound fast to the choroid's basal lamina.
   Its cuboidal cells bear numerous pigmented, cytoplasmic processes.
      These fringes extend between the rods and cones of the nervous retina.
      Such interdigitation, however, effects only a weak adhesion.
2. *Rods and cones.*
   These are the light-sensitive end-portions of the *rod-* and *cone cells.*
      The cells, known collectively as *visual cells,* are a neuro-epithelium.
      They are arranged vertically and parallel, palisade-fashion.
   The rods are slender cylinders; cones are shaped like long-necked flasks.
      Each is some 60 μ long; rods outnumber cones 130 million to 7 million.
      Both possess a slender *outer segment* and a thicker *inner segment.*
         The outer segment consists largely of stacked flat sacs, 0.014 μ thick.
         The inner segment is mostly an *ellipsoid,* containing many mitochondria.

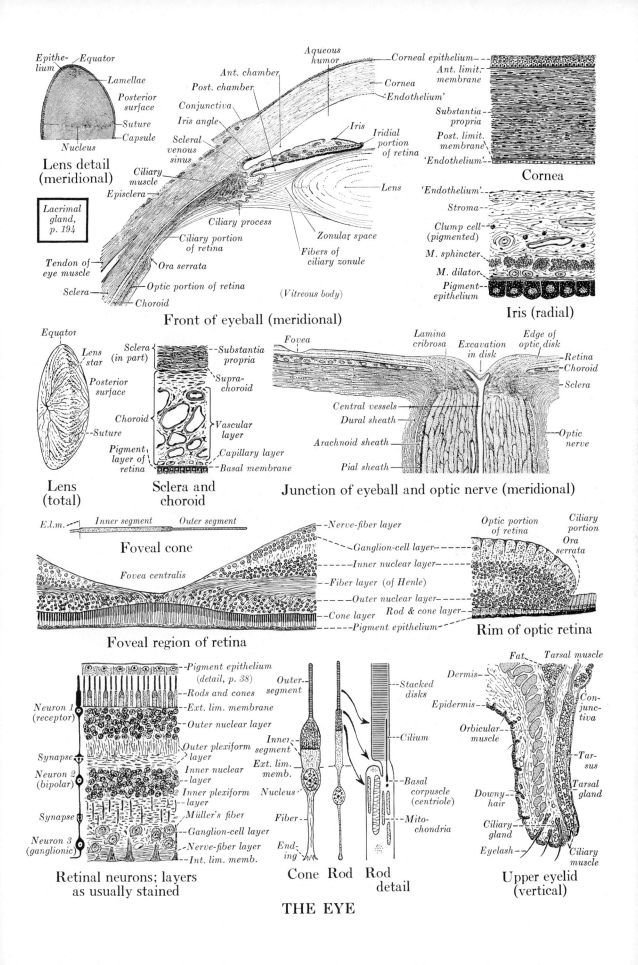

Lens detail (meridional)

Epithelium — Equator — Lamellae — Posterior surface — Suture — Capsule — Nucleus

Front of eyeball (meridional)

Ant. chamber — Post. chamber — Conjunctiva — Iris angle — Scleral venous sinus — Ciliary muscle — Episclera — Aqueous humor — Iris — Iridial portion of retina — Lens — Ciliary process — Zonular space — Fibers of ciliary zonule — Ciliary portion of retina — Ora serrata — Optic portion of retina — Choroid — Tendon of eye muscle — Sclera — (Vitreous body)

Lacrimal gland, p. 194

Cornea

Corneal epithelium — Ant. limit. membrane — Cornea — 'Endothelium' — Substantia propria — Post. limit. membrane — 'Endothelium'

Iris (radial)

'Endothelium' — Stroma — Clump cell (pigmented) — M. sphincter — M. dilator — Pigment-epithelium

Lens (total)

Equator — Lens star — Posterior surface — Suture

Sclera and choroid

Sclera (in part) — Choroid — Pigment layer of retina — Substantia propria — Supra-choroid — Vascular layer — Capillary layer — Basal membrane

Junction of eyeball and optic nerve (meridional)

Fovea — Lamina cribrosa — Excavation in disk — Edge of optic disk — Retina — Choroid — Sclera — Central vessels — Dural sheath — Arachnoid sheath — Pial sheath — Optic nerve

Foveal cone

E.l.m. — Inner segment — Outer segment

Foveal region of retina

Fovea centralis — Nerve-fiber layer — Ganglion-cell layer — Inner nuclear layer — Fiber layer (of Henle) — Outer nuclear layer — Cone layer — Pigment epithelium — Rod & cone layer

Rim of optic retina

Optic portion of retina — Ciliary portion — Ora serrata

Retinal neurons; layers as usually stained

Neuron 1 (receptor) — Synapse — Neuron 2 (bipolar) — Synapse — Neuron 3 (ganglionic) — Pigment epithelium (detail, p. 38) — Rods and cones — Ext. lim. membrane — Outer nuclear layer — Outer plexiform layer — Inner nuclear layer — Inner plexiform layer — Müller's fiber — Ganglion-cell layer — Nerve-fiber layer — Int. lim. memb.

Cone — Rod

Outer segment — Inner segment — Ext. lim. memb. — Nucleus — Fiber — Ending

Rod detail

Stacked disks — Cilium — Basal corpuscle (centriole) — Mitochondria

Upper eyelid (vertical)

Fat — Tarsal muscle — Dermis — Epidermis — Orbicular muscle — Downy hair — Ciliary gland — Eyelash — Conjunctiva — Tarsus — Tarsal gland — Ciliary muscle

THE EYE

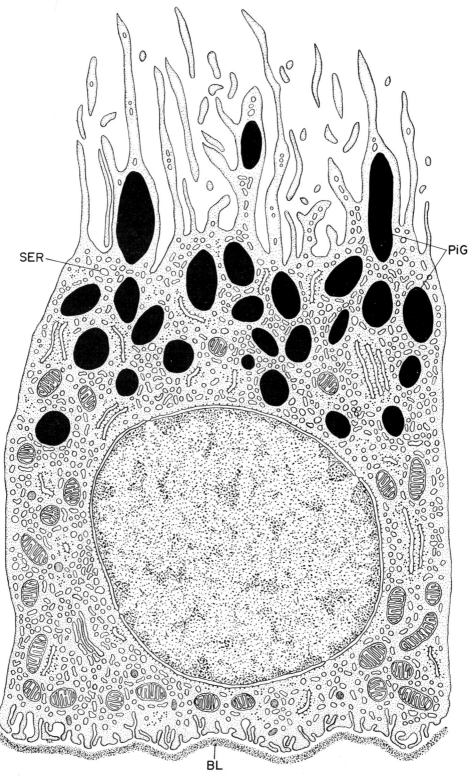

RETINAL PIGMENT CELL. The free surface of the cell bears numerous, long villous-processes. The basal surface is infolded and rests on a basal lamina (BL). The cytoplasm is poor in rough endoplasmic reticulum and free ribosomes, but is rich in smooth reticulum (SER). Mitochondria congregate in the basal half of the cell and pigment granules (PiG) in the apical half.

A modified cilium, with basal body, interconnects the two segments.
Both outer segments contain an unstable light-sensitive substance.
That of rods is *rhodopsin*, or visual purple; that of cones is *iodopsin*.
Both visual pigments play an important role in the process of vision.

3. *External limiting membrane.*
This sieve-like boundary is formed by junctional complexes that occur between the tops of tall *Müller's cells* (see below) and visual cells.
Above it extend the rods and cones, and microvilli from Müller's cells.

4. *Outer nuclear layer.*
The nucleated midregions of the *visual cells* comprise this layer.
Cone nuclei are ovoid, paler and lie just beneath the limiting membrane.
Rod nuclei are rounder, stain darker and lie at deeper, staggered levels.

5. *Outer plexiform layer.*
In this region the fiber-like basal portions of the visual cells terminate.
The *rod fiber* ends in a knob; the *cone fiber*, in a branched expansion.
Here *synapses* are made chiefly with the dendrites of *bipolar cells.*
These latter neurons lie mostly in the next deeper level.

6. *Inner nuclear layer.*
Here occur the cell bodies of *bipolar cells,* of *horizontal* and *amacrine cells* (association neurons) and of *Müller's cells,* which are supporting cells.
Bipolar cells are second, intermediate links in the neuron chains.

7. *Inner plexiform layers.*
This layer contains a second *synaptic region* in the system of neuron chains.
The chief synapses are between axons of bipolar cells and profusely branching dendrites of ganglion cells (belonging to the next deeper level).

8. *Ganglion-cell layer.*
In this layer are the nuclei and cell bodies of large, multipolar *ganglion cells.*
The ganglion cells furnish the third links in the neuron chains.
Also there are scattering neuroglial cells.

9. *Nerve-fiber layer.*
Here the *axons* of ganglion cells course radially toward the optic nerve.
This layer also contains the larger vessels entering from the optic nerve.

10. *Internal limiting membrane.*
It arises from the expanded ends and basal laminae of long *Müller's cells.*
These tall cells are vertical ependymal cells, supporting in function.
They extend as slender elements between the two limiting membranes.
They bear many recesses which shelter the bodies of the various neurons.

Two regions of the retina are modified in organizational plan.
Macula lutea.
An area in the direct optic axis is called the *macula lutea.*
This 'yellow spot' is nearly 5 mm. in diameter and yellowish when fresh.
Progressively toward its center, rods disappear and cones become slender and increasingly abundant.
Also the inner retinal layers spread aside, leaving a saucer-shaped pit.
This *fovea centralis,* in its central thinnest region, is only 0.6 mm. wide.
Its sole visual cells are 4000 slender cones, resembling rods in shape.
Their fibers slant obliquely from the fovea in peripheral directions.
That is, they pass toward the displaced bipolar and ganglion cells.
These last-named neurons are located more marginally about the pit.
The fovea is the region of clearest vision and greatest visual acuity.
The close packing of slender cones favors the resolution of details.
The absence of other neurons and vessels favors a sharp image.
Peripheral retina.
Near the ora serrata, nervous elements decrease; supporting elements increase.
Rods, especially, become sparser and disappear, leaving vacant spaces.

Ganglion-cell and nerve-fiber layers cease; the other nuclear layers blend.
(A somewhat similar loss of layers occurs next to the optic nerve.)

B. PARS CILIARIS.

The *ciliary body* bears a continuation of the retina on its internal surface.
Both here and on the iris the retina is wholly insensitive to light.
This blind expanse is sometimes called the *pars caeca.*
The *pigment epithelium* is represented by tall cells, with extreme pigmentation.
Only at the crests of the ciliary processes are the cells shorter and paler.
The so-called *ciliary epithelium* corresponds to the nervous layers of the retina.
It is a single layer of clear, tall, columnar cells; they face the vitreous.

C. PARS IRIDICA.

The continuation of the pigment layer onto the iris becomes modified further.
Most of its cells are *myo-epithelial*, spindle-shaped and radially oriented.
The cell body is epithelial in character and moderately pigmented.
Each end of the cell tapers into an unpigmented fiber-process.
This fiber-like process is myoid, both structurally and functionally.
A similarly fibrillated portion of the cell body lies next to the iridial stroma,
as do also the cell processes.
These modified cells constitute the *dilator muscle* of the pupil.
In the stroma of the iris, near its pupillary margin, lies a second muscle-mass.
It is the *sphincter muscle* of the pupil; like the dilator, it is involuntary.
It is a detached derivative of the primitive pigment layer.
The muscle fibers are typical, except for their ectodermal origin.
They are arranged in a flat ring that encircles the pupillary margin.
The insensitive continuation of the nervous retina also shows modification.
Its tall cells (clear in the pars ciliaris) again become heavily pigmented.
Nuclei and cell boundaries are both obscured.

D. VESSELS.

Vascularity is maintained chiefly by the middle, or vascular, tunic.
Its vessels do not enter the retina, but this tunic benefits from seepage.
The inner half of the pars optica is supplied by optic-nerve vessels (see beyond).

4. Optic nerve.

Both the embryonic optic cup and stalk are extensions of the brain wall.
Hence the optic 'nerve' is a central tract, and not a true peripheral nerve.
The *meninges* (dura; pia-arachnoid) of the brain cover the optic nerve also.
At the eyeball the *subdural space* and *subarachnoid space* end.
Here also the two sheaths merge into the sclera of the eyeball.
Continuations of the *pia mater* extend into the substance of the optic nerve.
Inside the nerve they subdivide the fiber-content into bundles of nerve fibers.
At the eyeball, this framework thickens by additions chiefly from the sclera.
The result is a sieve-like membrane, continuous with the sclera.
It is the *lamina cribrosa*, through which bundles of nerve fibers pass.
The *optic-nerve fibers* are axons of the ganglion cells of the retina.
At first, these fibers course radially in the nerve-fiber layer of the retina.
Near the posterior pole of the eyeball they turn 90° and enter the optic nerve.
The fibers enter at the circular nerve head, known as the *optic disk.*
This is a bulging disk that bears a central depression, or *excavation.*
The disk is insensitive to light; it is the 'blind spot' on the retina.
Once in the nerve, the fibers continue without interruption to the brain.
Just brainward of the lamina cribrosa the naked axons acquire myelin sheaths.
Consequently the nerve doubles its diameter here rather abruptly.
Glial cells and fibers (but not neurolemma sheaths) embed the nerve fibers.
The nerve fibers in each optic nerve total one million.
This is more than three times the number in all other cranial nerves.
A *central artery* and *vein* enter the optic nerve more than midway toward the eyeball.

They proceed to the eyeball in a central strand of supporting tissue.

In the retina they spread fan-wise within the nerve-fiber layer.

Turning at right angles, they extend through the inner nuclear layer.

(The only other vascular supply is fluid escaping from choroidal capillaries.)

5. Refracting media.

Behind the *cornea*, which is the strongest refracting agent, are four other media.

They are: *lens*; *ciliary zonule*; *vitreous body*; *aqueous humor*.

These fill the interior of the eyeball and co-operate in image formation.

A. LENS.

The *lens* is a transparent, plastic, biconvex disk situated just behind the iris.

Its posterior surface is more convex than the anterior surface.

The two surfaces meet at the rounded-off edge, or *equator*.

A homogeneous, elastic *capsule* encloses the entire lens.

A *lens epithelium* of single-layered cuboidal cells provides an anterior surface.

All the rest of the lens consists of transparent, refractile *lens fibers*.

These are altered cells in the form of elongated, hexagonal prisms.

The fibers are united by virtual fusion and by occasional desmosomes.

New fibers are added slowly throughout life from the epithelium at the *equator*.

Daughter cells elongate and become transparent; old nuclei no longer show.

Hence all but the central lens substance is arranged in concentric *lamellae*.

Also the cortical layers are softer than the older, central *lens nucleus*.

Fibers added about the fetal nucleus do not extend from pole to pole.

Their ends abut along *lens sutures* which radiate from the two poles.

On both back and front there results a branching pattern, the *lens star*.

The lens hardens with age, thereby losing its power of accommodation.

B. CILIARY ZONULE.

The lens is held in position by a system of fibers known as the *ciliary zonule*.

This radially arranged set of fibers serves the lens as a suspensory ligament.

It extends from the capsule at the lens margin to the ciliary body.

Individual *zonular fibers* are fine, seemingly homogeneous, inelastic elements.

Some fibers attach in front of the actual lens equator; others, behind it.

Hence there is a space, bounded by these two sheets and the lens margin.

This region is named the *zonular space*.

Actually each fiber is a bundle of finer *microfibrils*.

Images of near objects are brought to focus when the lens becomes more convex.

This accommodation is produced by the *ciliary muscle* and *zonular fibers*.

When the eye is at rest, the zonular fibers and lens are under tension.

This is because elastic sheets in the choroid pull on the ciliary body.

The resulting pull of fibers on the lens capsule stretches the lens.

Accommodation occurs when the muscles of the ciliary body contract.

The ciliary body then moves forward and also bulges toward the lens.

These shifts release tension on the zonular fibers and lens capsule.

The elastic capsule then relaxes and takes a more spherical shape.

The plastic lens substance also conforms to this new contour.

C. VITREOUS BODY.

This transparent, semisolid jelly fills the large space behind the lens and zonule.

In addition to its refractive role, it supports the lightly attached retina.

A *hyaloid canal* runs through it from the head of the optic nerve to the lens.

This was the course taken by the fetal hyaloid artery to the lens.

After fixation the jelly shows fibrillae, and a *vitreous membrane* can be seen.

The so-called membrane is merely a peripheral, fibrillar condensation.

The jelly is 99 per cent water, taken up into a hydrophilic polysaccharide.

D. AQUEOUS HUMOR.

The *ocular chamber* is the space between the cornea and vitreous body.

It is incompletely divided by the iris into two parts.

The *anterior chamber* lies between the cornea, iris and front of the lens.

The *posterior chamber* is a small ring-shaped space, triangular in section.
It is bounded by the iris, ciliary body and vitreous body.
The chamber contains *aqueous humor*, which is a clear, lymph-like fluid.
It originates in the ciliary processes as a secretion or transudate.
It finds outlets through the spaces of Fontana and the scleral venous sinus.

6. Accessory organs.

A. EYELIDS.

These are movable folds of skin, protecting the eye and shutting out light.
The thin skin of the outer surface of the lid is modified on the inner surface.
Here it becomes a transparent mucous membrane named the *conjunctiva*.
The epithelium is stratified columnar, and mostly but 2 to 3 cells thick.
Some of the superficial columnar cells specialize into goblet cells.
This membrane also continues, by reflection, over the front of the eyeball.
The number of epithelial layers increases and the surface cells flatten.
It has been described previously where it covers the cornea (p. 299).
The shape of a lid is maintained by an internal fibrous plate, the *tarsus*.
To its proximal border attaches the involuntary *tarsal muscle* (of Müller).
Embedded in the plate are numerous sebaceous *tarsal glands* (of Meibom).
Each gland has an axial excretory duct, into which open many alveoli.
The ducts discharge on the free, outer margin of the lid and lubricate it.
A thin sheet of muscle, the *orbicularis*, acts to close the eyelids.
The upper lid is raised by the *levator muscle*, which inserts on the tarsus.
Eyelashes, or *cilia*, are coarse hairs, with large sebaceous glands (of Zeis).
Between cilia are large, spiraling sweat glands (of Moll).

B. LACRIMAL GLAND.

This gland grows out from the upper lateral margin of the conjunctival sac.
There is a superior and inferior gland-mass, imperfectly separated.
Actually a group of individual units is drained by about 10 ducts.
Each unit is a compound, tubulo-alveolar *serous gland*.
The *alveoli* have tall cells, whose height varies with their functional state.
Resembling the parotid, they have narrower cells and a wider lumen.
Their cytoplasm contains large, pale secretion granules and fat droplets.
The cells are provided with *secretory canaliculi*.
Between the cells and basement membrane are stellate, myoid *basket cells*.
Lymphoid and other cells tend to collect in the stroma of the gland.
The secretion supplies the clear, salty *tears* that are somewhat bactericidal.
Tears flush the conjunctival sac and reach the inner angle of the eye.
Here they are collected by a *lacrimal canaliculus* in each eyelid.
Thence via the *naso-lacrimal duct* they reach the nasal cavity.

C. BULBAR MUSCLES; FIBROUS SHEATHS.

Six voluntary *bulbar muscles* (four recti; two obliques) insert on the sclera.
Only one movement (direct lateral) is produced by one of the muscles.
All other movements result from the combined effort of at least two muscles.
Fibrous *sheaths* invest the muscles and continue into the *bulbar fascia*.
The latter is a fibrous cup ('Tenon's capsule') in which the eyeball sits.
It is attached loosely to the sclera by collagenous fibers.

C. REGENERATIVE ABILITY:

The *corneal epithelium* heals its wounds by cell migration and subsequent mitosis.
The *substantia propria* restores losses by producing ordinary, opaque scar-tissue.
The *sclera* acts like any fibrous capsule in the formation of new repair-tissue.
The *choroid* replaces destroyed areas by differentiating fibrous scar-tissue.
It is not so well vascularized as before, but may contain many pigment cells.
The *iris* is notable in not repairing traumatic injuries inflicted on it.
There is perhaps a suppressive influence exerted in some way (by aqueous humor?).

At least, tissue from the iris can grow when cultivated in artificial media.
The *lens epithelium* will repair a locally destroyed area.
At the equator this restored epithelium can even lay down new lens fibers.
The *retina* heals local injuries by glial proliferation and replacement.
After interruption of the optic nerve, the retina persists remarkably well.
Only some of the ganglion cells perish within the ensuing weeks.
Possibly this is owing to the loss of blood supply rather than to direct trauma.
Lost vitreous substance can be replaced.

D. Diagnostic Features:

A meridional section through the eyeball is unmistakable, even to unaided vision.
Sections through *local regions* would include one, at least, of the following parts:
Cornea; iris; lens; ciliary body; pars optica and overlying coats; optic nerve.
Each of these is distinctive, especially if some neighboring region is included.
Sections through *accessory organs* would probably include the eyelid or lacrimal gland.
Each is unique, although the *lacrimal gland* must be distinguished from the parotid.
Positively, the alveoli have a wider lumen; negatively, they lack secretory-type ducts.

E. Functional Correlations:

Mechanical support and protection are furnished by the fibrous external coat.
The vitreous body and aqueous humor maintain a pressure within the eyeball cavity.
This keeps the lens in place, the retina from separating and the eyeball turgid.
Light regulation is accomplished through the automatic action of the iris.
Unique dilator and sphincter muscles control the size of the pupil.
In this way the intensity of admitted light is regulated.
Image formation is accomplished jointly by the cornea, aqueous, lens and vitreous.
The variable component that permits changes in focus is the lens.
The lens changes shape (accommodates) in maintaining sharp focus in near vision.
The manner of operation is the reverse of what might be expected (p. 303).
Optical isolation of rods and cones is aided by processes of the pigment epithelium.
The pigmented cells also prevent confusing back-reflection of light rays.
Sensory reception is a function of the visual rods and cones.
The image is brought to focus at the level of their outer members.
Bright-light vision (keen vision) is a function of the relatively insensitive cones.
In the fovea alone is high resolution and color discrimination obtained.
The retinal modifications here are adapted to these ends (p. 301).
Dim-light vision is a function of the extremely sensitive rods.
Yet the resolution of detail is poor, and color discrimination is lacking.
The different capabilities of the rods and cones correlate in part with their synaptic relations to neurons of the second and third order.
The rods connect with the bipolar cells in groups, and respond in groups.
The cones link with bipolars and ganglion cells by individual synapses.
Especially is this true in the fovea, where independent responses are desirable.

IV. THE EAR

The 'organ of hearing' is really a compound organ with different functions.
It is receptive to sound waves, which is the basis of the *auditory sense*.
It also responds to the effects of gravity and to movements of the head.
These trigger the sensations known as *static* and *kinetic*.
The organ consists of three related parts, lying mostly within the temporal bone.
These parts are distinct in origin, structure and function.

A. Structural Plan:

One portion is the *external ear*, which shows three subordinate divisions.
The *auricle* is a shallow appendage situated on the lateral surface of the head.

The *external acoustic meatus* is a short tube, leading inward to the ear drum.

The vibratory *tympanic membrane*, or ear drum, closes the deep end of the meatus.

A second component is the *middle ear*, which is a membranous chamber largely within bone.

The main *tympanic cavity* connects with the naso-pharynx by an *auditory tube*.

In an opposite direction leads off an auxiliary chamber, the *mastoid antrum*.

The latter communicates with many irregular spaces called *mastoid cells*.

A chain of three *ear bones* (*auditory ossicles*) crosses the tympanic cavity.

The set connects the ear drum with the internal ear.

A third part, or *internal ear*, is the receptive apparatus—also contained within bone.

It is extremely irregular in shape and, for this reason, is called the *labyrinth*.

Two different component parts have the same general configuration.

The *bony labyrinth* is an external shell of bone that encases the whole.

The *membranous labyrinth* is a fibrous, epithelium-lined, internal compartment.

As the actual sensory mechanism it consists of interconnecting sacs and ducts.

These are suspended in fluid and are filled with fluid.

The *utricle* and *saccule* are small sacs contained within a bony *vestibule*.

Three *semicircular ducts* are surrounded by bony *semicircular canals*.

The snail-like *cochlear duct* is encased within a bony *cochlea* of similar shape.

B. DETAILED STRUCTURE:

1. External ear.

A. AURICLE.

This is shaped and supported by an internal plate of *elastic cartilage*.

It is covered on all exposed surfaces by typical, thin *skin* (with hairs and glands).

Six *intrinsic muscles*, all vestigial, extend between portions of the cartilage.

Three *extrinsic muscles* pass from the skull to the cartilage.

They are rudimentary, and only rarely under voluntary control.

B. EXTERNAL ACOUSTIC MEATUS.

The outer one-half of the tube is supported by *elastic cartilage*.

The remainder is a tunnel through the temporal bone.

A continuation of auricular *skin* lines the inch-long, slightly tortuous tube.

In the *cartilaginous portion* there are fine hairs and large sebaceous glands.

Coiled, tubular *ceruminous glands* are a characteristic feature.

They are modified sweat glands, of the apocrine type.

The lumen is large; myoid *basket cells* are prominent.

The specialized gland cells contain coarse brown pigment granules.

Their discharged yellowish secretion mixes in the external meatus with sebaceous secretion and desquamated cells.

Drying of this mixture produces a thick waxy product, the *cerumen*.

In the *bony portion* the skin is very thin.

Hairs and glands occur only along the upper wall.

C. TYMPANIC MEMBRANE.

The *ear drum*, set at a strong slant, closes the external meatus at its deep end.

It serves as a common partition between the meatus and tympanic cavity.

The membrane is about 0.1 mm. thick and consists of 4 sheet-like layers.

The *outer surface* is very thin skin, continuous with that of the meatus.

Next deeper is a radiate fibrous layer and then a circular fibrous layer.

In an upper, triangular *flaccid region* these 2 layers are lacking.

The *inner surface* is a mucous membrane, with a low cuboidal epithelium.

It is a part of the lining of the tympanic cavity.

2. Middle ear.

The *tympanic cavity* is a flattened cleft contained within the temporal bone.

It is an air-space, traversed by the ear bones, their ligaments and a nerve.

A *mucous membrane* lines its walls and wraps about the ear bones and other contents.

The *epithelium* is simple; in most regions it is low cuboidal and nonciliated.

The *lateral wall* is the tympanic membrane and an encircling ring of bone.

The *medial wall* bears the *vestibular window* (oval) and the *cochlear window* (round).

The first is an opening into the vestibule, closed by the base of the *stapes.*

The second is closed by the fibrous, mucosa-covered *secondary tympanic membrane.*

Three jointed *auditory ossicles* extend, like a chain, across the tympanic cavity.

The *malleus,* or hammer, is firmly attached to the ear drum by its long limb.

The *stapes,* or stirrup, is fixed (at its basal plate) into the vestibular window.

It is in direct contact with the perilymph fluid of the internal ear.

The malleus and stapes are each supplied with a tiny tension-maintaining muscle.

The *incus,* or anvil, has a middle position and articulates with the other two.

The *mastoid antrum* (and mastoid cells) is lined with a thin mucous membrane.

This membrane is continuous with that of the tympanic cavity.

The *auditory* (or *Eustachian*) *tube* has a bony and a cartilaginous portion.

Both portions are lined with a *mucous membrane* whose epithelium varies in type.

Near the pharynx it is pseudostratified and ciliated.

Nearer the tympanic cavity it is simple columnar and ciliated.

Some *lymph nodules* occur in the lamina propria.

The submucosa contains mixed *sero-mucous glands.*

The *cartilaginous wall,* nearer the pharynx, supports two-thirds of the tube.

Its *cartilage* (elastic in part) is a plate, J-shaped in transverse section.

The major limb of the plate supports the medial wall of the tube.

The *bony wall,* nearer the tympanic cavity, surrounds one-third of the tube.

Its mucous membrane is continuous with that of the tympanic cavity.

3. Internal ear.

This portion of the auditory mechanism is also enclosed within the temporal bone.

But, unlike the tympanic cavity, it contains a system of sensory tubes and sacs.

The greatest length of this apparatus is about 0.8 in.

Externally there is the *osseous labyrinth* — a set of bony canals and chambers.

They are named the *semicircular canals, vestibule* and *cochlea.*

Their lining is periosteum whose free surface is mesenchymal epithelium (p. 34).

They contain a watery fluid, named the *perilymph.*

(Only the bony cochlea demands further description, p. 308.)

Internally there is a much slenderer *membranous labyrinth.*

It comprises a series of continuous, closed tubes and chambers.

Their general arrangement and shape follow the bony labyrinth that contains them.

They have a fibrous exterior and an epithelial lining.

Such membranous passages are anchored to the periosteum of the bony labyrinth.

They are surrounded, except for attached regions, by the fluid *perilymph.*

They are filled with a similar, but wholly separate, fluid *endolymph.*

The membranous labyrinth has two divisions, different structurally and functionally.

One deals with the *static* and *kinetic senses*; the other, with *hearing.*

The *static* and *kinetic senses* are served by five major constituent parts.

(1-3) Three *semicircular ducts* are set in planes at right angles to each other.

Each lies within a bony canal and bears a swollen *ampulla* at one end.

(4) The ellipsoidal *utricle* receives both ends of each semicircular duct.

(5) The spheroidal *saccule* communicates with the utricle by a slender tube.

From this tube the slender *endolymphatic duct* extends through the bone.

The duct ends in a dilatation, the *endolymphatic sac,* located between the temporal bone and the dura mater of the brain.

Its taller epithelial cells are specialized for absorbing endolymph.

Both the utricle and saccule occupy a middle chamber in the osseous labyrinth.

This *vestibule* lies between the semicircular canals and the cochlea.

The *auditory sense* is served by a tube, named the *cochlear duct.*

This tube is coiled in a tight spiral, like a snail's shell.

Near its base it communicates with the saccule by the slender *ductus reuniens.*

Its tip ends blindly at the apex of the coil.

The lining *epithelium* of the entire membranous labyrinth is largely simple squamous.

Certain local areas are specialized as thicker, sensory *neuroepithelia.*

There are six of these areas, innervated by branches of the acoustic nerve.

They occur in the semicircular ducts, utricle, saccule and cochlear duct.

A. MACULAE.

Both the utricle and saccule bear a thickened sensory area, named the *macula*.

The macula of the utricle is oval; that of the saccule is heart-shaped.

Their columnar epithelium has two kinds of cells—sensory and supporting.

Some sensory *hair cells* are shaped like short flasks with a rounded base.

They sit in a cupped nerve ending and do not reach the basement membrane.

Other short sensory cells are columnar: their bases are beset with nerve end-bulbs.

The nuclei of both cell-types lie at a middle level in the epithelial sheet.

Both types bear many hairlike processes that extend from the cell apex.

There is one modified cilium, and many microvilli of graded lengths.

These are anchored in a *terminal web* (formerly called a cuticular plate).

The *supporting cells* are slender elements whose nuclei lie at a deep level.

The narrower, upper portion bears a terminal web and sparse microvilli.

The surface of the macula is covered with a gelatinous *otolithic membrane*.

The 'hair tufts' project into slender recesses in this substance.

The recesses, like the general lumen, are filled with watery *endolymph*.

Toward the upper surface of the membrane occur particles named *otoconia*.

These are minute crystals, densely packed.

They are composed of calcium carbonate and a protein substance.

B. CRISTAE.

Each *ampulla* of the three semicircular ducts bears a *crista*.

This is an elongate crest oriented transversely to the long axis of the duct.

A crista has much the same structure as a macula.

Supporting cells, hair cells (and their 'hair tufts') are similar in both.

Over the crest is a striated, somewhat gelatinous mass called the *cupola*.

Into it project the ciliary tufts of the hair cells.

It is comparable to the otolithic membrane, but it lacks otoconia.

C. OSSEOUS COCHLEA.

The total mechanism for the organ of hearing is rather complicated.

For this reason the bony *cochlea* requires some preliminary attention.

It resembles a snail shell, with a broad base and narrow apex.

A spiraling, bony case makes about $2\frac{1}{2}$ turns around a central pillar.

This axial pillar is the *modiolus*; it is made of spongy bone.

A bony shelf projects from the modiolus into the cavity of the spiraling shell.

This flange, resembling the thread of a screw, is the *spiral lamina*.

From its free border a fibrous *basilar membrane* continues to the outer wall.

Together they divide the *spiral canal* of the cochlea into main compartments.

Above the lamina-partition is the perilymphatic space named the *scala vestibuli*.

One end communicates with the perilymphatic space of the vestibule.

At the other (apical) end it joins the tip of a similar, parallel scala.

This second passage is the *scala tympani*, located beneath the lamina.

Both scalae are lined by a simple layer of mesenchymal epithelium.

The *scala tympani*, beneath the lamina, requires some further description.

Its fibrous lining, at the beginning of its basal turn, helps to close the *cochlear window* (an aperture in the adjacent, bony tympanic wall).

Closure is made by the thin secondary *tympanic membrane*.

Its components are periosteal tissue of the scala and the mucosal lining of the tympanic cavity of the middle ear.

The membrane separates perilymph from the air of the tympanic cavity.

Nearby is the opening into the *perilymphatic duct*.

This canal extends from the scala tympani through bone to the subarachnoid space about the brain.

D. COCHLEAR DUCT.

The *duct* is a membranous tube, much smaller than the bony cochlea containing it.

One end is blind; the other end communicates with the saccule.

The latter connection is made by the slender *ductus reuniens.*
Externally there is fibrous tissue; internally, a lining of epithelium.
The duct is something of a right triangle in transverse section.
The more acute angle points toward the modiolus.
The leg opposite this angle attaches to the bony shell of the cochlea.
The base rests on the spiral lamina and its membranous extension.
The hypotenuse is the vestibular membrane, bounded on each surface by fluids.
The *upper surface*, or roof, of the duct is the slanting *vestibular membrane.*
This thin membrane (of Reissner) separates the perilymph of the scala vestibuli from the endolymph of the cochlear duct.
The membrane contains a thin middle layer of nonvascular connective tissue.
The outer surface is bounded by mesenchymal epithelium of the scala vestibuli.
The inner, free surface is bounded by squamous epithelium of the duct.
The *lateral surface* blends with thickened periosteum of the bony cochlea.
This thickening, more extensive than the duct, is the *spiral ligament.*
Its more internal part contains many capillary vessels.
Loops even invade the thick pseudostratified epithelium of the duct.
(This is the only good example of such epithelial invasion in mammals.)
The thickened epithelium and subjacent connective tissue comprise a unit.
The combination is a vascular complex named the *stria vascularis.*
It apparently is the source of endolymph.
The *basal surface,* or floor, of the duct is lined with a varying *epithelium.*
Part of it is greatly elevated and specialized for sensory reception.
This is the *spiral organ* (of Corti), the receptor for hearing.
The epithelium rests upon the periosteum of the spiral lamina, and upon its fibrous continuation (basilar membrane) to the outer cochlear wall.
The fibrous component of the floor of the duct is specialized locally.
Medially the periosteum is thick where it approaches the spiral organ.
This thick *limbus* serves for the attachment of the tectorial membrane.
Laterally, beneath the spiral organ and beyond it to the spiral ligament, stretches a specialized fibrous layer, known as the *basilar membrane.*
The membrane varies in width progressively along the duct.
It is widest at the extreme apical end of the cochlear duct.
It is narrowest at the beginning of the basal turn of the duct.
The basilar membrane consists of three layers.
Facing the spiral organ, the border layer is thin.
It is a homogeneous ground substance.
Facing the scala tympani, the border layer is thicker.
It is a delicate fibrous tissue.
The intermediate stratum is the most important component.
Its main feature is a set of 25,000 *basilar fibers,* strung like harp strings.
They are fine threads, or auditory strings, made of scleroproteins.
The fibers are embedded in sparse, homogeneous ground substance.
E. SPIRAL ORGAN.
The *spiral organ* has a number of special components.
These will be described in order, from the periphery toward the modiolus.
1. *Peripheral cells.*
Close to the stria vascularis is a groove, the *external spiral sulcus.*
Its floor consists of cuboidal *cells of Claudius and Boettcher.*
Within the border of the spiral organ itself the cells gain height steadily.
They make several rows of supporting elements, named the *cells of Hensen.*
2. *Outer hair cells.*
These outermost sensory cells occur in rows, 3 to 5 cells wide ascendingly.
Their total number is about 20,000.
They are short prisms that do not extend halfway to the basilar membrane.
A *terminal web* (formerly called a cuticular plate) occurs at the cell top.

Many sensory 'hairs' embed in this web and project free above it.

The so-called hairs are large, stiff microvilli of different lengths.

They broaden progressively toward their tips. Cilia are lacking.

The rounded base of the cell receives nerve endings.

A space between the nearest hair- and Hensen cell is the *outer tunnel.*

3. *Outer phalangeal cells.*

These are tall supporting cells (of Deiters), one for each outer hair cell.

The round base of a hair cell sits in the cupped side of its phalangeal cell.

Above this level the phalangeal cell narrows to a slender stalk.

At the surface it expands greatly.

4. *Outer pillar cells.*

Each has a broad base and an expanded top or 'head.'

The head bears a convexity on its medial side (see beyond).

Nuel's space lies between these pillars and the nearest of the outer hair cells and phalangeal cells.

5. *Inner pillar cells.*

An inner cell resembles an outer pillar cell but its head bears a concavity.

The convexity and concavity of each outer and inner cell-pair fit together.

The arrangement resembles a ball and socket joint.

From this union the two cell columns diverge greatly basalward.

The resulting gable-shaped space is the *inner tunnel* (of Corti).

6. *Inner phalangeal cells.*

There is a single row of these cells, narrowing greatly toward their tops.

All phalangeal and pillar cells contain a thick, axial bundle of microtubules.

These expand at the cell apex and become a plate (formerly 'cuticular plate').

The flat plate is a type of specialization known as the *terminal web.*

7. *Inner hair cells.*

These make a single row of flask-shaped cells, similar to the outer hair cells.

Their total number is about 3500; microvilli are less numerous.

The rounded cell base is supported by pillar, phalangeal and border cells.

8. *Border cells.*

Inward of the inner hair cells is a single row of columnar *border cells.*

9. *Limbus and tectorial membrane.*

Thick periosteum over the bony spiral lamina makes an elevated *limbus.*

It is covered by simple columnar epithelium.

These cells are capped by a prominent cuticular membrane.

Continuous with this cuticular membrane is the imposing *tectorial membrane.*

It projects outward peripherally, hanging free over the spiral organ.

It is thickest midway and tapers toward its attached and free ends.

Between the tectorial membrane, limbus and spiral organ is the prominent *internal spiral sulcus.*

The *tectorial membrane* is an epithelial derivative, cuticular in nature.

It is a delicate, flexible, fibrillar, gelatinous substance.

When fresh, it fills about one-fourth of the spiral duct.

Fixation brings shrinkage and distortion.

The lower surface rests upon the tips of hairs from the hair cells.

10. *Surface pattern.*

Each supporting cell in the spiral organ bears at its top a dense plate (see above).

All of these plates constitute a sheet named the *lamina reticularis.*

In surface view it comprises a mosaic, regular in pattern but containing gaps.

Each gap in the mosaic contains the top of a hair cell with its dense plate.

4. Vessels and nerves.

The arteries and veins pursue different courses.

Arterial blood is distributed through three branches.

One branch supplies part of the saccule, utricle and semicircular ducts.

A second branch supplies the remainder of the saccule, utricle and ducts.

It also supplies one-third of the basal turn of the cochlea.

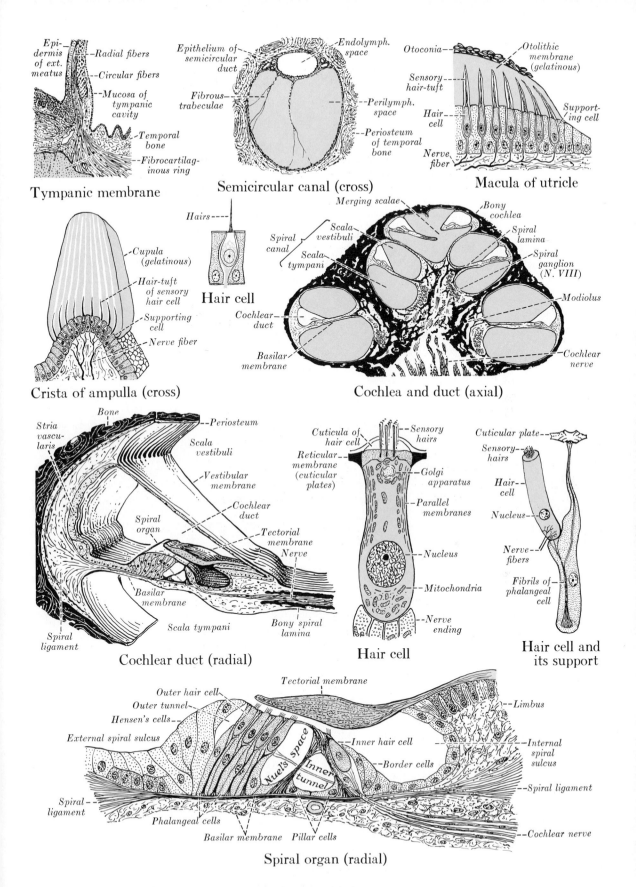

Epi-dermis of ext. meatus — Radial fibers
— Circular fibers
— Mucosa of tympanic cavity
Temporal bone
Fibrocartilag-inous ring

Tympanic membrane

Epithelium of semicircular duct
Endolymph. space
Fibrous trabeculae
Perilymph. space
Periosteum of temporal bone

Semicircular canal (cross)

Otoconia
Otolithic membrane (gelatinous)
Sensory hair-tuft
Hair cell
Support-ing cell
Nerve fiber

Macula of utricle

Hairs
Cupula (gelatinous)
Hair-tuft of sensory hair cell
Supporting cell
Nerve fiber

Crista of ampulla (cross)

Hair cell

Merging scalae
Bony cochlea
Scala vestibuli
Spiral lamina
Spiral canal
Scala tympani
Spiral ganglion (N. VIII)
Modiolus
Cochlear duct
Basilar membrane
Cochlear nerve

Cochlea and duct (axial)

Stria vascu-laris
Bone
Periosteum
Scala vestibuli
Vestibular membrane
Cochlear duct
Spiral organ
Tectorial membrane
Nerve
Basilar membrane
Bony spiral lamina
Scala tympani
Spiral ligament

Cochlear duct (radial)

Cuticula of hair cell
Sensory hairs
Reticular membrane (cuticular plates)
Golgi apparatus
Parallel membranes
Nucleus
Mitochondria
Nerve ending

Hair cell

Cuticular plate
Sensory hairs
Hair cell
Nucleus
Nerve fibers
Fibrils of phalangeal cell

Hair cell and its support

Tectorial membrane
Outer hair cell
Outer tunnel
Hensen's cells
External spiral sulcus
Limbus
Inner hair cell
Nuel's space
Inner tunnel
Border cells
Internal spiral sulcus
Spiral ligament
Spiral ligament
Phalangeal cells
Basilar membrane
Pillar cells
Cochlear nerve

Spiral organ (radial)

THE EAR

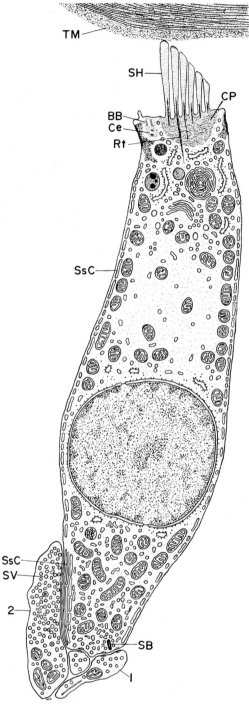

HEARING CELL.   This figure represents an outer hair cell of the spiral organ (of Corti). The cytoplasm contains mitochondria, especially basally; along the sides of the cell they are aligned just interior to rows of smooth endoplasmic reticulum. Apically there are a Golgi complex, centriole (Ce), basal body (BB), dense bodies (some lysosomes), a few rough cisternae and many smooth tubules. The tallest club-shaped sensory hairs (SH) touch the fibrillated tectorial membrane (TM). The basal end of each hair contains an axial core that continues, as a rootlet (Rt), through a terminal web, formerly called a cuticular plate (CP). The base of the cell is in contact with sensory end bulbs (1), both plasma membranes showing local thickenings; a synaptic bar (SB) and vesicles are near by. A larger efferent ending (2) faces subsurface smooth cisternae (SsC) in the hair cell. Both types of ending contain synaptic vesicles (SV). Flattened cisternae (SsC) underlie the plasma membrane.

A third branch supplies the modiolus and bony spiral lamina.

It also passes to the outer wall of both scalae and to the stria vascularis of the spiral duct.

Veins likewise have three lines of drainage.

Some come from the semicircular ducts and part of the utricle.

Others come from the utricle, saccule, spiral lamina and stria.

Still others come from the bony spiral lamina and its spiral ganglion.

There are no vessels in the vestibular membrane.

The same statement is true for most of the basilar membrane.

Probably endolymph from the stria vascularis nourishes the spiral organ.

All vascular arrangements are such as to minimize sounds from pulsating blood.

Lymphatics are lacking; the perilymphatic spaces collect and remove excess fluid.

The *auditory nerve* has a vestibular and a cochlear division.

Its ganglion cells are bipolar, with a peripheral and a central process.

Peripheral processes are functional dendrons; central processes are axons.

The peripheral fibers, after a short course, lose their sheaths and branch.

The *vestibular division* supplies the maculae and cristae.

Its *vestibular ganglion* lies at the outer end of the bony internal meatus.

The dendrons terminate by forming baskets and end-bulbs about the hair cells.

The *cochlear division* courses in the modiolus and supplies the spiral organ.

Its *spiral ganglion* lies in the thick base of the bony spiral lamina.

Bundles of *nerve fibers* pass outward in the spiral lamina.

Some fibers are distributed to the inner hair cells.

Each fiber ends about one or, at most, two cells.

More fibers cross the tunnel and Nuel's space to reach the outer hair cells.

Each fiber supplies only a single hair cell of these rows.

All fibers terminate by arborizing about the hair cells.

C. REGENERATIVE ABILITY:

The *external ear* heals as skin (p. 190) and cartilage (p. 75) do elsewhere.

The ear drum will heal perfectly after surgical incision or septic perforation.

Only in unusual circumstances does scar tissue develop.

The *middle ear* promptly resurfaces defects made in its mucosa.

The *internal ear* will repair injuries inflicted on its nonsensory membranous labyrinth.

Unlike taste buds, whose innervation is similarly related to secondary sense cells, the spiral organ does not degenerate following destruction of its nerve.

D. DIAGNOSTIC FEATURES:

The *auricle* is characterized by thin skin on both surfaces.

Internally, elastic cartilage occurs and skeletal muscle may be included.

The *external meatus* (outer half) retains the cartilage; bone supports the inner half.

Large sebaceous glands and prominent, coiled ceruminous glands are diagnostic aids.

The *middle ear* presents a variety of appearances, depending on the plane of section.

The *tympanic cavity* has a thin mucosa, with simple epithelium, applied to bone.

Its cavity may include cuts through one or more small ear bones.

Such bones are covered with reflected mucous membrane.

The *tympanic membrane* is a very thin partition between two cavities.

It has thin skin on one surface and low cuboidal epithelium on the other.

The mucosal side may attach or adjoin a slice of bone (the malleus).

The *auditory tube* (ciliated epithelium) is characteristic in its course outside the skull.

Its wall contains mixed glands and a cartilage, hook-shaped in transverse section.

The *membranous labyrinth* is unique by being partly free and partly attached.

It is largely bordered by a space, outside of which is bone.

Specific identifications of some parts are difficult, except in fortunate sections.

Semicircular ducts are easily identified, but not by exact names.

Easiest of all to recognize, when seen by itself, is the cochlea.

If cut in a radial plane, its modiolus and chamber-pattern are unmistakable.

The *spiral organ* is easily diagnosed when cut in a radial plane.

Sections cut in other planes tax interpretative ingenuity.

E. FUNCTIONAL CORRELATIONS:

The *auricle* evolved as a sound-collecting appendage.

It is most effective in mammals whose auricle is deeply cupped and movable.

Cerumen protects the skin of the external acoustic meatus from drying.

Its bitter taste is said to repel insects and other intruders.

The *ear drum* is a vibratory membrane, set in motion by sound waves.

The chain of *ear bones* acts like a bent lever in transmitting vibrations.

They convert the movements of the drum into intensified thrusts.

The foot plate of the stapes, set in the vestibular window, acts like a piston.

It transmits vibrations directly to the perilymph.

The incompressible perilymph, thus 'pushed in,' is enclosed within a bony capsule.

It compensates by 'pushing out' the secondary tympanic membrane.

The *auditory tube* permits pressures in the tympanic cavity and outside air to equalize.

This takes place when the tube opens during swallowing.

The open communication, however, presents a potential avenue of infection.

The *semicircular ducts* inform concerning any *rotational movements* involving the head.

Any degree of rotation of the head leads to stimulation of the cristae.

Displacement of the endolymph against the cupola disturbs the hairs of hair cells.

The ensuing information is a part of the kinetic and proprioceptive senses.

The responses lead to compensatory movements of the eyes, head and limbs.

Each crista is stimulated by movements occurring in the plane of its canal.

The *utricle* informs concerning the *position of the head* in space and linear acceleration.

This static function depends on a shifting in the position of the otolithic membrane.

Gravitational-pull acts on the otoconia, and the hair tufts are moved.

The stimulus thus transmitted initiates compensatory postural reflexes.

The utricle also informs concerning *linear acceleration*, either positive or negative.

Evidence on the *saccule* is conflicting but tends to discredit vestibular function.

It seems to be associated with the cochlea by receiving slow *vibrational stimuli*.

The *spiral organ* (and specifically the hair cells) is the receptor for *sound*.

Perilymph vibrates at the same frequencies as those of the air-borne sound waves.

Pressure changes in the scala vestibuli are transmitted across the vestibular membrane.

Induced pulsations in the endolymph displace the basilar membrane correspondingly.

These sympathetic vibrations affect the relation of sensory hairs to the tectorial membrane, which rests directly upon them.

Such bending of hairs is the basis of an effective stimulus.

Pitch is said to be correlated with the variable width of the basilar membrane.

This membrane is a narrow ribbon (high tones) in the basal cochlear turn.

It grades into its greatest width (lowest tones) at the apical end.

There is evidence pointing to a difference in function among the hair cells.

The outer hair cells are more effective in responding to feeble stimuli.

The inner hair cells are more effective in discriminating pitch accurately.

Index

Entries are under nouns, single or compound, rather than under adjectives or other qualifiers. An exception is where eponyms are involved.

Bud, irruptive, 89, 92
 taste, 209, 297
Bulbo-urethral glands, 274
 functions of, 275
Bulbs, end (of Krause), 294
Bundle, atrioventricular, 107, 138
 tendon, 56
Bursa, 190
 functions of, 190

CALCIFICATION of cartilage, 74, 91, 93
Calcination, 77
Calcitonin, 97, 173, 175
Calcium, amount in bones, 77
 in teeth, 206
 deposition of, in bone, 89
 in cartilage, 74, 91, 93
 level of, in plasma, 97, 173, 175
 parathyroid glands and, 97
 turnover of, 83, 97, 173, 175
Callus, bony, 96
 temporary, cartilaginous, 96
Calvarium, 91
 growth of, 91
Calyx, of kidney, 259
Canal, alimentary, 213
 anal, 226
 Cloquet's, 303
 Haversian, 80
 Hering's, 237
 hyaloid, 303
 portal, 236
 root, 207
 Schlemm's, 300
 semicircular, 307
 spiral, of cochlea, 308
 Volkmann's, 80
Canaliculus, bile, 237
 dentinal, 206, 207
 lacrimal, 304
 of bone, 78, 80, 81
 secretory, of glands, 166, 167, 217, 233, 237, 304
Capillary, 127
 arrangement of, 127
 bile, 237
 false types of, 129
 functions of, 128
 lymph, 139
 secretory, of glands, 166, 167, 217, 233, 237, 304
 sinusoidal, 129
 size of, 127
 structure of, 128
Capsule, cartilage, 73, 75
 Glisson's, 236
 glomerular (Bowman's), 254
 joint, 85
 lacunar, of bone, 79, 88
 of lens, 303
 of organs, 125, 149, 153, 236, 253, 264
 Tenon's, 304
Carbohydrates, 15
 absorption of, 228
 in cytoplasm, 23
Carbohydrate balance, suprarenal cortex and, 183
Cardia, of stomach, 216
Cardiovascular system, 127
Carotid body, 134

Cartilage, 72
 articular, 85, 93
 calcified, 91
 elastic, 74
 epiphyseal, 93, 94
 fibro-, 75
 functions of, 76
 growth of, 74
 appositional, 70
 interstitial, 70
 hyaline, 72
 asbestos transformation of, 74
 calcification of, 74
 nutrition of, 73
 of bronchi, 246, 248
 of larynx, 245
 of trachea, 246
 regeneration of, 75
 regressive changes in, 74
 types of, 72
Cartilage capsules, 73, 75
Cartilage cell groups, 72
Cartilage cells, 72, 75
Cartilage lacunae, 73
Cartilage matrix, 72, 73
 chemical composition of, 73
 physical structure of, 73
Cartilage territory, 73
Castration, effects of, in male, 268
 on prostate, 274
 on seminal vesicles, 273
Catabolism, 17
Cavernae, of penis, 276
Cavity, joint, 85
 marrow, 84, 93, 94
 nasal, 243
 functions of, 244
 olfactory region of, 244
 respiratory region of, 243
 vestibule of, 243
 oral. See *Mouth.*
 pulp, of tooth, 207
 tympanic, 306
Cecum, and valve, 225
Cell, A, of pancreas, 234
 acidophil, of hypophysis, 177
 acinar. See *Cell, alveolar.*
 adipose, 48, 54
 aging of, 29
 albuminous, 166
 alpha, of hypophysis, 177
 of pancreas, 234
 alveolar, of lung, 249
 argentaffin, of appendix, 225
 of gastric glands, 218
 of intestine, 221
 autolysis of, 29
 B, of pancreas, 234
 band, 63
 basal, of glands, 168
 basket, 168, 202
 basophil, of blood, 63
 of connective tissue, 47
 of hypophysis, 176
 beta, of hypophysis, 177
 of pancreas, 234
 binucleate, 24
 bipolar, of retina, 301
 blood, 59, 67